Thieves of Virtue

Basic Bioethics

Arthur Caplan, editor

A complete list of the books in the Basic Bioethics series appears at the back of this book.

Thieves of Virtue

When Bioethics Stole Medicine

Tom Koch

The MIT Press
Cambridge, Massachusetts
London, England

MIT Press books may be purchased at special quantity discounts for business or sales promotional use. For information, please email special_sales@mitpress.mit.edu or write to Special Sales Department, The MIT Press, 55 Hayward Street, Cambridge, MA 02142.

This book was set in Sabon by Toppan Best-set Premedia Limited. Printed on recycled paper and bound in the United States of America.

Library of Congress Cataloging-in-Publication Data

Koch, Tom, 1949–
Thieves of virtue : when bioethics stole medicine / Tom Koch.
p. cm.—(Basic bioethics)
Includes bibliographical references and index.
ISBN 978-0-262-01798-5 (hardcover : alk. paper)
1. Bioethics—History. 2. Bioethics—Political aspects. 3. Bioethics—Philosophy. 4. Medical ethics—Political aspects. 5. Medical ethics—Philosophy. I. Title.
QH332.K63 2012
174.2—dc23
2012004932

10 9 8 7 6 5 4 3 2 1

Contents

Series Foreword

Glenn McGee and I developed the Basic Bioethics series and collaborated as series coeditors from 1998 to 2008. In fall 2008 and spring 2009 the series was reconstituted, with a new editorial board, under my sole editorship. I am pleased to present the thirty-third book in the series.

The Basic Bioethics series makes innovative works in bioethics available to a broad audience and introduces seminal scholarly manuscripts, state-of-the-art reference works, and textbooks. Topics engaged include the philosophy of medicine, advancing genetics and biotechnology, end-of-life care, health and social policy, and the empirical study of biomedical life. Interdisciplinary work is encouraged.

Arthur Caplan

Acknowledgments

Like philosophy, writing is popularized as a solitary endeavor, the work of the individual to be completed in solitude. But like the ethics that philosophy promotes writing—at least writing for publication—is a decidedly communal enterprise. From conception through publication, it is the result of the labors of many and not the author's alone.

I have been informed, for example, by presenters at the American Society of Bioethics and the Humanities (ASBH) and other meetings, not the least by those with whom I have most strongly disagreed. My library is filed with the writings of those authors, noted and underlined, a paper communion with their thinking. Those authors, and others, have served as peer reviewers whose critical comments have improved the journal articles that I in turn have written and that served as building blocks for this book.

I have learned much, and more, perhaps, from the students who like the fellow in the Bob Marley tee shirt, have challenged my understanding over the years. In medicine, I've been privileged to work with a group of medical students at the University of British Columbia who meet most weeks to discuss medical ethics and ethical practice at the home of Drs. Margaret and Robin Cottle.

It was through my conversations with students at an ASBH meeting that I first met MIT acquisitions editor Clay Morgan. He found my dialogue with students interesting and encouraged me to submit a proposal based on those student discussions. Series editor Art Caplan approved it and this book was begun as a result. The original, draft manuscript benefited greatly from the critical comments of peer reviewers, the unsung heroes of publishing. Their observations were most important where they were least complimentary and I am grateful to them all.

At the MIT Press I was fortunate to have the assistance of Kathleen A. Caruso, the production editor who brought Julia Collins on board as text editor. Together they identified problems and helped assure the result would be if not error-free (what book ever is?) then as error-free as possible. It was through Kathleen's good offices that I was able to employ Tobiah Waldron as an indexer. I believe in indexes but am talentless in their construction. Tobiah served ably where my own efforts would have failed.

In clinic and hospital I have been privileged to learn from and work with a series of nurses and physicians. These include, in a partial list, the late William McArthur of Vancouver, a friend and teacher; Dr. Harvey Pasternak of Toronto and Dr. Margaret Cottle of Vancouver, BC. Earlier in my career I had the opportunity to work at The Hospital for Sick Children with caring and talented physicians like Dr. Arlette LeFebvre and Dr. Jonathan Hellmann.

The most important thing I learned from them all was that the real lessons come from patients and their families, from those in distress who seek help when confronting serious illness. It is those persons who time and again emphasized to me the messy, emotional, and interpersonal nature of issues of care and caring. I admit that when I am not dealing with people facing difficult treatment decisions that questions of ethics seem pretty straightforward if not always simple. But in the crucible of another's distress, the complexity of real choices is continually made clear.

Finally, I am most grateful to Professor Walter Wright for his continuing advice and support. I was a freshman in the first class he taught in philosophy at Clark University in the late 1960s. Since then he has been for more than forty years a friend, mentor, and always a teacher I could turn to with questions whose solution seemed impossible.

Teaching, like medicine, is less a profession than an act of faith. The real test of a teacher's mettle is not a student's performance in Philosophy 204 or Philosophy 301. It has little to do with grade point averages or acceptance to graduate studies. Rather, the excellence of the teacher is evidenced in the person who results, the one who in maturity integrates classroom teachings and worldly activities over time. Walter Wright never doubted the potential of us students to become better and more moral people who, sooner or later, would reflect on the ethics and philosophy he taught.

I hope he'll like this work. At the least, I hope he'll see in it my attempt to combine the learning that began in his classroom with the experiences of medicine and its practice that are central themes in this book. This book is dedicated to him and his efforts across a long career of teaching those too young to really appreciate the materials he presented to generations of students, year after year after year.

Introduction

Bioethics was supposed to be about you and me, about people and the medicine they receive, or desire. It was to be a tool with which individuals and the societies they inhabit could answer questions of medical practice and the research that sometimes put those politely called "human subjects" at risk. Born in the 1960s, it was to be a public service that brought a specific kind of analytic, moral philosophy to questions of medical care and healthcare delivery. In the end, bioethics was an experiment in a method of philosophically grounded, practical ethics that promised simplicity in a world that is multilayered, messy, and complex. The result would be, its progenitors promised, a set of generally applicable, universally accepted ethical guidelines at once intellectually and morally robust.[1] The realities of patient care and treatment (or nontreatment) were the medium of that experiment rather than the focus of its principals' passionate concern. Medicine is about how to do things; bioethics was forged to decide whether we should do them and if so, when and to whom. The result was what Albert Jonsen called a "demi-discipline,"[2] an applicable ethical perspective based on philosophical principles that put philosophy at the service of social medicine.

There was something out of joint from the start. Bioethics began with citizens engaged in a public debate over healthcare but quickly became a profession whose members spoke a language generally inaccessible to the average person. The bioethics profession trumpeted the right of patient choice but did so without considering the many ways in which those choices would be limited by its assumptions. Bioethics set up the medically untrained, philosophical adept as the adjudicator of clinical choices and the social organization that determined their boundaries. From the start those adepts were distanced from the bedside and the complexities of care. From the start bioethics promoted individual agency as an article of faith without attention to the socioeconomic constraints on individual choice. Experience as either a reality check or a teacher was not required. Who needs experience as either a reality check or a teacher? In situations fraught with ambiguity, emotion, and uncertainty, bioethics offered the philosopher's stock in trade, a dispassionate rationality, as a panacea.

"One of the most remarkable and resounding features of this field is the extent to which the matters with which it deals have spread beyond the spheres of the contributing intellectual disciplines of which it is composed," write Fox and Swazey in *Observing Bioethics*, "and the professional milieus in which their members usually operate, to pervade the public domain."[3] Understanding how moral philosophers became practical ethicists who served as adjudicators of medical practice and planning is one of the goals of this book. There have been other histories of bioethics, other studies of its ideas.[4] Most have been by bioethicists who believe in their demi-discipline and its place in the world. This is an alternate history by an ethicist and gerontologist working in medicine who believes in ethics and philosophy—who believes in principles of care—but not in bioethics. It is at one level a social critique of bioethics, its promises and its premises. At another it engages a critique of bioethics' deployment of philosophy as a legitimating ideal. That necessitated the frequent quotation from a range of foundational works, especially those of Immanuel Kant. If one accepts the argument that a philosophical approach is important it is fair to ask if that philosophy is both adequately employed and correctly applied.

The Necessity

Since the 1960s, bioethicists have sought to displace a traditional ethic of medicine that, age to age and culture to culture, was the bedrock of medical practice and research until bioethicists decided it was not. This was necessary, bioethicists claimed, because the older ethics' inherent paternalism was inimical to contemporary notions of individual liberty. And, too, the advance of radical new medical technologies required a means of address beyond that of the older ethic. The new, philosophically grounded ethic would enlarge the range of "virtuous actions," providing a definition of morally right goods and values in a manner permitting their application to questions of medical practice and research. Those goods were to be revealed through a specific methodology and an associated set of essential values grounded in the work of Enlightenment philosophers. This approach would permit philosophers-cum-ethicists to critique the old ethic and direct medical practice and research to the eventual benefit of all.[5]

Strangely, at least to me, bioethics' foundational claims have been assumed but not, in the past, carefully considered. Are the foundational claims of bioethics, the basis of its legitimacy, credible? Was the older ethic of medicine so illiberally paternalistic as to require replacement? Was it truly incapable of treating advancing medical sciences? And from another perspective, the question is whether the abstract and thin philosophical approach of the philosopher-ethicist serves (indeed, has it *ever* served?) in the mediation of complex realities?

Because bioethics is grounded in a philosophy, in this critique-cum-history I make fairly frequent reference to the works of philosophers central to bioethical thinking and writing, especially Immanuel Kant. In doing so I seek not to debate the utility of these works but rather to argue for a test of consistency: *If* bioethics is grounded in Enlightenment philosophies and methodologies, as interpreted today, *then* one may expect a congruence between the ideas presented by the older philosophers and those offered by contemporary bioethicists who quote them. If the practice conflicts with those grand ideals then something is seriously out of joint.

The argument that results is necessarily "messy," in the language of the sociology of science and technology.[6] Because the elements that shape and promote medicine and medical practice occur within a context that is both cultural and social, attention must be paid to the socioeconomic and political backcloth within which medical practice and research are (and have always been) promoted. Seeing things from this perspective, what Andrew Pickering called the "mangle" of practice[7] is a necessary focus because medical practice and research are cooperative enterprises at once economic, political, and social as well as clinical and scientific. One of the signal failures of bioethics, I will argue, is its woeful inattention to these interrelated histories in their effect on medicine and on bioethics itself.

This text therefore does not move handily from simple thesis to simple conclusion followed by a limited set of recommendations. Indeed, one of the book's central conclusions is that the simplicity of that form is a part of the problem. It assumes dilemmas of care and noncare can be narrowly defined and then easily resolved within the existing paradigm. I argue bioethics' artificial and narrow system of ethical thinking imposes an artificial simplicity upon issues that are inherently complex. The result, I argue, too often results in a disservice to many people, and especially to those most fragile and at risk. This does not mean there are no answers. The answers to complex problems will not be found, however, in a reflexive reliance on simplistic arguments, definitions, or principles.

This is not an argument against philosophy as an intellectual endeavor. It does, however, question the assumption that high philosophy is a necessary groundwork for a practical guide to the dilemmas that arise at the bedside of the ill or at the workbenches of researchers. Nobody carries Kant to a clinical consult. Nobody quotes Hegel (or Feuerbach) to the members of an Institutional Review Board meeting.

Organization

A general outline of this book's chapters will explain how its themes are developed. Chapter 1 begins with a student who questions the relevance of classic philosophy and philosophers to contemporary ethical concerns. If an ethic is not to be a terror imposed upon a population at the least it must be comprehensible (and ideally acceptable) to the average person. The student in his Bob Marley tee shirt symbolizes that need and serves, across subsequent chapters, as a reminder of that necessity. Ethics as a general enterprise is then narrowed to the consideration of bioethics; the "demi-discipline" whose "foundation myth" presents a core set of ideas that both differentiates and legitimates bioethicists. The axioms of the myth are then used as the subject of succeeding chapters.

Because the foundation myth asserts bioethics was necessitated by the failure of traditional medical ethics, chapter 2 reviews the ethical tradition that began with Hippocrates of Cos (460 BC to ca. 370 BC) and served across millennia into the last half of the twentieth century when the first generation of bioethicists judged it in need of replacement. To simplify this complex history I focus on the famous Hippocratic oath as an ethical covenant. Across subsequent chapters this provides a backcloth against which other bioethical claims can be assessed.

Chapter 3 traces the birth and early growth of bioethics beginning with the debate in the 1960s over the scarcity of beds in then-new dialysis programs. This was a seminal event both in the history of bioethics and in a more general social history that saw the idea of social abundance replaced by that of resource scarcity as a naturally occurring and generally limiting condition. By the 1990s the assumption of scarcity was popularly and professionally presented by bioethicists as a continuing and chronic problem of "lifeboat ethics" in which some necessarily must die (or be left untreated to die, or be killed) that others might survive.

Chapter 4 considers the assumptions of the lifeboat and of scarcity as a natural condition. Scarcity, I argue, is rarely natural but more typically the result of prior choices whose effects almost always are predictable. A lifeboat ethic that pays no attention to antecedent conditions, I argue, is an ethical and moral failure. In its stead I propose an ethic *of* the lifeboat in which antecedent conditions are the principal moral concern. A signal failure of bioethics, I argue, has been that its authors and practitioners almost universally ignore the second ethic while focusing exclusively on the first.

Chapter 5 argues that the assumption of scarcity as a necessary limit requiring ethical triage has been a central theme in bioethical development. This perspective was responsible for the shift in bioethics from the traditional medical ethics' focus on patient care, and the physician's responsibility for it, to a neoliberal ideology in which care and caring become products of individual consumption rather than communal and thus interpersonal responsibility. In a market-based argument the preeminent good is economic. From this perspective, the advance of the "knowledge industry" becomes more critical than the needs of the person who becomes important only as a research subject or product consumer.[8] In thinking about this I focus on *The Belmont Report* as the framework within which this ethical shift was advanced.

Chapter 6 considers the second foundational work of the demi-discipline, *Principles of Biomedical Ethics* (shortened for convenience, here, to *Principles*). Since 1979 *Principles* "has served as groundwork for the training of countless students and professions in medicine and biomedical ethics."[9] With *Belmont*, *Principles* sought to define, justify, and then apply a philosophically grounded "systematic analysis of the moral principles that should apply to biomedicine."[10] Its importance extended, and extends today, well beyond the thinly principled ethics it in fact promotes. Considered together, *Belmont* and *Principles* created a general argument whose practical application, I argue, has directed bioethical teaching and thinking for two generations.

Chapters 7 and 8 separately consider two different areas of contemporary bioethical debate. The focus of chapter 7 is the famous meeting between disability rights lawyer Harriet McBryde Johnson and Princeton philosopher and ethicist Peter Singer.[11] The lawyer and the philosopher-ethicist separately proposed issues of normalcy and difference in a non-debate whose real subject was the promotion or reduction of human diversity. That meeting juxtaposed two very different philosophies, two different philosophical methods. That there *were* two distinct approaches insists that bioethics' specific, philosophical perspective is neither inevitable nor necessary. Rather, it is only one alternative whose adequacy (or inadequacy) can be assessed on the basis of different but at least equally valid persepectives (personal, philosophical, social, scientific, and so on).

Similarly, chapter 8 considers arguments by contemporary bioethicists advancing genetic "enhancements" and "engineering" as welcome overtures to the possibility of a self-directed transformation of humankind. This dream is not peripheral to bioethics, I argue, but central to its historical goals. This eugenic argument is, I argue, not simply ethically unpalatable but scientifically naive. In its stead I offer a different version of what "human flourishing" might mean were it to be grounded not only in the complexities of science but also in a humanist ideal of care and caring among persons.

It is frequently argued that even if bioethics has failed in its promise of a unified set of ethical values, it has served as a champion of individual freedom and the liberty of individual choice in the arena of medical care. That claim, first considered briefly in chapter 3, is treated extensively in chapter 9. If one sees paternalism as an evil, I argue, it is one promoted today less by working physicians and nurses than by bioethicists. And, too, I argue, bioethics has been instrumental in promoting a perspective that reduces choice. The failure of its promise of choice and freedom are, I suggest, inherent in the real source of bioethical imagining, the lifeboat ethics that it has promoted from the start.

Chapter 10, the last chapter in this book, begins with discussion of a series of recent articles whose authors, all well-known bioethicists, lament the state of their demi-discipline as dying, dead, or at least in serious trouble. All insist that some new ethic must be developed that will repair the failed or failing bioethics that has evolved over the last half-century. Their obituary for the field that has employed them and their predecessors serves primarily to argue what the previous nine chapters attempted to demonstrate: the bankruptcy of bioethics as a practical ethic. A reformation (or transformation) requires first an understanding of the systemic failures of the bioethics that has, these authors say, run its course. It is that understanding that I attempt to argue in this book and summarize in chapter 10.

The problem cannot be remedied by a new set of simplistic principles or maxims because, I argue, issues of medical practice and research are not easily resolved through reference to a thinly philosophical method. In a real sense there is no ethics of medicine, and no bioethics. Medicine is one example of practice occurring within a broader ethic of social care (or noncare) and valuation operative at a range of scales: personal, familial, historical, and social. To ask about an ethics of medicine is to ask about a general ethic within a culture whose framework is economic, political, and social. One may use medicine as a focal point for those discussions but its treatment must occur within the broader framework of social conscience and development.

This does not mean questions of ethical care and practice are unanswerable but instead that questions need to be posed differently and considered through a very different reference system. Is our primary focus to be, as it once was, the life and safety of the patient or is it to be—as some bioethicists seem to suggest—the needs of the research community and its "knowledge industry"? Is the care of the fragile to be an essential practical good, or is medicine to be simply another commodity whose delivery is predicated on the basis of economic efficiency? What do we say to those who our policies and priorities leave with no good choices, to those "in the lifeboat," because of prior decisions that made that unhappy situation inevitable?

How we answer these questions will depend on our response to a prior set of questions. These include the degree to which we see ourselves as isolates or as members of a community. To the extent we perceive these as community issues, how do we define the relationship between individual "rights" and societal obligations of the community to the person (and vice versa)? And at a different scale, do we understand society as principally an economic enterprise in which the citizen is merely a consumer, or does society constitute a kind of social covenant in which all are to participate, to the best of their abilities, irrespective of their physical abilities? What degree of difference—cognitive, physical, sensory, and social—will we tolerate in the society we hope to promote?

This book suggests answers but does not promote them. Its primary goal is to free us, or begin to free us, from the assumptions of an ethic that, I argue, has been more an impediment than a boon to the ethical practice of medicine, and thus to society at large. My hope is that this book will serve as a stepping-stone to the carving out of an ethic that is humanist, responsible, and defensible. That end is not, however, the goal of this book: its utmost aim is prepare the field for a better—by which I mean a clearer, more consistent, more transparent, and certainly more rigorous—ethic than the bioethics we have today.

1

Dead Germans and Other Philosophers: Ethics as a Professional or a Public Occupation

The most interesting students are in the middle rows, slouched in aisle seats from which they can make a rapid escape from the classroom if the lecture is intolerably dull. In front of them are well-socialized notetakers content to record whatever is said so it can be repeated on an exam page. They do not question overmuch and are never excited about the issues. In the back rows are mainly students whose interest is limited to passing a course with the minimum of study. They are about, as their parents would say, "getting the job done," and in the main could not care less about the content of a lecture or its subject. Rarely taking notes, they rely instead on first-row friends for a cram session early in exam week ("What was that guy's point?"). The real potential is in the middle rows, the kids who will get excited if only given a chance.

This day the room was filled with sixty-five undergraduates gathered for my lecture on the ethics of mapping and data analysis.[1] Because the area of my interest is medical—the nature of disease as a public phenomenon and a personal threat—the examples I used were disease- and health related. The student who captured my attention was a tall, gangly fellow in a faded Bob Marley tee shirt topping fashionably torn designer jeans. A splendid head of long, blond dreadlocks completed the look. He did not volunteer a comment or question, of course (how uncool that would be!), but when asked his opinion responded with a compellingly righteous certainty. Fear and frustration when mixed in equal measure often sound like that.

After the lecture a few students, mostly front-row notetakers, stopped to chat on their way to lunch. The Bob Marley fellow, as I thought of him, hands sunk in his jean's back pockets, waited until the others had gone before approaching. "I like this ethics stuff. It's, uh, real," he began.

"But I don't want to have to read a lot of dead Germans. Can I do this ethics stuff without them?"

I had referenced Kant, mentioned Heidegger's *Being and Time*, disparaged Wittgenstein's "a picture is a fact," and casually dropped a passing reference or two to Foucault who while not German qualified as a dead authority. "What's wrong with the dead Germans?" I asked. "Man, what do they know about earning a living," he laughed, "about genetics, or about automobiles? They had their day and the question is how do we get ours."

Life is too short, he told me, to spend endless hours deciphering arcane works written in foreign languages by those whose conclusions encouraged, directly or indirectly, a range of social evils: colonialism, imperialism, misogyny, slavery, and so on. Who were *they* to talk to *us* about good and bad, right or wrong? For the student in the Bob Marley tee shirt, reading dead Germans (or Greeks, or French thinkers) wasn't the prelude to an informed consideration of ethics but merely one more form of indoctrination, one not to be endured. As James Wood put it, "School tutors the adolescent in repression and the rectitude of the bourgeois order, at the very moment in life when, temperamentally and biologically, one is most Dionysiac and most enraged by the hypocritical ordinances of the parental league."[2] For this student, and for others, the distance between high moral argument and the conclusions drawn from them indict the old philosophies, whose study will therefore have no place in his university schedule.

I tried to explain that philosophy is not a map to correct behavior but more like a compass that, if read accurately, gives a sense of orientation and purpose. There is, however, no magnetic north, fixed and unchanging, in philosophy. At their best, as Michael Ignatieff wrote, philosophers seek to argue no more than "the permanent or semi-permanent categories in terms of which experience is conceived and classified."[3] Ethicists attempt to apply those philosophical categories in a pragmatic transformation of ideals into ideas of correctness in the world. History reviews the result, often harshly.

Of course, the ideas organized into those categories are rarely new. They always come from . . . somewhere. As Ignatieff put it: "No abstract or analytical point exists out of all connection with historical, personal thought."[4] And so in their review, I continued, in my conversation with the student, we need to know the history of past thinkers if only to understand their conceptual and practical failures. "We all of us inherit everything, and then we choose what to cherish, what to disavow, and what to do next, which is why it's worth trying to know where things come from," wrote Jill Lapore in an article on the history of American eugenics.[5] For those interested in ethical orienteering that means knowing something about the philosophers who thought about right and wrong, about humanness and what it means. To ignore this intellectual inheritance is to give up the game from the start.

I thought I was pretty eloquent but the student was at best only half-convinced. I suggested he take a course in applied ethics. "Will I have to read those dead Germans?" he asked. "Yes," I said, "but not too many and only in translation."

This book starts with a student's questions as a reminder—to myself as much as to the reader—that an ethic's rationale must be not merely comprehensive but also comprehensible to those whose lives will be affected by its application. For me, the problem was not the student's insistence that an ethics grounded in traditional philosophies is tainted by historical failures, but that those philosophers are difficult to understand and formalized in a way that is largely inaccessible to those who, like him, seek practical engagement without long tutelage and indoctrination. The very idea of practical ethics demands that it, and the moral perspective that underlies its categories, be not merely comprehensive and consistent but also explicable both to those who will apply it, and equally important, to those whom its judgments will affect.

The deeper problem was one the dreadlocked student perhaps intuited but could not articulate: the route from philosophy to ethics to practice is often obscure. "Philosophers are often like little children," Wittgenstein wrote in the *Tractatus* (4.112), "who first scribble random lines on a piece of paper with their pencils, and now ask an adult, 'What is that?'"[6] Ethicists take those scribbles and say, "It is a category of the world we make and use just so." The student in the Bob Marley tee shirt wanted not scribbles but a clear frame in which questions of right and wrong could be considered on the basis of propositions consistent in their application and transparent in their formulation. Who doesn't?

And, too, the problem with philosophy as a basis of an applicable ethic like bioethics is that at best it only suggests an orientation, never a system of problem resolution. Again with Wittgenstein: "Philosophy does not result in philosophical propositions but rather in the clarification of propositions" whose verity is always up for grabs (*Tractatus* 4.112). With their "If . . . then" construction, propositions are not take-it-to-the-bank associations but rather ideas about potential relations based on shifting, often disputed definitional statements. We thus may present but cannot state as necessarily true the contingent associations we too often proudly assert as philosophically precise, ethically applicable certainties. And yet, in courses with names like "Applied Ethics in Medicine 330," and "Introduction to Bioethics 205," ethical propositions are typically presented not as subjects for consideration but as principled conclusions of more or less truth, near philosophical absolutes with universal currency. The result is a blinkering rather than a widening of the field of moral inquiry.

We do this all the time, cloaking suppositions as unquestioned—or worse, unquestionable—verities. This violates the very spirit of the philosophical enterprise (still with Wittgenstein), however, in which "philosophy is not a body of doctrine but an activity" (*Tractatus* 4.112). Ethics and its philosophical underpinnings are, or should be, a platform from which we can challenge existing propositions rather than a reflexive assertion of a set of philosophically grounded ideals and their attendant values. The question is whether any of it matters in a practical way. As Larry Churchill put it, baldly but not incorrectly, perhaps, "philosophical theorizing might be considered harmless entertainment, which if taken too seriously would look ridiculous."[7]

The ridiculous becomes deadly serious, however, when distilled into an ethic that purports to serve as a practical guide to appropriate behavior in complex situations. Bioethics is an example of the way in which philosophical theorizing can be stepped down (or stepped up, depending on one's point of view) to create a practical guide to issues of treatment or nontreatment affecting persons who are sick. And, as an ethics of medicine based on a philosophical perspective, bioethics is taken very seriously indeed,[8] dictating decisions of patient care or noncare as well as institutional and legislative agendas that advance or retard areas of medical care and treatment.[9] Where specific questions of appropriate care arise, they do so under the umbrella of bioethical assumptions advanced in law and advocated as a guide to practice. In short: "The way in which medical professionals engage in bioethical issues ultimately reflects the type of care patients are likely to receive."[10] The question becomes what is bioethics and who are those ethicists who define its categories and construct its propositions?

Bioethicists

Bioethicists like to think of themselves as a diverse group of opinionated individuals with a wide range of political views who cannot be easily characterized without caricature. As philosophers, or at least philosophically trained, adepts, they serve, writes a former president of the American Society for Bioethics and Humanities (ASBH), as surrogates for the general public when issues of ethical uncertainty arise.[11] The tool they bring to public service is a kind of analytic thinking that can be variously applied and interpreted. Those variations, the potential of multiple interpretations, in no way belies, however, the unity of bioethics as a perspective and a profession, "in the MacIntyrean sense of being a specialized, skilled, activity with its own set of standards and intrinsic goods."[12] Those standards are set forth in a set of core competencies members are expected to possess and are taught to bioethicists in training in university courses. And, too, there is a specific ethic, a code of conduct and behavior, to which bioethicists are expected to adhere.[13]

Thus beneath the appearance of diversity exists a unanimity of definition and purpose. As former ASBH president Mark Kuczewski wrote in 2010: "We have become a professional and academic community that engages in practices that include shared narratives, values, and virtues."[14] It is *as* bioethicists that ASBH members are academically situated (in university departments), practically employed (in hospitals and on research review boards), professionally identified (as contributors to and editors of bioethical journals), and socially organized (at annual meetings, for example). It is not as individuals but as bioethicists that ASBH members testify in court cases and are interviewed as experts on TV.

"What does your Dad do?" the child asks. "He's a bioethicist and teaches philosophy," says the child's friend.

It is *as* a bioethicist with training and credentials, and thus a bioethical point of view, that one becomes not simply a lonely scholar but also an employed specialist and thus a political actor and social participant.

There is nothing special here; it is the way of all experts in modern society. "The privilege of creating and holding knowledge increases our capacity, our freedom to act," cautions Audrey Kobayashi, "but [thus] enhances the responsibility of action."[15] That action and its attendant responsibilities are, for bioethicists, based on adherence to a central ideal of bioethics and the methodology of its actualization. From the start, bioethicists have promoted their "demi-discipline," as Albert Jonsen first called it, as "an intellectual enterprise aimed at giving moral guidance.[16] And here, too, one may see bioethicists as an activist group rather than merely a set of diversely opinionated, variously political scholars. Again this is merely particularizing the general social form. "Moral enquiry," writes Alistair McIntyre, "always and everywhere involves particular communities engaged in particular practices ordered toward particular notions of human flourishing."[17]

The object of bioethics, and thus bioethical practice, the thing that distinguishes its practitioners in their apparent diversity, is the application of a philosophically grounded methodology facilitating a moral inquiry into "notions of human flourishing" in the arenas of medical practice, organization, and research.

If one seeks answers in these areas—some kind of moral truth and a program for its attainment—bioethics' first half-century has been an abysmal failure. The last half-century of bioethical engagement has not produced what early bioethicists promised, a "single and canonical moral vision" applicable to medical practice and research.[18] From continuing debates over the appropriateness of abortion to questions concerning the ethics of zenotransplantation there is not one subject that all or even a majority of bioethicists agree will serve a singular notion of humanness or human flourishing. Instead bioethicists in their diversity have created, as physician and philosopher Tristram Engelhardt put it, an "intractable moral pluralism . . . that brings into question many of the aspirations of bioethics, especially those of its founding."[19]

If bioethicists have failed spectacularly in the construction of a single, broadly acceptable moral vision, they are united in promoting a specific kind of philosophical training as the methodology by which the moral and ethical questions of medicine are to be addressed.[20] This methodology is expressed in a shared and specific formal language employed in bioethical articles, lectures, and position statements. Its instruction is promoted through an accepted canon of philosophical texts (the "dead Germans") taught to all bioethicists and commonly referenced in their writings. Underlying that language is a set of assumptions assumed to be true by most bioethicists if not necessarily by all philosophers. It is in the canonical textbooks of bioethics—for example, Beauchamp and Childress's *Principles of Biomedical Ethics*—that one sees the methodology and its underlying assumptions promoted in a language that argues its necessity as well as its potential, albeit as yet unfulfilled, to uncover necessarily truthful notions of humanness and human flourishing.

Foundation Myth

Foundation myths legitimate a movement, a people, politic, or profession by defining a raison d'être in relation to the greater society. In this way they create a community of persons whose shared attributes make of them an "x" (bioethicist, lawyer, physician, and so on). It is through allegiance to the myth that individuals with little personal standing become members of a collective with moral weight and stature in society.[21] Foundation myths thus define a common persona for those collectively engaged in a singular activity through the expression of a specific expertise.[22]

Bioethics' foundation myth, which legitimates its community of bioethicists, is stated in the opening pages of Beauchamp and Childress's *Principles of Biomedical Ethics* (discussed here in chapter 6) and more or less explicitly in the works of a diverse range of practitioners including, in a very partial sample: communitarian Daniel Callahan;[23] critics like Renée Fox and Judith Swazy;[24] disciplinary historians like Albert Jonsen;[25] and humanist practitioners like Margaret Somerville[26] and physician-ethicist Howard Brody.[27] The myth can be summarized as follows:

> In the 1960s and 1970s a traditional ethics of medicine was shown to be insufficient in the face of an unprecedented series of advances in medical science and technology unfolding in an era of socioeconomic scarcity. Bioethics arose as a replacement capable of confronting these new realities. Grounded in a Western philosophical tradition (especially the writings of Immanuel Kant), bioethics would better serve in the evaluation of these technologies. Further, bioethics was necessitated as a champion of individual freedom and patient choice in the

face of illiberal and paternalistic practices common under the older ethics of medicine.

With the rise of bioethics a new class of medical professional came into being. This was the bioethicist, an expert in valuation uniquely qualified to apply philosophical systems of thought to ethical questions arising in areas of medical care, delivery, and research.

The importance of this myth lies not in its factuality but in its acceptance. That is, it matters less whether the specific elements of the myth are demonstrable than that they are believed. This myth presents a set of assumptions, all of which are disputable and most of which are challenged across the subsequent chapters of this book. I propose here that bioethics was necessitated neither by the failure of a traditional medical ethic nor by its inability to address issues uniquely arising in mid- and late twentieth-century medical science. The argument will be that the singular vocational focus of traditional medical ethics, the needs of the patient, was inimical to a progressively neoliberal agenda in which patient care and treatment were defined as secondary to a separate set of social and economic priorities. Bioethics arose as a way of furthering those priorities. The traditional ethics was not incapable, I argue, merely unsympathetic to a kind of consumerist accountancy that bioethics embraced from the start.

"Ethicists have been a guest in the house of medicine," wrote Mark Kuczewski with admirable frankness, "and in order to survive in that environment have had to align themselves with money and power."[28] In that alignment the real hero of bioethics, wrote Charles Peters, in a seminal article in the early 1980s, was never the medical caregiver engaged with his or her patient's care but instead "the risk-taking entrepreneur who creates new jobs and better products."[29] And as Daniel Callahan, an elder statesman of the demi-discipline, wrote in *Why America Accepted Bioethics*, bioethics triumphed because it was conducive to liberal sensibilities advanced within the progressively neoliberal climate of American politics and its market place.[30]

"The true terror of this new order has to do with its being ruled—and observed to be ruled," writes T. J. Clark, "by the sheer concatenation of profit and loss, bids and bargains: that is, by a system whose focusing purpose or compelling image or ritualization is of that purpose."[31] Its principal focus was never really medicine and the complexities of its practice but, instead, the application of a consumerist economics and ideology—more libertarian than liberal—to medicine.[32] It is disputable whether only an ethic accepting this ordering could have won popular and professional acceptance. That is, bioethics was an answer but not necessarily the only one possible. It is, I think, indisputable that bioethicists of all stripes have generally embraced, at least in North America and Great Britain, Clark's "concatenation" and continue to see it as natural rather than constructed and thus a perspective to be accepted reflexively rather than critiqued.

In this read bioethics becomes a modernist hijacking of the traditional ethics of medicine and its injunctions for personal (and interpersonal) care as a primary vocational, social good. It is a "hijacking" to the degree that bioethicists rejected a traditional medical ethics not because of its inadequacies but rather because its priorities were seen as incompatible with those of a neoliberal, modernist order. By modernist I mean, "A social order which has turned from the worship of ancestors and past authorities to the pursuit of a projected future of goods, pleasures, freedoms, forms of control over nature, or infinities of information."[33] The specific order advanced by bioethics is neoliberal, one in which consumerism and transactional thinking are advanced, in the name of individual autonomy, over values of community and communal responsibility. The result is not morally rich but instead ethically blank, a bookkeeper's recording rather than a moralist's accounting. It is simplistic but not inaccurate to argue, as does British physician and bioethicist Miran Epstein, that: "Bioethics owes its historical success primarily to the service it has done for the neoliberal agenda"[34]

That many and perhaps most bioethicists will not easily see themselves in this way is not surprising. Modernism in general "is a process that deeply misrecognizes its own nature much of the time."[35] Bioethicists will certainly prefer to see themselves as defenders of individual choice and freedom rather than protectors of corporate profits and governmental economic priorities. Certainly most would find distasteful the idea that they are tools of a socioeconomic agenda many would, if asked, reject. They might find comfort in the long history of philosophers and ethicists who, with the best of intentions, proposed solutions to problems that hindsight found wanting. As even the student in the Bob Marley tee shirt knew, history is replete with examples.

Bioethics: Moral Folk Theory

Allied to bioethics, sometimes leading and sometimes following, is a body of laws developed by legislatures and applied by jurists to specific cases. The conjunction of bioethical thinking and legal judgment is one source of bioethics' continuing importance.[36] Jurists and lawmakers cite bioethical texts and their ideas in court judgments and the formation of laws. Bioethicists cite legal cases, where data on individual circumstances is carefully preserved, in their arguments. The difference between the two is critical, however. Jurists and legalists apply statute to practice without necessarily arguing the ideals that laws promote. Bioethicists seek immutable principles based on moral law or, at the least, a morality based upon a "set of norms shared by all persons committed to morality."[37] In other words, they promote as real and universal a moral perception whose end is moral action.

The ethics that results in bioethics, irrespective of the bioethicists' particular allegiance (communitarian, feminist, principalist, utilitarian, etc.) is a version of what Mark Johnson calls "the Moral Law folk theory," a set of ideas with broad applicability: "Reason guides the will by giving it moral laws. . . . Moral reasoning is thus principally a matter of getting the correct description of a situation, determining which moral law pertains to it, and figuring out what action that moral law requires for the given situation."[38]

The roots of this folk theory lie deep in the Western philosophical tradition. It assumes, first, that there exists a discernable, singular, and applicable moral law "out there" and second that it can be discovered by the rational, logical individual intent on its discovery. Once perceived, that law is assumed to serve as a practical guide to contemporary dilemmas. As understood through a range of Enlightenment thinkers into the present, the moral reasoning permitting this kind of rational discovery is assumed to be untainted by emotion, desire, physical circumstance, or narrow self-interest. Was it otherwise it would not be the product of pure reason. From this comes an emphasis on the rationally self-conscious being who must be free to choose but, one must add, whose moral choices are not to be eccentric. The law is not anarchistic so there is only one law and one ethic derived from it. It is philosophy's test to order the reason that perceives it, the ethicist's job to apply it. Divergence from the law that results is unethical, or at the least nonrational.

At the heart of this folk theory, some might call it this grand illusion,[39] are the works of Immanuel Kant (figure 1.1). His is the name we give to a waypoint in Western philosophy in which the old moralities were refashioned into a modern form during the Enlightenment. In Kant's work we hear the echoes of earlier moral philosophers' debates on the nature of humankind and its societies reaching from the Greeks to other Enlightenment authors like Hobbes, Locke, and Rousseau. And in the way of intellectual history Kant's ideas in their turn have been the bedrock on which later thinkers, from Hegel to Marx and beyond, built their ideas.[40] Kant's name is thus a legitimating groundwork for the folk theory's rational ideal and its notion of a kind of discoverable universal moral truth. It is also central to the perspective that bioethics sought to bring to medical thinking.[41] No philosopher is more frequently quoted in the literature or more consistently taught in bioethics classes.[42]

Kant presents, and bioethics promises what Johnson's folk theory insists is possible, what Isaiah Berlin described as a kind of "secularized Protestant individualism, in which the universal law [reason] replaces God as an organizing principle."[43] In place of the soulful search for the deity through adherence to revealed scriptures we have the individual in his or her reason dispassionately seeking the true universal morality, the immutable law accessible to unemotional reason. From this perspective ethics in general and bioethics specifically becomes a largely instrumental trade whose practitioners identify moral universals and then apply them to a specific problem of medical care, research, policy, or treatment.

All this assumes, of course, the existence of moral laws that are absolute and not contingent, bound by circumstance. It further assumes that morality will be revealed to the disinterestedly rational, philosophical, adept seeker. Finally, the assumption (and they do pile up) is that once understood these morals can be confidently applied to explicate an ethically complex problem. In all this neither the specifics of individual circumstance nor the social context in which they exist are assumed to be relevant.

Kant's argument for the transcendent, independent, isolate, free individual who through reason perceives the moral law—it's out there,

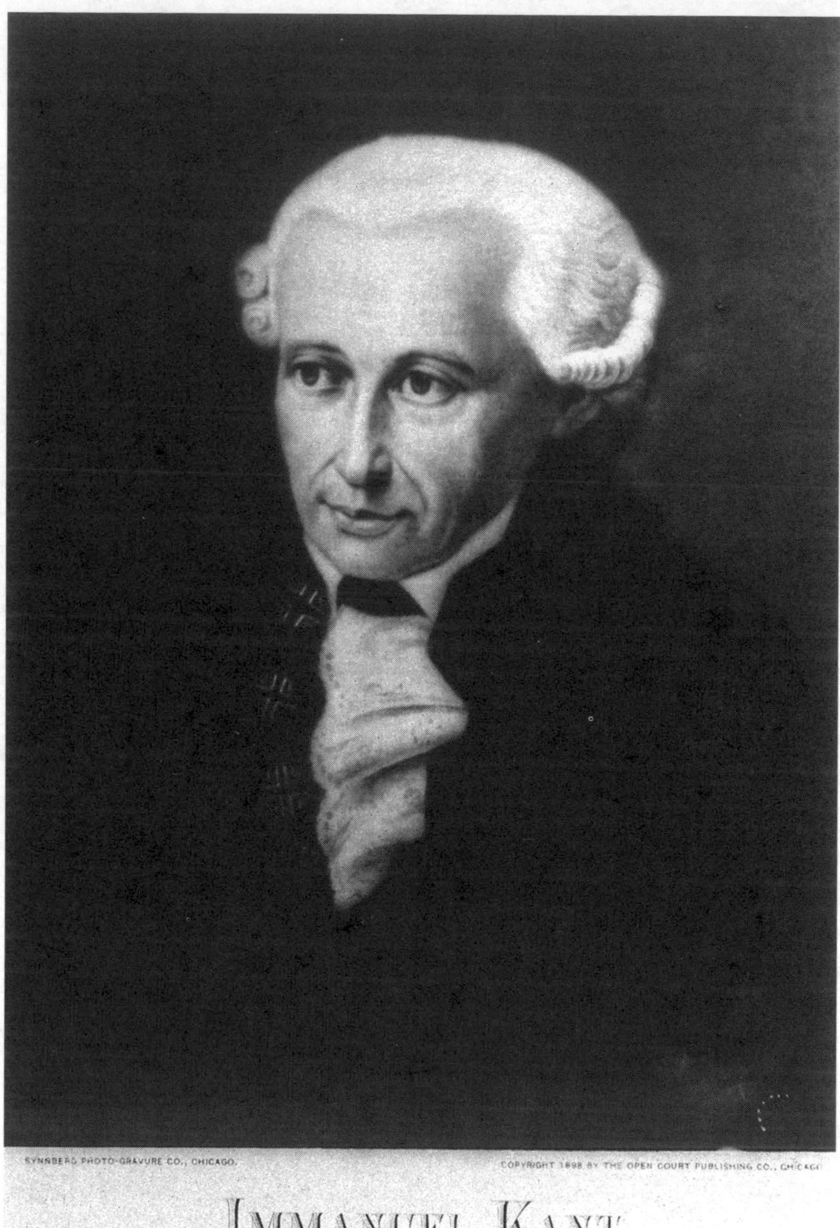

Figure 1.1
Immanuel Kant is the name we give to both the works of the philosopher and a waypoint in Western philosophy. His focus was on unbridled reason, distinct from emotion and experience, with which the individual could find the universal law and its principles. *Source*: National Library of Medicine, Bethesda, MD.

somewhere, awaiting rational discovery—is a wonderful imagining well beyond the world of any experiential reality. It was also, of course, a glorious failure that, as Alasdair MacIntyre, put it, divorced reason from everything that gives it meaning.[44] The result is not moral vision but fragmentation; not grounded ethics but an emptiness outside any social or ethical tradition.

The reason is simple: We do not live outside history in a moment of pure reason but within a history whose antecedents define our culture and our world. We live not alone but in society and the issues of ethics are as much about communal activities or impediments as they are about personal preferences and reasons. Our problems and our lives, to put it another way, are not singular and theoretical but complexly interpersonal and indivisibly constructed of a multiplicity of richly layered socioeconomic histories that all contribute to the specific circumstance. "My individual self is not something which I can detach from my relationship with others, or from those attributes of myself which consisted in their attitude toward me," writes Isaiah Berlin.[45] The solitary thinker is not really independent; the freedom of the individual is always bounded by interpersonal and social attachments, histories, and strictures.

The problem is fundamental. As others from Hegel to Charles Taylor have made clear, there *is* no clear route from the transcendent to the mundane, from Kant's rational, isolated imaginings to the complex choices occurring in a society with multiple and often conflicting beliefs and goals (figure 1.2).[46] The practical default for most bioethicists, as it was for Kant, is typically a retreat to a kind of simplistic utilitarianism that (oh irony!) for the ostensible good of the majority reflexively denies the preferences of individuals whose freedom to independent, rational choice bioethicists insist is or should be preeminent.

The problem lies not in the writings of long-dead philosophers like Immanuel Kant who, as the dreadlocked student noted, had no experience or interest in the modern issues that confront us. Nor, in their own day, were they practical ethicists seeking to find a better way to govern and be governed. The problem lies in the vainglorious attempt to apply these philosophers' general ideas of humankind as if they provided a simple map through the mire of social complexity that is the modern condition. They ignore the absolute disconnect between thin principle and the complexities of choice that occur in situations where clinical

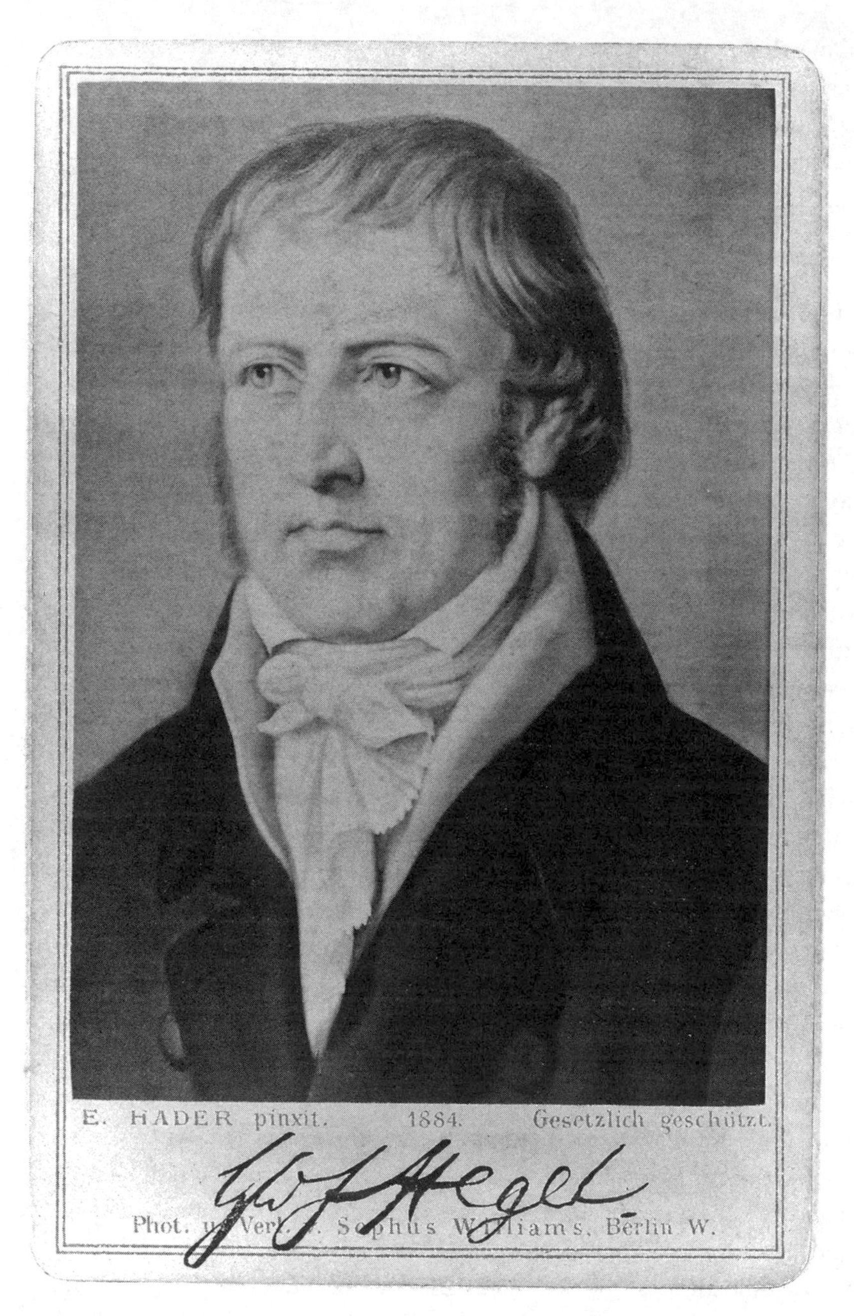

Figure 1.2
G. W. F. Hegel both critiqued and advanced the work of Kant, imposing a dialectic dynamic that made of reason's search for the universal a matter of historical progression. *Source*: National Library of Medicine, Bethesda, MD.

facts are at best tentative, the familial situation emotionally conflicted, and the social context of care limiting.

Put baldly, in its application of Johnson's folk theory bioethics is a simple perspective that ignores complexity and its causes. "There is complexity if things relate but don't add up, if events occur but not within the processes of linear time, and if the phenomena share a [cultural, geographic, or social] space but cannot be mapped in terms of a single set of three-dimensional coordinates."[47] My job is to show that in bioethics things don't add up and that the realities that bioethics pretends to map across an ethical landscape cannot be located easily along the philosophical coordinates bioethicists propose as accurate and firm.

Evaluation and Standards

As Hegel argued and Wittgenstein knew, history—like philosophy and its ethics—is continually contested, a subject of ongoing revision. The history of bioethics presented here differs in its parts from those offered by other bioethicists. How is the reader to choose? One way is simply to test the assertions of a history and if they are false, then the history's validity becomes suspicious. For example, is it true, as Beauchamp and Childress insist, that in the second half of the twentieth century the traditional medical ethics was found to be incapable?[48] If it is then the claim that it needed replacement gains weight. If it is disproved the claim is weakened.

Another test is whether there is a demonstrable consistency between a propositional predicate and its logically necessary conclusion (if . . . then). The better the history and its attendant argument, the more consistent its propositions. If a theory promises freedom and liberty but empowers enslavement, the result is a contradiction that impeaches the substance of that theory. This was, in essence, the criticism of the dreadlocked student in his designer-torn jeans (those from the Greeks into the nineteenth century who favored slavery and the marginalization of women but talked about individual freedom, etc.) and it is not wholly without merit.

In the end, however, these tests are insufficient, if only because discerning "falsehoods" is almost as hard as discovering "truths." And, too, consistency is never itself a wholly reliable test. Psychotic fantasies, to take the extreme, may be extremely consistent but based on the illusion that, in fact, persons from Mars captured the patient and implanted invisible listening devices in that person's left parietal lobe. "If" one accepts the assumption of alien implantation then everything makes sense. Much of my work here focuses on the propositional predicate, assumptions of circumstance or fact that lead to conclusions that seem logical, and indeed inevitable if, but *only* if, one accepts its predicate statement. Focusing on the "if" rather than the "then" of bioethical statements requires an approach that is necessarily interdisciplinary, ranging across not simply the philosophy and sociology of science but also the science itself. There is no other recourse if the fantastic assumption is not to be accepted reflexively as factual and thus consequential.

In the world of the concrete, "every statement of fact is haunted by questions of motive, origin, and ideology."[49] Facts stand not alone but in a context that give them meaning. Thus to think seriously about medical ethics means to consider not simply the individual proposition but as well the motive, origin, and ideology that contributed to its construction. In this way I seek an external context against which the received history (and its attendant philosophy) can be assessed. From this perspective, to anticipate the conclusion, bioethics spectacularly fails.

Consider bioethics' organizing ideal of "autonomy" and the resulting instrumental advocacy of individual choice in medical decision making: as Tom Beauchamp says, "Kant would have rejected the way the notion of autonomy has been treated in the most significant accounts of autonomy in applied [bio] ethics."[50] Indeed, he almost certainly would have rejected much of the ethics that bioethics promotes today, often in his name. Kant, who promoted humanity as precious and unique, certainly would have rejected Peter Singer's "All Animals Are Equal,"[51] and Margaret Nussbaum's morally equivalent species rights that include animals within the justice paradigm of her capabilities approach.[52]

We know Kant rejected graft organ transplantation—in his time it was the teeth of the poor being transplanted to the mouths of the rich—that today bioethicists almost universally promote as an unquestioned good.[53] Can we then indeed imagine in Kant's name a "duty" to provide organs for others, as Jean-Christophe Merle insists we must?[54] And how do we credit, giving Kant's belief in the radical freedom of the individual, bioethicist Rosamond Rhodes's insistence upon the (to her) enforceable duty of all to participate (whatever the individual might wish) in research test programs that carry real risk without any potential benefit to the human subjects involved?[55]

The real question becomes not, as Nicole Gerrand described it, the misuse of Kant in bioethical debates,[56] but whether Kant (and by extension other old philosophers in the Enlightenment tradition) is any use at all. And if Kant is not, then the methodology he promoted and which is the heart of bioethics allegiance to folk theory must go at as well. And then . . . what is the point of bioethics?

Social Evaluations

Another, more pragmatic way to think about bioethics is to forget philosophical niceties entirely and apply more general, instrumental definitional standards. To do this one finds a definition of bioethical purpose, and service, and then asks if the work of bioethicists meets that definitional promise. Bioethicist and physician Howard Brody, who won a lifetime award for his contribution to the field in 2009,[57] proposed one such test: "Is bioethics succeeding in speaking truth to power? Is bioethics effectively taking the side of the relatively less powerful, or siding with those who would exploit them?"[58] If the answer to the first part of the question is yes, then bioethics serves. If the answer to its second clause is yes, then it does not.

There is no reason to believe most other bioethicists share or have ever shared Brody's definition of bioethics as a thing that stands against exploitation of the weak by the strong. Some, for example Hilde Lindemann, have suggested this might serve someday as a general goal but is certainly not a yardstick by which the discipline could be judged.[59] Assessing bioethics' ability or interest in speaking truth to power is perhaps best understood as a way of asking what and whom does bioethics serve in the world of the sick and those who care for them? To find an answer it is necessary first to restate Brody's questions, noted in the preceding paragraph, as a proposition: *if* bioethics is not first and foremost a servant of the powerful and the status quo, *then* its measure must be its ability to act against the exploitative and oppressive. At the least, this is the type of statement the student in the Bob Marley tee shirt would have understood, one whose specific parts can be investigated.

Another bioethicist cited approvingly by Brody, Judith Andre created a related but more modest operational definition. Her bioethics, following upon the writing of Margaret Urban Walker,[60] is about "keeping moral space open, providing language and skills within it, identifying moral problems and helping create solutions for them."[61] Here the hope is that the methodology of bioethics will promote an arena in which social and philosophical discourse might lead to a careful examination of problems, their origins and solutions, in a way that is broadly accessible. Again, this can be stated as a proposition: *if* bioethics seeks to create transparently acceptable solutions to moral problems, *then* it must provide a language for their consideration that is applicable across a broadly deliberative process. The questions that result are, first, is bioethics designed to create solutions to moral problems? Second, if so, does it provide the language and means for its application (the "moral space") in a broader rather than narrower fashion?

It is in part in service of Andre's moral space that I chose a title drawn from Confucius. He warned us about the village worthies with "fine words and an insinuating appearance" who made virtue their own domain rather than a common good. Confucius wanted everyone to think about what is right and wrong, to think about what is correct and appropriate in a manner that was broadly conceived and popularly understood rather than narrowly construed. Defining a virtue or social good for their own benefit, Confucius's thieves were those who hid behind professional positions and a specialist language to make intelligent, practical virtue seem like a special virtue rather than a general good.

To promote a broader rather than narrower arena of moral deliberation I have labored to keep the text as free as possible of medical, legal, or philosophical jargon. Hopefully, the result will be as easily accessible to the student in his Bob Marley tee shirt as it is to the professor in his or her office, or the treating physician taking an hour for lunch at the clinic. In the same spirit, footnotes have been kept at a minimum to improve the readability of the whole. I have relied instead on a rather dense bibliography whose citations reflect the groundwork on which I both tear down and build. This is not a polemic but a critique, after all.

It will soon be clear, if it is not already, I find Brody and Andres at once wonderfully sincere and hopelessly naive. There is no evidence that either bioethics' progenitors or their inheritors have ever been concerned principally with speaking truth to power. In the main (there are always exceptions) they were and are interested in finding positions of power—in academics, in hospitals, or in government—in which their analytical and rhetorical skills will find favor. I think the sociologist John Evans was spot on when he argued, on the basis of a detailed study of documents and writings, that bioethics was created at least in part to shut down public deliberation that researchers feared would result in stronger regulations or funding cuts.[62] And more generally, I will argue, bioethics developed not to argue issues of care but to justify a specific vision of economic priorities within a neoliberal politic. Because a moral space is promised and not delivered bioethicists have become thieves of virtue and that, to me, is a pity.

All this boils down to a single, easily stated argument: bioethics' legitimacy rests on premises that that cannot be supported and a philosophical tradition at best tangential to its practical assignments. Despite its apparent allegiance to Kantian philosophy, and its attendant methodology, it takes a radical's knife to the heart of Kant's approach and the body of his conclusions. The structure and content of that wonderful, if failed, Enlightenment argument were debased through the piecemeal appropriation of his (and other philosopher's) complex works to serve ends that have little to do with the philosophical enterprise in which Kant and his successors were engaged. Maybe this book should have been titled, "*Who* killed Immanuel Kant and why did they do it?" That, however, would have been both too precious and too limited in its focus. The real subject is the means by which care of the fragile and sick is advanced or withheld. The real question is the degree and nature of our communal responsibility for the care of this or that individual.

2

Something Old: A Brief Review

There is nothing particularly mysterious about ethics, an attempt to formulate principles of conduct and practice in our lives. As a noun the word "ethics" tumbles down the language tree from the old Greek word *ēthos*, sometimes translated as "moral custom"[1] and sometimes as "character."[2] Is this or that choice the act of a "good" character, a person whose behavior we admire? The things we admire are those adhering to a moral custom, to ideas about the goodness or badness of specific acts. As custom, ethics and its moral valuation carry a shared meaning and a social history. Because we are all so engaged in custom and the assessment of character we are also engaged in philosophy, the name we give the framework of categories and definitions with which we organize our perspective on the world as a moral place. The word "philosophy," in its turn, means "loving wisdom" and wisdom is what we call the astute ability to navigate through the ethics and morals that develop from a specific philosophy as we struggle, alone and together, to navigate the landscape of appropriate or inappropriate action.

We think these thoughts as individuals educated within a culture whose ideas, language, and history shape—and are at the same time shaped by—our ethics, moralities, and philosophies. Our perspective is informed first by what we learn as children, then as students like the dreadlocked fellow in the Bob Marley tee shirt. Still later, these ideas are tested by our experiences as members of this or that community. Whatever one may think, for that judgment to have validity beyond the eccentric self it needs the agreement of others. The goal of the ethicist is to try and hack out an area of common agreement about the value of acts based on a shared morality grounded in a philosophy whose propositions are broadly accepted in a society at a specific point in time.

Professional ethics is no more mysterious. Its object is to define the parameters of appropriate action for a group of people with a singular set of skills that are plied in a society that values those skills.[3] Professional ethics never exists apart from the ethics of the society in which its practice takes place. It is instead the particular application of a general ethic to a singular arena of activity. In that application it both reinforces the broad, general morality (the "custom") and gains legitimacy from its application ("character"). As such the ethics of a specific trade has a critical role in a society's organization, enforcing its morality and demonstrating its application.[4]

Others have focused on the idea of a general professional ethic[5] and, separately, of a specific ethic of medical practice.[6] As a general or specific code, the result defines as appropriate (or inappropriate) the way in which a specific set of skills is applied while certifying *as* professionals those who agree to apply them in an approved manner. The famous Hippocratic oath, written sometime around the fourth century B.C.E., is the most famous, indeed the archetypical example of a professional ethic. For all that is to come later the Hippocratic tradition needs to be reviewed for two reasons. First, it is this tradition that bioethics sought to replace as outmoded, paternalistic, and unserviceable in the face of modern technologies. If these criticisms are true, when and how did it come to fail? And, second, if the criticism is insupportable, what does that say about the bioethics based on the older ethic's critique? At the least, a review of the Hippocratic tradition presents an alternative ethic against which the new one can be compared.

Across this history are two very different perspectives on the role of the physician and of medicine in general. First is the classical Hippocratic perspective in which the physician's principal role is the care of the patient as a member of a community and society, a person whose worth is not questioned. Beginning in the nineteenth century a new perspective arose that saw the physician as first and foremost a servant of the state, and of state economics. Future chapters will argue that bioethics might have embraced either ethical viewpoint as primary but from the start adopted the second. Its principal allegiance as an arbiter of medical practice has never been the patient in need of care but the state and its economic future. As such it has sought continually to restrain the traditional moral agency of the Hippocratic physician, or at least his or her focus on patient care as the primary good he or she is pledged to promote.

Hippocratic Ethics

The canon of Hippocrates of Cos (460 BC–ca. 370 BC) included a summary of the anatomical, biological, and theoretical medicine of his day (figure 2.1). The famous Hippocratic oath was a part of the whole, a social statement of the role of the physician in his or her society. A central claim of modern bioethics and a principal rationale for its creation is the presumed inadequacy of the traditional Hippocratic ethics of medical practice that it sought to replace.[7] The canonical *Principles of Biomedical Ethics* presents this as a necessity so obvious it needed little discussion.[8] The result, as Tristram Engelhardt politely put it, is that, "The Hippocratic vow to 'keep the ill from injustice' and a historical definition of the physician as a moral agent responsible to and for the patient have been diminished."[9] That implies a heady charge: the moral agency of medical practice, its ethical and social character, was diminished by a bioethics that opened the door, at least potentially, to injustices a Hippocratic ethicist would not have permitted. If true, the question becomes how this happened and the manner in which the bioethicist replaced the physician to the detriment of the patient. To answer that question first requires a review of the traditional ethic of medicine and its manner of service over centuries.

Hippocratic Ethics

Under the old, Hippocratic ethic medical professionals pledged themselves to a code of conduct and practice that was at once medical and social. "Greeks habitually thought of themselves as so indissolubly linked with their own particular city-state," writes Peter Singer, "that they did not distinguish between their own interests and the interests of the community in which they lived."[10] The Hippocratic oath was thus the obligation of a specific set of community members who saw their interests, those of their patients, and the interests of the community at large as inextricably entwined. Those who swore to the oath were acknowledged as moral agents whose income was derived from the sale of their services

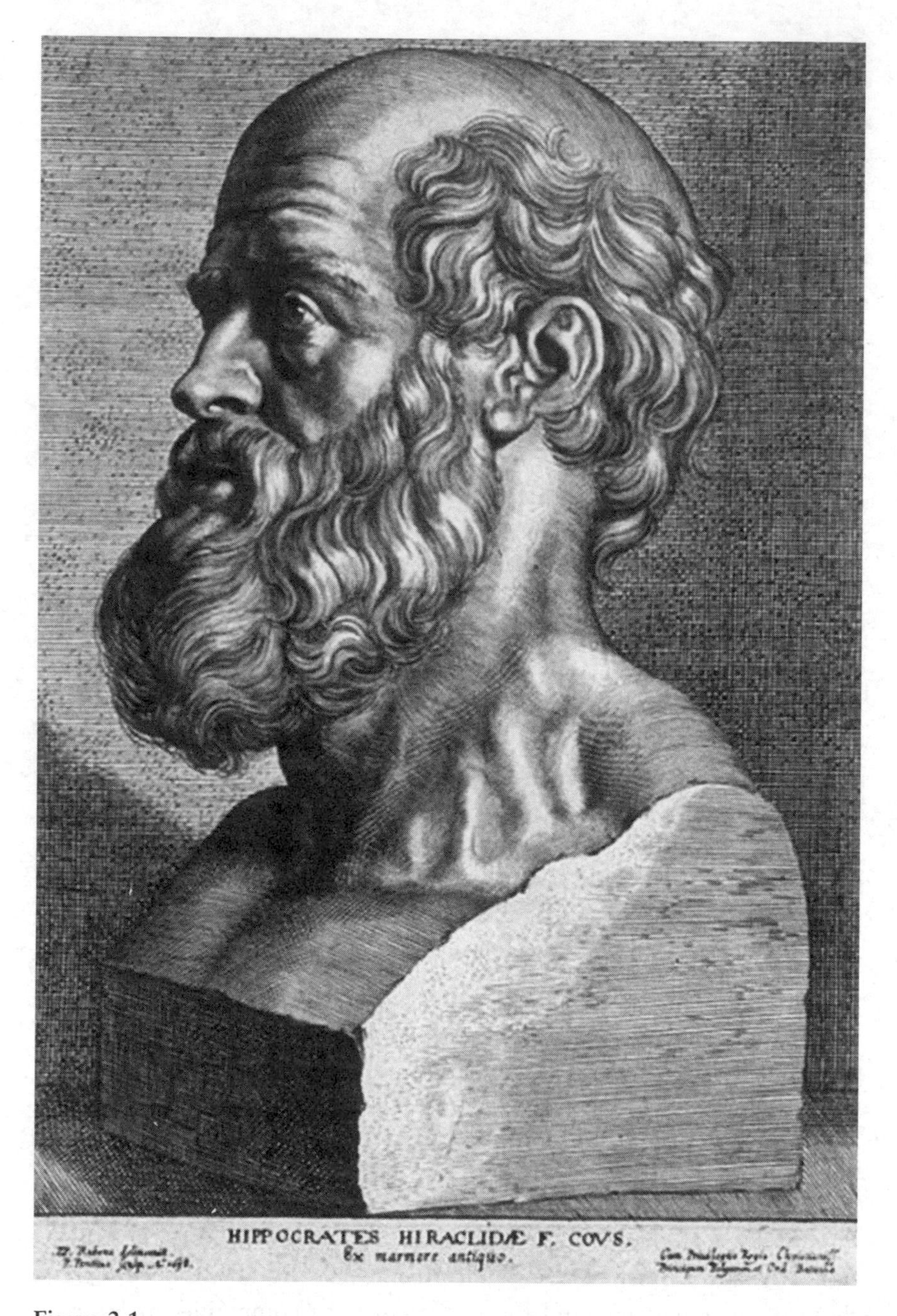

Figure 2.1
The "father of medicine," Hippocrates created a technical corpus and an ethical focus that served medicine until the 1960s when bioethicists declared it insufficient. Rubens crafted this bust of Hippocrates in 1638. *Source*: National Library of Medicine, Bethesda, MD.

to other citizens. As caregivers of the individual they thus also served the state at large.

While the oath named a pantheon of gods, its legitimacy was not derived from their invocation. Apollo, Asclepius, Health, Hygeia, indeed, "all the gods and goddesses," were evocations that tied the professional, and the profession itself, to society by invoking the cosmology in which its general morality was grounded (figure 2.2). This legitimized an ethical covenant operative at three levels. First, it bound the physician to his school of medicine and its general standards of practice in a compact of mutual assistance, cooperation, and learning. Second, the oath defined the goal of practitioners as the care of the sick irrespective of income or standing. Third, the oath tied the community of physicians to society at large. The reward for honorable practice came not from the gods but from the communities physicians lived in and whose citizens they were privileged to care for. The only promise the oath made was that those physicians who lived by its ethics would "enjoy life and the practice of the art, respected by all men."

Boiled down to its essential features there were really just two parts to the oath. In the first, medical practitioners swore to honor and respect their teachers ("hold him who taught me this art equally dear to me as my parents, to be a partner in life with him") and their fellow practitioners (it was, in those days, a male occupation). To equate medical teachers with parents—those from whom one learned how to live in society within its rules—served to create a hierarchical sense of familial allegiance (to teachers and then to colleagues), and thus by implication produced an ethical imperative of interpersonal, family-like mutual support among colleagues. This section of the oath thus enshrined a collegial value system essential to the advance of medical knowledge, the performance of the system of medical instruction, and the moral vision of the medical community. Out of this came a sense of professional solidarity and cooperation as well as an ethic that distinguished between appropriate and inappropriate behaviors.[11]

Hippocratic Practice

The second section of the oath defined the ethical responsibilities of the fee-for-service practitioner, an entrepreneur whose income was directly in relation to the sale of specific services. However, care, not income, was

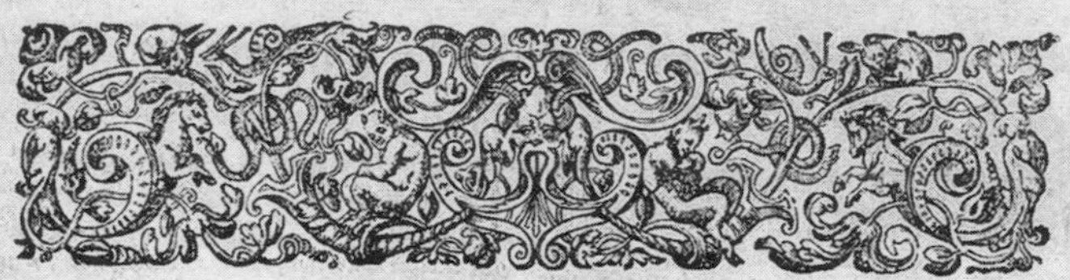

ΙΠΠΟΚΡΑΤΟΥΣ ΟΡΚΟΣ.

HIPPOCRATIS IVSIVRANDVM.

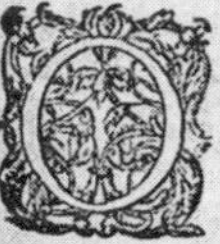

'ΜΝΥΜΙ [1] Ἀπόλλωνα ἰητρὸν καὶ Ἀσκληπιὸν καὶ Ὑγείαν καὶ Πανάκειαν, καὶ θεοὺς πάντας καὶ πάσας, ἵστορας ποιεύμενος, ἐπιτελέα ποιήσειν κατὰ δύναμιν καὶ κρίσιν ἐμὴν, ὅρκον τόνδε καὶ ξυγγραφὴν τήνδε. [3] ἡγήσασθαι μὲν τὸν διδάξαντά με τὴν τέχνην ταύτην, [4] ἴσα γενέτῃσιν ἐμοῖσιν, καὶ βίου κοινώσασθαι καὶ χρεῶν χρηΐζοντι μετάδοσιν ποιήσασθαι. καὶ γένος τὸ ἐξ ἑωυτέου, ἀδελφοῖς ἴσον ἐπικρινέειν ἄῤῥεσι. καὶ διδάξειν τὴν τέχνην ταύτην, ἢν χρηΐζωσι μανθάνειν, [5] ἄνευ μισθοῦ καὶ ξυγγραφῆς. [6] παραγγελίης τε καὶ ἀκροήσιος, καὶ τῆς λοιπῆς ἁπάσης μαθήσιος, μετάδοσιν ποιήσασθαι υἱοῖσί τε ἐμοῖσι, καὶ τοῖσι τοῦ ἐμὲ διδάξαντος. καὶ μαθηταῖσι συγγεγραμμένοις τε, καὶ ὡρκισμένοις νόμῳ ἰητρικῷ. ἄλλῳ δὲ οὐδενί. διαιτήμασί τε χρήσομαι, ἐπ' ὠφελείῃ καμνόντων κατὰ δύναμιν καὶ κρίσιν ἐμήν. [7] ἐπὶ δηλήσει δὲ καὶ ἀδικίῃ εἴρξειν. [8] οὐ δώσω δὲ οὐδὲ φάρμακον οὐδενὶ αἰτηθεὶς, θανάσιμον. οὐδὲ ὑφηγήσομαι ξυμβουλίην τοιήνδε. ὁμοίως δὲ οὐδὲ γυναικὶ πεσσὸν φθόριον δώσω. ἁγνῶς δὲ καὶ ὁσίως διατηρήσω βίον τὸν ἐμὸν καὶ τέχνην τὴν ἐμήν. οὐ τεμέω δὲ οὐδὲ μὴν λιθιῶντας. [9] ἐκχωρήσω δὲ ἐργάτῃσιν ἀνδράσι πρήξιος τῆσδε. εἰς οἰκίας δὲ ὁκόσας ἂν ἐσίω, ἐσελεύσομαι ἐπ' ὠφελείῃ καμνόντων, ἐκτὸς ἐὼν πάσης ἀδικίης ἑκουσίης καὶ φθορίης τῆς τε ἄλλης [10] καὶ ἀφροδισίων ἔργων, ἐπί τε γυναικείων σωμάτων [11] καὶ ἀνδρῴων, ἐλευθέρων τε καὶ δούλων. ἃ δ' ἂν ἐν θεραπείῃ ἢ ἴδω, ἢ ἀκούσω, ἢ καὶ ἄνευ θεραπείης κατὰ βίον ἀνθρώπων, ἃ μὴ χρή ποτε ἐκλαλέεσθαι ἔξω, σιγήσομαι, ἄῤῥητα ἡγεύμενος εἶναι τὰ τοιαῦτα. Ὅρκον μὲν οὖν μοι τόνδε ἐπιτελέα ποιέοντι, [12] καὶ μὴ ξυγχέοντι, εἴη ἐπαύρασθαι καὶ βίου καὶ τέχνης, δοξαζομένῳ παρὰ πᾶσιν ἀνθρώποις, εἰς τὸν αἰεὶ χρόνον· παραβαίνοντι δὲ καὶ ἐπιορκοῦντι, τἀναντία τουτέων.

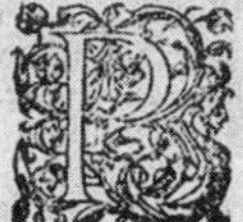

ER Apollinem Medicum, & Æſculapium, Hygiamque & Panaceam iureiurando affirmo, & Deos Deasq; omnes teſtor, me quantum viribus & iudicio valuero, quod nunc iuro, & ex ſcripto ſpondeo planè obſeruaturū. Præceptorem quidem qui me hanc artem edocuit, parentum loco habiturum, eique cùm ad victum, tum etiam ad vſum neceſſaria, grato animo communicaturum & ſuppeditaturum. Eiusque poſteros apud me eodem loco quo germanos fratres fore, eosque ſi hanc artem addiſcere volent, abſque mercede & ſyngrapha edocturum. Præceptionum quoque & auditionum, totiusque reliquæ diſciplinæ, cùm meos & eius qui me edocuit liberos, tum diſcipulos qui Medico iureiurando nomen fidemque dederint, participes facturum, aliorum prætereа neminem. Victus quoque rationem, quantum facultate & iudicio conſequi potero, ægris vtilem me præſcripturum, eosq; ab omni noxia & iniuria vindicaturum. Neq; cuiuſquam precibus adductus, alicui medicamentum lethale propinabo, neque huius rei author ero. Neque ſimili ratione mulieri peſſum ſubdititium ad fœtum corrumpendum exhibebo: ſed caſtam & ab omni ſcelere puram, tum vitam, tum ætatem meam perpetuò præſtabo. Neque verò calculo laborantes ſecabo, ſed magiſtris eius artis peritis id muneris concedam. In quancunque autem domum ingreſſus fuero, ad ægrotantium ſalutem ingrediar, omnem iniuriæ inferendæ & corruptelæ ſuſpicionem procul fugiens, tum vel maximè rerum venerearum cupiditatem, erga mulieres iuxta ac viros, tum ingenuos, tum ſeruos. Quæ verò inter curandum, aut etiam Medicinam minimè faciens, in communi hominum vita, vel videro, vel audiero, quæ minimè in vulgus efferri oporteat, ea arcana eſſe ratus, ſilebo. Hoc igitur iuſiurandum ſi religiosè obſeruaro, ac minimè irritum fecero, mihi liceat cum ſumma apud omnes exiſtimatione perpetuò vitam fœlicem degere, & artis vberrimum fructum percipere. Quòd ſi illud violauero & peierauero, contraria mihi contingant.

Figure 2.2

This is a 1595 version of the Hippocratic oath, in Greek and Latin, from the National Library of Medicine collection, Bethesda, MD. *Source*: http://www.nlm.nih.gov/hmd/greek/greek_oath.html (accessed December 12, 2011).

to be the primary virtue of Hippocratic practitioner. "Into whatever homes I go, I will enter them for the benefit of the sick, avoiding any voluntary act of impropriety or corruption." The famous injunction to "first, do no harm" reinforced this caring goal by naming harm as its prohibited corollary. This meant not giving poisons ("I will not give a lethal drug to anyone if I am asked, nor will I advise such a plan") or otherwise acting in a manner that would violate the sanctity of life that was a principal moral value underlying the oath and the society in which it was enacted.

The oath also prohibited a series of specific social improprieties, for example, having sex with patients or members of patient households. The goal here was multiple. First, it was to ensure the physician would have the help and support of family members necessarily engaged in the care of a patient. The promise to keep secret "All that may come to my knowledge in the exercise of my profession" assured the physician would not use personal knowledge gained in patient care inappropriately. And by promising to act morally rather than selfishly, the oath emphasized the goal of selfless service to the patient—slave or slave owner, rich or poor—by the Hippocratic practitioner. In his or her rejection of improprieties the physician was to be an exemplar of moral behavior as well as a practitioner whose goal was the health of the community through the care of its individual members.

Implicit in the oath was a principle of distributive justice: medicine might be a business whose paying clients were the slave owners and not the slaves, but the Hippocratic physician had a duty to care for the poor as well as the rich even when that care yielded little financial compensation. As Thomas Percival reminded his eighteenth-century contemporaries, physicians and surgeons were never to "suffer themselves to be restrained by parsimonious considerations from prescribing . . . drugs even of high price, when required in diseases of extraordinary malignity and danger."[12] Nor, Percival continued, were the obligations of Hippocratic physicians separate from those of hospitals or other social institutions: "No economy of a fatal tendency ought to be admitted into institutions founded on the principles of purest beneficence."

Care of the most needy social members thus was enshrined as a good beyond the economic priorities of society or the relative wealth of its members. Percival's restatement of the Hippocratic ideal warned against permitting "sordid financial pressures" to affect the obligation to care. As Michael Walzer put it, "The distributive logic of the practice of medicine seems to be this: that care should be proportionate to illness and not to wealth."[13] The ideal of care as a general communal virtue—"that people care about, and, where necessary, care for one another"[14]—thus was focused for the physician on the specific obligations of the professional.

Certainly this is idealistic and simplistic. There were always some whose medical practice was self-serving. There were always dilemmas and conflicts about what was right but, in the main, the Hippocratic ideal served as the ideal within which medicine was practiced in various cultures across centuries of epidemics and pandemics in which physicians did what they could for the sick even when that care, often uncompensated, put the physician's own life at risk. In the records of the Black Plague, and later of yellow fever, and later still, of cholera there were doctors who fled the danger but others who stayed in place to serve those who needed their help, often dying as a result. To not treat was to deny the categorical imperative of humanist duty and social service that were the moral heart of the Hippocratic oath as it had come down through the centuries.

This ideal of fiduciary responsibility over professional accountancy stood, at least in theory, into the second half of the twentieth century. In 1957, for example, the American Medical Association declared: "A physician should not dispose of his services under terms or conditions which tend to interfere with or impair the free and complete exercise of his medical judgment and skill or tend to cause a deterioration of the quality of medical care."[15] It was this sense of vocational virtue irrespective of personal gain, of care as an overriding noncommercial, social ethic that bioethics would seek to replace.

Medicine and Society

The attraction of the oath to the new practitioner was multiple. First it assured the doctor a place in a professional society whose members might be called upon for collegial counsel and support. A trace of that sense of mutuality is maintained today in, for example, the Fellowship Pledge of the American College of Surgeons whose members pledge to support and seek the support of others at need.[16] Second, the Hippocratic association engendered public trust in the Hippocratic practitioner: Patients might not know a doctor personally but would know and trust in the community of medicine to which the physician belonged. "Many of the writings in the Hippocratic corpus reflect the concerns of physicians traveling from place to place through Greece and Asia Minor."[17] There was little reason to trust the itinerant stranger as a person but every reason to trust the Hippocratic practitioner. Third, the oath set parameters of appropriate practice that gave the physician guidance. Some acts were encouraged, others were prohibited, and therefore if asked to perform an abortion or euthanasia the Hippocratic doctor could say, "No, I'm not allowed."

Equally important, the first part of the oath honoring the medical teachers and their instruction tied the physician to the knowledge base that was Hippocratic medicine. That corpus of knowledge, made available to society through its physicians, was formidable. Hippocrates was no armchair philosopher but a medical man setting out the state of then current knowledge—ethical, practical, and social. The ethic would have been less important if the medicine it instructed were less impressive. The Hippocratic canon was complete in its description of the nature and origin of disease. As importantly, it was clear in its focus on the human subject in his or her community and its physical environment. Together, the clinical, environmental, and social elements of the Hippocratic vision combined to describe how disease could be addressed and health promoted. Membership in the Hippocratic community meant membership in a community of knowledge that was the best of its day. This knowledge was at once environmental, social, and technical (figure 2.3).

We read today Hippocrates' description of an influenza epidemic and recognize it; we read his description of cancer and know it as the tumorous growth we might see today in surgery or under the microscope, sectioned and stained. Even if his explanations strike us as quaint Hippocrates was a close observer who understood the relationship between observed symptom and bodily dysfunction. Bubbles in the urine, he instructed, were a symptom of a kidney disease we know today as *proteinuria*. It results not from a "windiness" of the airs of the body, as he wrote, but from an excess of protein resulting in a decrease in the urine's surface tension. Still, symptom by symptom, disease by disease,

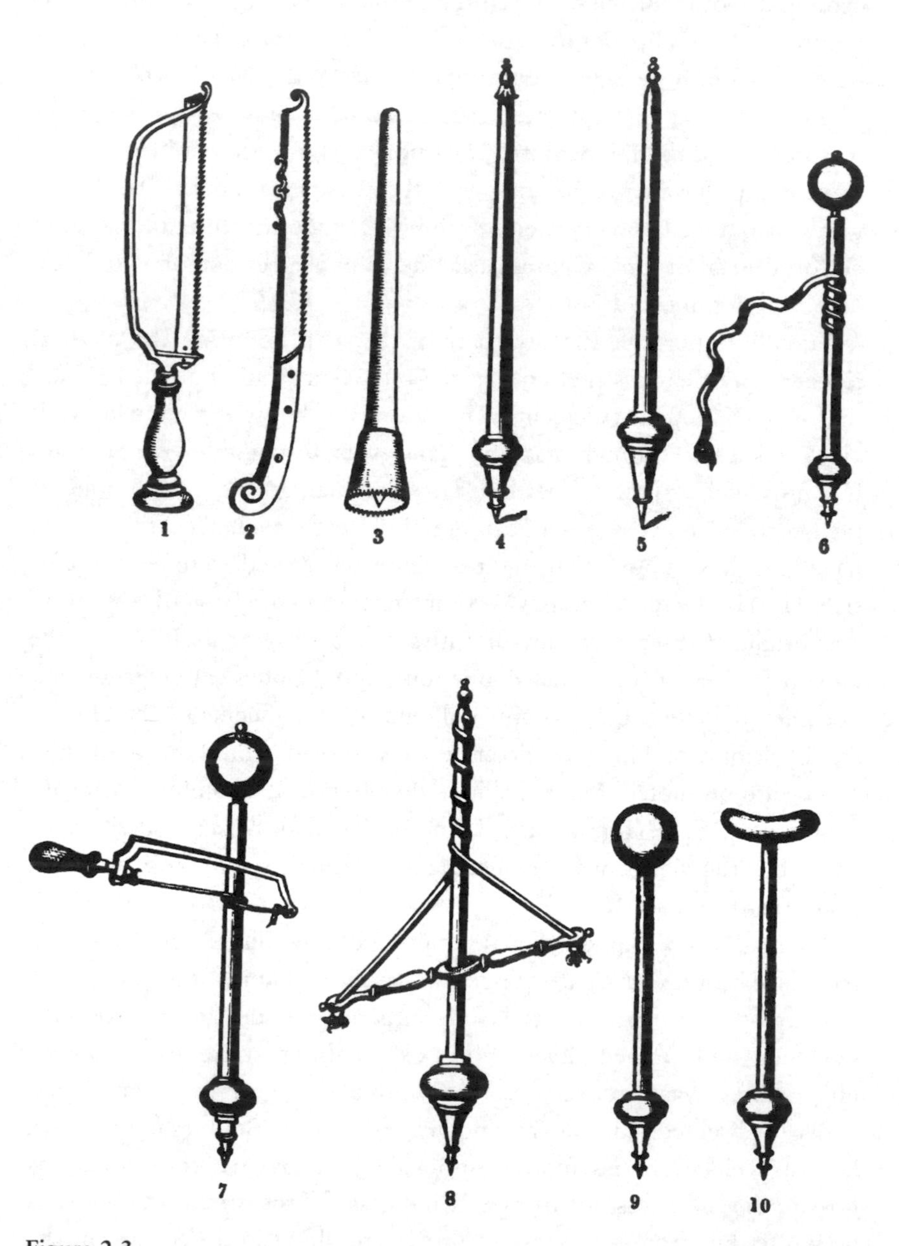

Figure 2.3
This plate of medical tools, from a nineteenth-century English translation of the works of Hippocrates, emphasizes not Hippocratic ethics but the practicality of the medicine he promoted. From Francis Adams's nineteenth-century *The Genuine Works of Hippocrates*. *Source*: http://www.chlt.org/sandbox/dh/Adams/ (accessed December 12, 2011)

Hippocrates cataloged the ills of the patient and then matched them to the treatment options of the day.

And, too, Hippocrates was perhaps the first medical environmentalist who saw the relation between disease and location clearly. He was as well an early advocate of "preventive medicine," urging appropriate diet and lifestyle as a way to promote good health. All in all, the Hippocratic corpus was an astonishing thing whose prestige has endured for more than two millennia and in a range of translations (Arabic, English, Greek, Latin, and so on). In taking the Hippocratic oath the physician took possession of this knowledge as his own, this perspective. The oath was the lynch pin in the total assemblage of knowledge that was at once clinical, practical, scientific, and social. Little wonder, then, that the oath remained a medical constant even as medicine advanced from its Hippocratic base into the sciences of the twentieth century. Indeed, it became a model for other oaths by which a range of professional associations sought legitimacy in the guild tradition of the Middle Ages,[18] and still later, in the industrializing world.[19] It was, at least until bioethics sought its replacement, the model of a community ethic by an association of persons whose skills distinguish them in a society willing to grant them exclusive rights to a range of technical practices.

Medical Symbolism: The Caduceus

The genius of the oath lay not in its specificity but its plasticity. Its injunctions to care and to community were not tied to any one God, not bound by the strictures of a single religion or society. Greek or Roman, Catholic or Jew, all could swear the oath without believing in the Gods of the Greek pantheon. What mattered was the promise to apply a technical body of knowledge to the general benefit of society through the care of its individual members. All else was malleable, to be interpreted and reinterpreted as the knowledge base, and the societies in which it developed, changed.

Consider the traditional symbol of the physician: Asclepius's staff around which a single snake was entwined (figure 2.4). Nobody really understands it. We call it Asclepius's staff because he was the Greek God of medicine, the son of Apollo and the Trikkaian princess Koronis. Perhaps its use suggested the Gods' approval of the physician's work

ἍΠΑΝΤΑ ΤᾺ ΤΟΥ͂
ἹΠΠΟΚΡΆΤΟΥΣ.

OMNIA OPERA
HIPPOCRATIS.

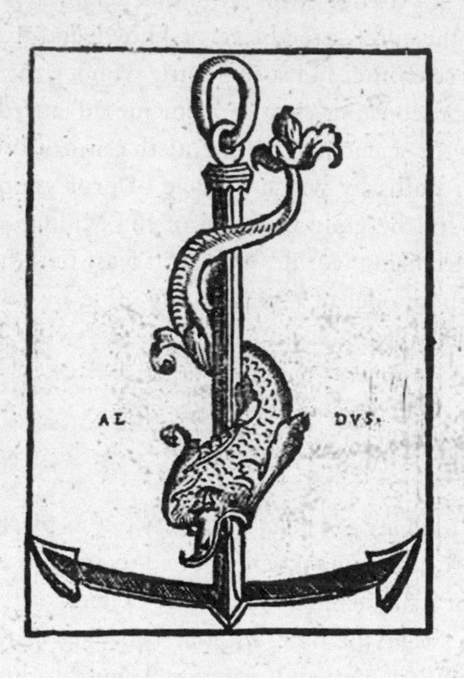

Ne quis alius impune, aut Venetiis, aut usquam lo-
corum hos Hippocratis libros imprimat, &
Clementis VII. Pont. Max. & Sena-
tus Veneti decreto cau-
tum est.

Figure 2.4
The traditional symbol of the physician was the single snake entwined around an upright staff. A second snake was later added, although the symbolism of either single or entwined snakes is somewhat unclear. *Source*: National Library of Medicine, Bethesda, MD.

and thus the godly nature of medical care. Or, perhaps, the staff merely symbolized the itinerant physician who carried a walking stick as he traveled from place to place. The snake may have symbolized rejuvenation, an idea that comes from its periodic shedding of its skin. Or, perhaps, it was not a snake at all but the filarial worm *Dracunculus medinensis* physicians would cut from under a patient's skin and wind on sticks in Hippocratic times.[20] Nobody really knows. Nor does it matter overmuch.

The symbol was suppressed in the first centuries of the Christian era because of its association with Asclepius, and thus the old pantheon of gods that Christianity sought to replace. It was reinstated in the Renaissance, however, when in the burst of new sciences and new thinking a grounding in antiquity seemed desirable. The symbol was then reinterpreted to signify not pantheistic allegiance but instead a tradition of socially responsible, practical medicine. Later, the single snake was given a companion in its eternal entwinement around the solid staff. Maybe this was an aesthetic addition to balance an image that seemed incomplete. Perhaps the entwined snakes were to suggest the duality of the human—mind and body—that nineteenth-century philosophies would later assert.

Some think the entwined pair a reference to Hermes, the swift messenger of Zeus, although it seems to have been introduced at a time when Hermes was no longer admired (figure 2.5). Still, as a bow to antiquity, the snakes' twinning made sense. Mythology told of how the once mendacious and thieving god-child (and thus the patron of the commercial marketplace) in maturity became a peacemaker, separating two fighting serpents who then entwined themselves in friendship around his staff, giving us the symbol we see today in the modern caduceus.[21] Just maybe, the entwined snakes were an early recognition of the need to resolve tensions between commercial realities and medical ideals in an ethical practice that was also a compensable trade.

We do know that Hermes' wings first were added to the staff and entwined snakes during the American Civil War to create the symbol of the U.S. Military Medical Corps. That symbol was emblematic of the speed with which the wagons of the service could reach the wounded on the battlefield. In the twentieth century that addition became a general symbol of swift service by, among others, ambulance companies, and of

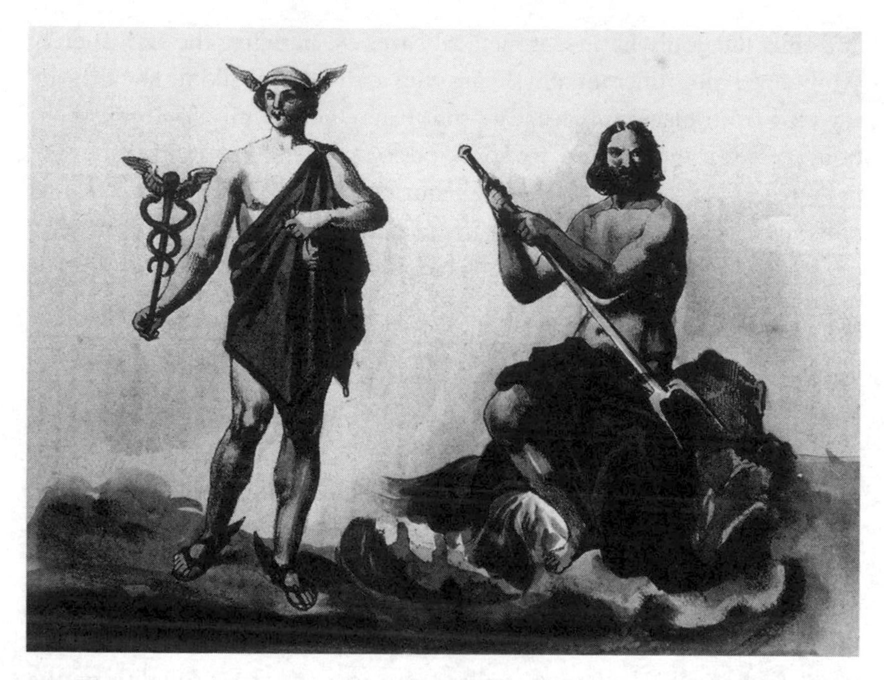

Figure 2.5
In this nineteenth-century lithograph by an unknown artist, Mercury is shown with the entwined snakes on his staff next to Neptune with his symbol of office, the Trident. *Source*: National Library of Medicine, Bethesda, MD.

appropriate and timely service by medical suppliers and pharmaceutical suppliers.

Social Medicine

Elements of the symbol of the physician changed but the essential message—care—did not. Across this same long history society changed and medicine changed as a result. With the growth of mercantilism medicine increasingly faced the challenge of dynamically epidemic diseases spread in the seventeenth century across the trading world by cargo ships and trading caravans.[22] With the urbanization promoted by vastly increased global trade and accompanying early industrialism came overcrowded cities whose populations were at increasing risk for a range of epidemic and pandemic diseases. To be a doctor and thus fulfill the oath came to mean, for some, a public role in which the physician's focus was not solely the individual patient but the body public. Given the profound entwining of individual and community in the older Greek ideal, this was less a transposition than a shift in emphasis, one that was preventive and general in nature.

By the end of the eighteenth century, for example, U.S. physician Benjamin Rush, a signatory of the U.S. Declaration of Independence, diagnosed poverty as a primary, disease-inducing ill. Poverty "exposes men to being soldiers and dying with yellow fever. It exposes women to diseases from hard labour, and to seduction, and both sexes to famine, strong drink to obviate hunger, and to the diseases from cold."[23] Why should cities be erected, asked Noah Webster during the savage yellow fever epidemics of the late eighteenth century, if they are only to be the tombs of men?[24] Dr. Samuel Latham, a contemporary of Rush and Webster, was equally eloquent. What was the point of caring for small-pox patients, he asked, if the poor were saved to endure conditions inimical to health and guaranteed to breed another, likely fatal disease? He asked the question time and again, first as a cofounder of the first U.S. medical journal, the *Medical Repository*,[25] then as a New York State assemblyman, later as a U.S. congressman, and finally as a U.S. senator.

At the end of the eighteenth and beginning of the nineteenth centuries, physicians like Latham increasingly perceived it to be their Hippocratic duty to act as citizens to reduce the causal factors promoting disease. If poor drainage and poor sanitation created areas of foul odors whose miasmas were the locus of infectious disease, as medical theory then insisted,[26] then as citizens entrusted with specialized knowledge it was the duty of physicians to argue for better sanitation. If poverty and its attendant ills promoted disease, then physicians were obliged to act as social activists for the good of all potential patients. After all, Hippocratic medicine was as much about wellness as it was about disease.

Here, perhaps, is another rationale for the caduceus's second snake, as a symbol of social medicine entwined with one symbolizing the duty to the individual patient. Certainly, as followers of Hippocrates, eighteenth-century physicians saw charitable care of the poor as a duty. But, which poor and how many were a doctor obliged to serve? Neither the Hippocratic canon nor Christian scripture (or Talmudic wisdom, for that matter) explained how much service a physician was obliged to give to those who could not afford to pay his or her fees. Certainly members of local families fallen on (hopefully) temporary hard times could not be turned away but what about the itinerant drunk, con man, laborer, or traveling wastrel who presented as needy? Was there an obligation to treat all these strangers? If they were not members of the immediate communities was their humanity sufficient to demand a physician's response to their needs? Where did duty end and the economics of the individual practice take over?

Cholera: Economic and Social

These tensions came to a head in the first cholera pandemic that began in 1817 in Paswar, India,[27] spreading into Europe in the 1920s and arriving in Britain in the autumn of 1831. In an attempt to prevent its arrival, in early 1831 the British government proposed quarantine measures refusing port entry to ships from areas where the disease was already active.[28] There was nothing new in this idea. Recurrent plague visitations had resulted early on in the assumption of disease as a dynamic traveler that accompanied pilgrims. Quarantines had been a consistent response to epidemic and pandemic disease at least since the repeated plague epidemics of the fourteenth and fifteenth centuries.[29] The assumption was that epidemic disease was a portable thing that traveled with merchant goods. To stop plague, or another epidemic, one stopped the travel (figure 2.6). The result, in the early years of cholera, was that three thousand ships seeking entry to British ports were delayed at a cost of thousands of pounds to merchants and shipping companies.[30]

Physicians writing in *The Lancet* in 1831 argued on ethical grounds against quarantine as an offensive restraint of the nation's lifeblood, trade.[31] It was, they wrote, a "savage system," a ruinous intrusion on the economic life of the nation. Irrespective of its efficacy, quarantine was a "visitation" worse than the plague itself. To insist that quarantine was worse than plague was to say that restraint of trade, even if it protected the life of citizens, was more serious than the death of thousands from pandemic disease. Here, perhaps for the first time, physicians were arguing a public policy to protect not the individual patient, not the population in which patient and physician together resided, but instead the economic lifeblood of the nation at large. Rush, Webster, Latham,

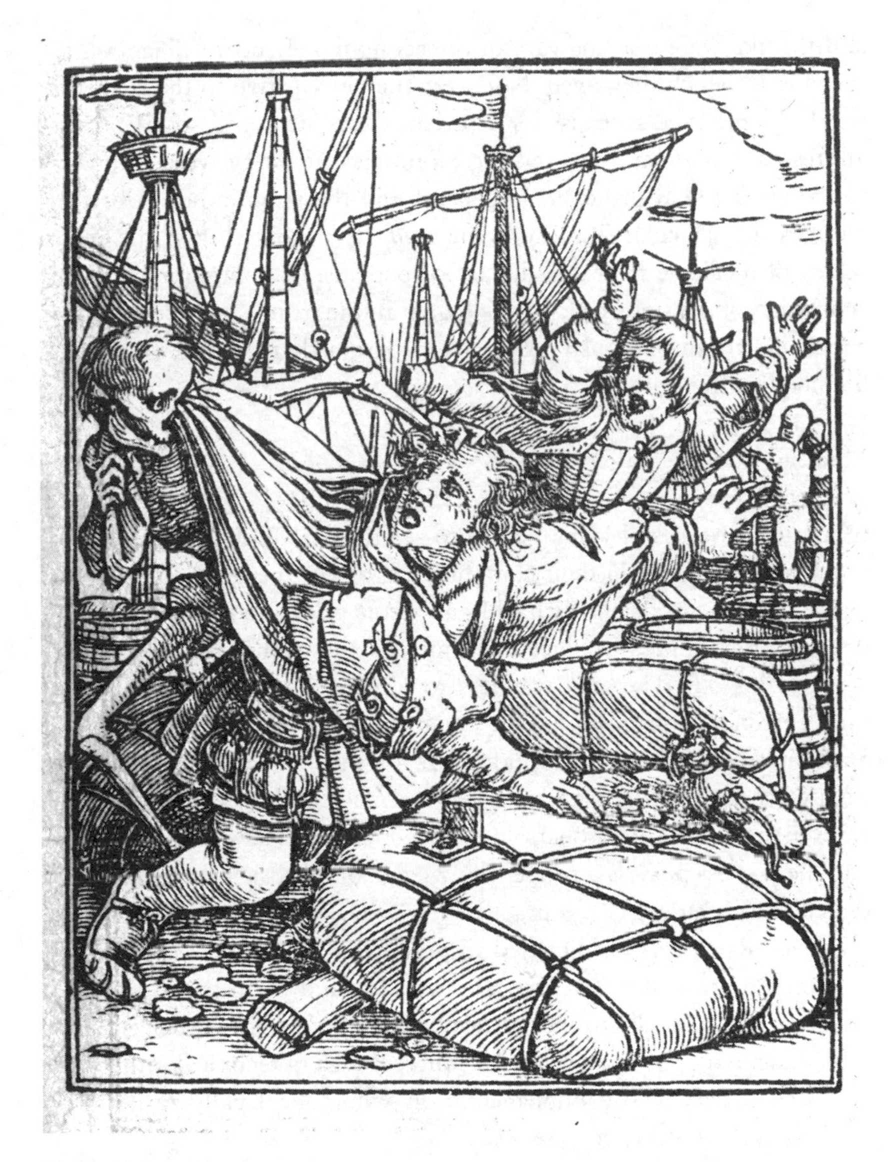

Figure 2.6
In Holbein's *Death of Death*, merchant ships and their cargo carried plague from place to place. *Source*: Tom Koch, *Disease Maps: Epidemics on the Ground* (Chicago, IL: University of Chicago Press, 2011).

and the like were not unaware of the economic effects of illness on the societies in which they lived. Nor were they insensitive to the costs that would be incurred were issues of urban cleanliness and social poverty addressed. For them, however, the economics of safety were secondary to the ethical goal of health in general and the specific health of their patients in particular. Radically, the *Lancet* authors shifted the moral center of medicine from the disease of persons, or communities, to the economics of the state, transforming quarantine from a method of citizen protection to an onerously expensive program that impinged upon the lifeblood of the state: its trade.

Medicine and the State

In a range of areas physician came to see themselves as servants not of the ill and the needy in their communities, but of the state. In 1836, for example, Irish physician Michael Ryan wrote a text on medical jurisprudence that attempted to place medicine practice within the legal framework of his day. The goal was less to inform medical practitioners of their personal or professional duty than to put medical practitioners in authoritative positions as adjudicators of medico-legal disputes. "We peruse the most absurd and unscientific medical evidence, more especially in the reports of coroners' inquest, which could never have appeared had the witness possess a proper knowledge of forensic medicine, or had the coroner been a medical practitioner."[32] The physician jurist was not a healer—Ryan was not licensed to practice in England—but instead a legalist and scientist whose first allegiance would be to the forensics of medicine and secondly to the articles of law that governed society. In his jurisprudential opus Ryan argued a coherent idea of technical rather than social standards whose implementation would be legally rather than professionally supervised.

Eugenic Medicine: 1890–1907

This shift in moral focus from patient care to state necessities was fundamental. By the late nineteenth century, a number of medical researchers sought to advantage society through the identification of burdensome social deviants who, they believed, could and should be removed from the public.[33] Critical here was the work of nineteenth-century neuroanatomist Franz Joseph Gall (1758–1828), who claimed his findings would permit medical experts to describe precisely the innate intellectual and moral capacities of individuals and thus permit the exclusion of those who were found deficient (figure 2.7). The diagnostic he proposed was called phrenology and based on the observable shape of the person's skull.

Here the goal of medicine, in the guise of fundamental research, was the definition of the acceptable person within a population whose composition could be controlled to the advantage of the state and its economies. The result was what in 1888 Sir Francis Galton named eugenics, a process of social selection in the interests not of today's patients but instead of a better, future state. The assumption was that medical science had the knowledge to identify the inborn characteristics of individuals and the ability to distinguish between those that were burdensome and those that could be valued as socially productive. Practitioners had a social duty to apply that knowledge in a manner that would eliminate future generations of unproductive and thus economically burdensome social misfits. Physicians who had sworn first to do no harm and to treat all who required care were now asked to participate in harmful judgments and practices. Those who accepted this duty for the good of the economic state would help cull those judged medically deficient from the population.

Some physicians took to the role of medical judge, and sometimes executioner, with alacrity. Famously, in the early twentieth century Chicago surgeon Harry J. Haiselden refused to treat "defectives." These were infants he might have saved but whose limitations were so severe he thought they would be better off dead and society would be better off without them. Arguing his views in the newspapers of the day, "he hoped to demonstrate that his ideas enjoyed widespread support among those who had no previous chance to express their opinions in public, and to compel those who previously had no opinions to choose sides."[34] The national debate that resulted was, in many ways, a precursor to contemporary disagreements on physician-assisted suicide[35] and separately, the eugenics of genetic testing discussed here in chapter 8.

Here the old Hippocratic ethic came into direct conflict with an ethic whose focus was state economics. A series of coroner inquests reviewing deaths attributed to Haiselden condemned his actions as reprehensible,

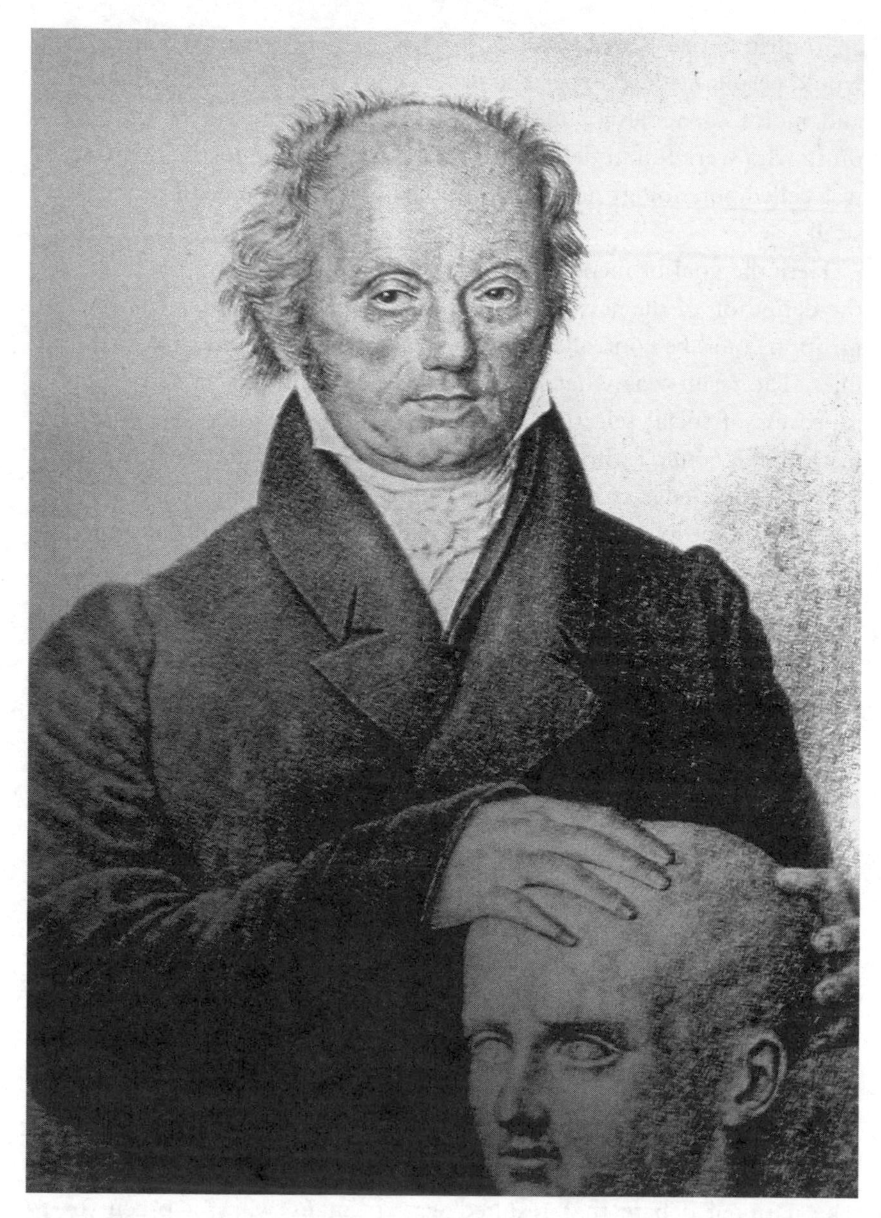

Figure 2.7
This portrait shows Gall with his hands on the bust of a head whose characteristics he believed he could interpret through the science of phrenology he proposed as a medical science. *Source*: University of Sidney, Dr. Niko Tiliopoulos.

because "a doctor's duty is to 'save or prolong life,'" but not legally actionable.[36] The Illinois attorney general demanded indictments that the state's attorney, a supporter of Haiselden, refused to file. The legal, medical, and social codes were in this struggle seen as distinct and separate (a medical decision could be socially reprehensible but legal).

For its part, the medical community was divided. The Illinois State Board of Health refused to revoke Haiselden's medical license while the Chicago Medical Society expelled Haiselden for unprofessional behavior. The behavior it condemned was not Haiselden's violation of the Hippocratic oath but rather his habit of arguing his position in the newspapers of the day. To his medical contemporaries, Haiselden's failure was not in the noncare of his patients but in a public stance that bypassed his professional community. For their part, the newspapers of the day happily weighed in on one or another side of the controversy. Some thundered that to let a patient die was a violation of the physician's duty irrespective of the person's cognitive, physical, or sensory limits. Others insisted that regardless of what medicine said, such behavior violated the social mores that governed medicine as a social practice.

More practically, some asked how individuals could be assured a treating physician would not see them as useless (had they been blinded, disfigured, paralyzed, and so on) and thus unworthy of not only care but also continuance. And if physicians were to be allowed to practice nontreatment for the benefit of society at the expense of patient lives, would they not inevitably be allowed then to take lives in the name of social necessity? These questions were ways of struggling with another, fundamental one: do we value persons based on their productive capacities or as fellow human beings irrespective of any cognitive, physical, or sensory limit? Justice Oliver Wendell Holmes rendered the American answer in his famous (and infamous) 1927 Supreme Court opinion, *Buck v Bell*. There he argued society had the right to eliminate from its body those who, through incurable and inherent deficiencies, "sapped the strength of the State."[37] In this case that person was "a feeble minded white woman," Carrie Buck, who was to be involuntarily sterilized so she could not breed more feeble minds who would diminish the strength of future generations.

In effect, Haiselden's eugenic vision had won in what Stephen J. Gould later called "one of the most famous and chilling statements of our

[American] century."[38] For all that followed it is important to see this decision clearly. Holmes's majority opinion interpreted the U.S. Constitution in such a way as to give to the state ultimate control of Carrie Buck's reproductive capacity. In doing this he argued that the protection of individuals was secondary to the needs of the state as an economic entity. Even more radically, Holmes argued that a future economic necessity could serve as the grounds for a contemporary choice of action or inaction. His famous declaration—"Three generations of idiots is enough" was a declaration that state resources would soon be insufficient to assure the care of the unproductive without sacrificing resources needed elsewhere. Idiots like Carrie Buck should willingly sacrifice for the good of the state (what else could they do for it, after all?), Holmes wrote, and if they selfishly declined, the state had the right to impose its will upon their bodies in the name of a future economic good.

In his opinion Holmes assumed (correctly) that at least some physicians would willingly participate first in the identification and then in the sterilization of "defectives." This willingness was a fundamental challenge of the Hippocratic promise to "do not harm." After all, Carrie Buck did not ask to be sterilized. The physicians who performed her tubal ligation did so not for her health or welfare but for the perceived benefit of the future of the economic state. She was thus defined not as citizen, person, or patient, but in effect as a mere polyp on the body public to be excised to prevent future, similar abnormalities. The state *was* the patient; its economic needs paramount.

The Unworthy Life

Just as bioethicists tend to dismiss Hippocratic ethics as irrelevant, they similarly insist the eugenic history of the late nineteenth century through the mid-twentieth century is a "dark and distant past" without contemporary relevance.[39] Ignoring its U.S. roots, most assume the lawful sterilization of some and the termination of others was a principally German aberration occurring during the years of the Third Reich. Bioethicist Art Caplan, for example, insists the eugenic underpinnings of Nazi euthanasia and eugenic practices "have little to do with contemporary ethical debates about science, medicine, and technology."[40] Similarly, Jonathan Glover asserts that those who use the history of Nazi eugenics as an argument in contemporary medical debates "do so at some distance from any serious knowledge of what the Nazis did."[41]

And yet it was the United States, not Germany, that was the redoubtable major exporter of eugenic policies in the 1920s and early 1930s.[42] It was with Haiselden that the Hippocratic imperative to care was transformed into at best a secondary concern. It was with *Buck v. Bell* that the state's economic interests were defined in law as more important than those of the patient. This transformation restricted the idea of patients as a protected class served by physicians solely dedicated to their well-being.

Where before medicine had seen all patients as equal in their need for care, the eugenicist, armed with the science of the day, sought to parse humans as biologically and thus socially distinct on the basis of characteristics judged productive or prohibitively expensive. "You do not have to treat people equally," Ian Hacking observed, "if they are sufficiently different."[43] Medical practitioners in the employ of the state were to be the experts judging when differences were sufficiently manifest to define the patient as the disease to be contained if not excised. It was this idea, and the ethical structure on which it was based, that fueled the excesses of German and other eugenic programs in the 1930s.

In the 1920s Karl Binding, a German professor of law and philosophy, and Alfred Hoche, a psychiatrist, sought to produce a moral, medico-legal argument advancing euthanasia. Read carefully today, their *Permitting the Destruction of Unworthy Life*[44] seems benign in comparison to the language of *Buck v. Bell*. In the context of late-twenty-first-century bioethical debates over euthanasia and "futility" in a context of resource scarcity, Binding and Hoche's arguments seem less sinister than quaint. In the spirit of Michael Ryan, who in 1836 had attempted to introduce a jurisprudential medical guide to British law, Binding and Hoche sought to produce a similar guide to practice in Germany, stating: "The young physician enters practice without any legal delineation of his right and duties—especially regarding the most important points. Not even the Hippocratic Oath, with its generalities, is operative."[45]

The lawyer and the physician together hoped to provide specific guidance that would permit physicians (and the state) to distinguish between worthy and unworthy lives. They argued that patients who might be saved to an at least moderately normal life be distinguished from those whose lives would be better ended on both humanist and socioeconomic grounds. Those whose termination they advocated included, first, persons "irretrievably lost as a result of illness or injury who, fully understanding their situations, possess and have somehow expressed their urgent wish for release." Second were those who, following a severe injury, were rendered persistently unconscious with little hope of a return to consciousness.

Writing in what he knew to be the last year of his life, Binding sought to gain for terminally ill patients the option of a physician-assisted death at the time of the patient's own choosing. Hoche's more general focus was the "mental incurables," and here his language was judgmental and intemperate in precisely the manner of Holmes's several years later. What most modern readers forget is that his argument was grounded in a specific dilemma well known to his contemporaries. At the end of World War I a lack of sufficient food supplies resulted in the mass starvation of institutionalized mental patients in Germany. The patients were sacrificed not because they were deemed unworthy of care but because a national famine meant there was not enough food for all. In a very real way, Hoche's argument was an attempt to if not justify then at least rationalize the homicidal triaging of resources that resulted.[46]

Binding and Hoche insisted that the acts they promoted were too weighty to be left to the judgment of any single patient or medical professional. Requests for termination by a patient or patient's family, they agreed, were to be adjudicated by a board or council of physicians who could speak to a patient's physical state, a psychiatrist (in the case of mental illness), and "a lawyer who looks to the laws." In no case was this to be an act of state expediency, they insisted, but instead and in every case an informed response to the suffering patient's, or a competent surrogate's, request. Still, their argument insisted that these were not issues of solely medical determination but instead areas of state judicial responsibility.

Although Binding and Hoche denied the Hippocratic oath offered physicians guidance, what they sought was a way around the oath's prohibition against euthanasia without losing its sense of general patient duty. They did this by asserting that in a small set of cases the objectives of Hippocratic medicine were best served through the relaxation of prohibitions that had served a far simpler medical reality. Modern technologies permitted the maintenance of those who would, in more primitive times, have died. Maintaining those lives was not, they argued, necessarily to the patient's benefit. Not for the last time, advancing medical technologies were used to justify the noncare, and in some cases, the self-conscious medical termination of the patient.

German professional and medical associations initially rejected these arguments as beyond the Hippocratic pall. In 1935, however, Dr. Gerhard Wagner of the National Socialist Physicians League revived *Permitting the Destruction of the Unworthy Life* at a Nazi Party Congress.[47] He combined the general argument of the unworthy life with a Holmesian economic rationale that asserted the right of the state to avoid "the 'burden and unexcelled injustice' that the cost of care for the mentally ill 'placed on normal, healthy members of the population.'"[48] In effect, German Nazism caught up with the kernel of Holmes's majority opinion eight years after *Buck v. Bell*, advancing it to its logical conclusion.

In 1939, two weeks after the invasion of Poland that began World War II, the German Committee for the Scientific Treatment of Severe, Genetically Determined Illness ordered the registration of all children with chronic conditions, especially those that were hereditary (for example, Down syndrome). Based on this registry, state physicians were to identify those unproductive persons whose termination would save the state the cost of their care. In addition to the genetically "defective" the list was later expanded to include almost anyone with a debilitating, degenerative condition (for example, multiple sclerosis), the persistently unconscious, and others whom physicians selected as being unproductive and thus social burdens. From there it was a very short walk to the racial cleansing of all those with an ancestry the state deplored.

Experimental Objects

At the same time a related debate was engaged on both sides of the Atlantic. To what extent was it appropriate for physicians to use the superfluous—the so-called degenerates, orphans, indigents, idiots, the poor, and so on—as objects of medical research? In the nineteenth century ethical debates revolved around the theft of corpses—most famously the case of Burke and Hare in England—for medical instruction and research.[49] In that conflict the needs of medical students for corpses to dissect, and for pathologists to study, was opposed by social assertions of the sanctity of the dead. In England, the Anatomy Act of 1832 offered, at least in theory, protection to the remains of the deceased.[50]

The twentieth-century battle over the need for living research subjects was structurally identical. The question was (and remains) the balance between the needs and protection of the patient and the need of researchers for subjects of study. In all cases the argument pits a potential future good (anatomy insights, well-schooled practitioners, new medical products) against the immediate good of patient care and protection. Transforming protected patients into research objects makes a mockery of the sanctified caring relationship of patient and physician, and thus of society's old ethic of the value of the person irrespective of position. But . . . it happened. Orphans living in state homes and "incurables" in institutions were broadly seen, as later chapters here detail, as social surpluses that might be appropriately put to use as research objects in a manner that would benefit medical science.

This use of the patient as research object, and especially the socially marginal patient, began at the latest in the last decades of the nineteenth century. In a 1907 lecture to the Congress of American Physicians and Surgeons on the "Idea of Experiment in Medicine," William Osler addressed the issue (figure 2.8). Perhaps the most famous physician of his day, he acknowledged the need for human subjects in medical research. He acknowledged, too, the potential future good that research might return. But he insisted that the potential of future knowledge must never trump the needs of the patient under care. "Absolute safety and full consent are the conditions which make such tests allowable. We have no right to use patients entrusted to our care for the purpose of experimentation unless direct benefit of the individual is likely to follow. . . . Risk to the individual may be taken with his [or her] consent and full knowledge of the circumstances."[51]

For Osler, the assemblage of advancing knowledge was ethically secondary to the Hippocratic focus on patient care and support. A person might *choose* to accept the dual roles of patient and subject, Osler argued in what is perhaps the first articulation of the idea of "informed consent," but the impersonal employment of the fragile as research objects violated the very essence of medical ethics, as Osler understood it. At stake was the ethics of care that gave physicians their moral grounding. When the

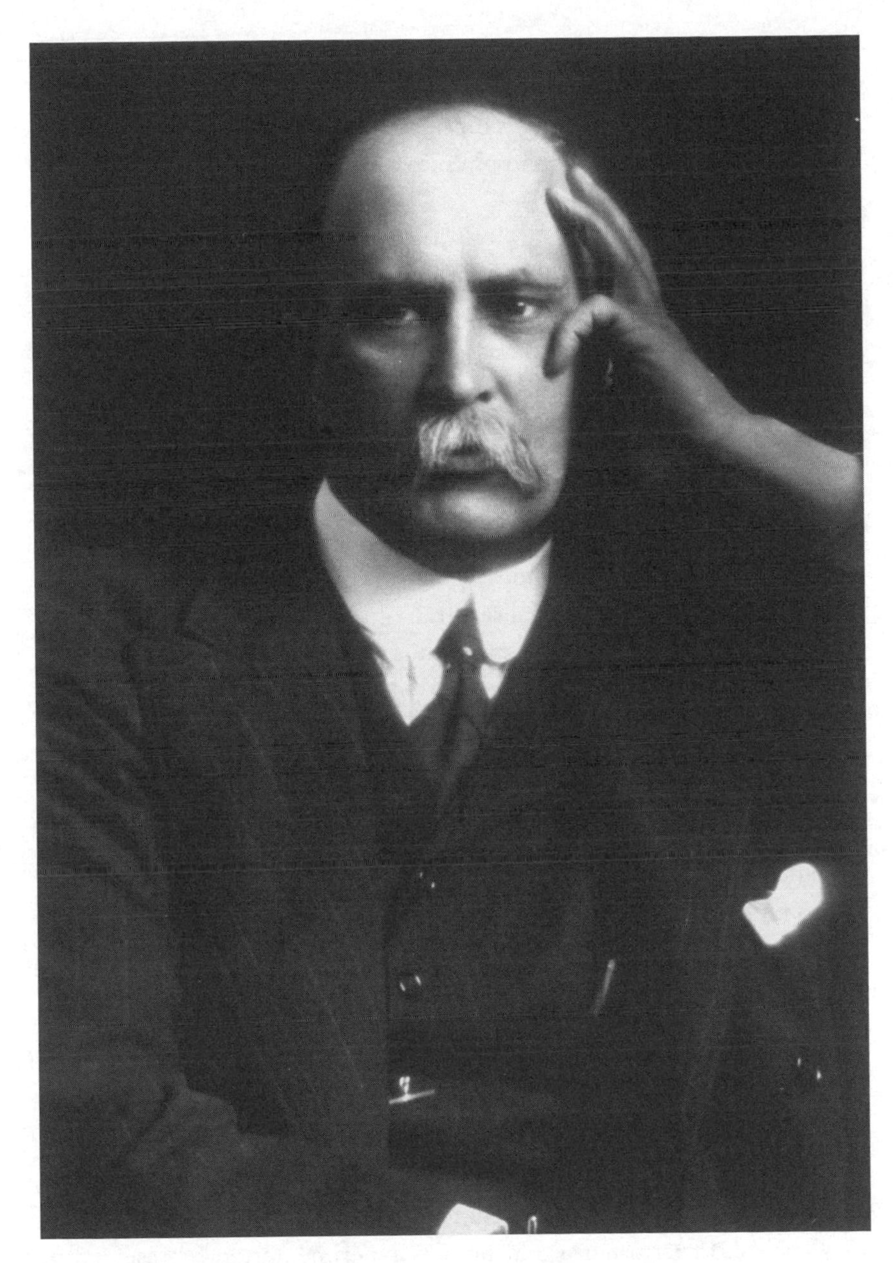

Figure 2.8
One of the great figures of evolving medicine, William Osler argued the Hippocratic primacy of physician responsibility to patient care over the potential needs of researchers. *Source*: National Library of Medicine, Bethesda, MD.

priorities of research overrode the necessities of care all was lost, "for without that the sacred cord which binds physician and patient snaps instantly."[52] At risk were not simply the lives of patients but also the whole ethic of trust that bound physician and patient together in society.

Nuremberg

In 1930s Germany the Nazi state defined, on the basis of a review by medical professionals, whole classes of persons as mentally, physically, racially, and therefore socially unworthy. The protection that the state, and thus the medicine practiced in it, in theory offered (and owed) its citizens was lifted, excluding these "undesirables." To simply exterminate the socially unproductive would be wasteful, however. Thus the Nazi program of medical experimentation began as a social recovery project transforming socially superfluous, economically burdensome human subjects into serviceable and useful research objects. The participating physicians' client was the military state, their goal the advancement of the science of medicine itself.

The use of persons as research objects was widely condemned at the end of World War II with the trial of Nazi physicians-researchers for "crimes against humanity."[53] The most terrifying thing for many was that those who perpetrated these horrendous acts in violation of their Hippocratic oath appeared, in the dock, as anything but monstrous.[54] They were simply employees of the state following, as good employees do, the directives of their superiors. They were in the main sound medical professionals pursuing with the encouragement of their superiors the advance of a clinical science they believed would serve future generations. Most did not see their actions as evil, immoral, or unethical. Half-starved detainees worked at manual labor until they could no longer stand. Why not *learn* from them in a manner that would advance medical science, benefiting future generations? Yes, the Hippocratic oath said, first "Do no harm," but didn't the long-term good of knowledge assemblage outweigh the short-term harm that human experimentation represented to socially unwanted patients likely to die soon anyway?

Nuremberg was the basis of a postwar movement that defined the objectification of patients as research objects as a violation of both medical ethics and the general morality protecting the individual social member irrespective of his or her position in society. This sense of protected humanity was enshrined in documents like the charter of the United Nations in 1945 and the General Declaration of Human Rights of 1948. The same values have been restated time and again in other international agreements and covenants, perhaps most recently in the Universal Declaration on Bioethics and Human Rights.[55] In this manner respect for all human life (and here again, echoes of the old Hippocratic ideal of community can be heard) was asserted, and with it came a promise of freedom from exploitation, stigmatization, or violation.[56] This, in turn, reaffirmed the old Hippocratic insistence upon patient care and the caring relationship as the guiding ideal of medicine irrespective of commercial or state interests.

American Medicine

The objectification of the patient as a research subject was not a uniquely German aberration. American physicians similarly used their patients as objects of experimentation in a range of research programs. They did so not furtively but in state-supported projects whose results were reported in the medical and scientific literatures. The argument for this followed logically from *Buck v. Bell.* If the interests of the economic state trump those of the socially superfluous patient, then the right of those patients to care and protection is diminished. Permission to invade their bodies for the purpose of sterilization (as a move to save the future state money) is only a little different from using their bodies in research whose result, hopefully, will add to science and thus provide future benefit.

In 1932 the U.S. Public Health Service began an unremarkable project to first identify and then study African Americans with syphilis in Macon County, Georgia. The discovery that a "considerable portion of the infected Negro population remained untreated during the entire course of syphilis" was described in the 1936 *Journal of the American Medical Association* as a research opportunity too good to miss.[57] Rather than treating the subjects to the best of the physicians' ability they became instead ciphers in a decades-long program of clinical study.[58] From 1936 until 1972 the Tuskegee researchers followed the course of the untreated disease in 399 impoverished, African American, syphilitic sharecroppers. Available treatment protocols were largely ineffective when the study began but by 1947 penicillin was widely recognized as an effective treatment. Tuskegee researchers did not deploy it, however, preferring instead to simply study the patients' degeneration. The attending physicians, employed by the state, saw themselves primarily as servants of what would be called, a generation later, the "knowledge industry." The needs of the patients, the necessity of their care, were simply irrelevant when compared to what might be learned from passively documenting their degeneration from a treatable condition.

There was also, famously, the infection with hepatitis of fragile orphan children at the Willowbrook State School: "In 1956, Dr. Saul Krugman—with the sanction of the New York State Department of Mental Hygiene, the New York State Department of Health, the Armed Forces Epidemiology Board, and others—began an experiment at the Willowbrook State School, a state-supported institution for mentally handicapped children. In this experiment Willowbrook residents were intentionally infected with live hepatitis virus so the effect of gamma globulin treatment could be observed."[59] Physicians defended their actions on the grounds that because hepatitis was rampant at the institution most residents would be infected anyway, sooner or later. Deliberately infecting them thus did no real harm and provided a social benefit in the knowledge that might be gained in the experiment.

These were the most spectacular examples of what was fairly common practice in the postwar era. In the early 1950s, for example, it was common for physicians treating poorer patients, typically African Americans, to see them as research objects. "Many scientists believed that since patients were treated for free in the public wards, it was fair to use them as research subjects as a form of payment."[60] Here the distinction was made between the well-to-do patient paying for services, and thus protected, and those who because of poverty were considered fair game as research objects.

In 1966 Henry Beecher published a well-documented, much-discussed article detailing twenty-two research projects in the United States that violated basic principles of medical ethics and socially acceptable research.[61] Nor was the United States alone in its often cavalier use of fragile and impoverished humans for research purposes. The practice was common in England and other victor nations at the end of World War II.[62]

When a group of moral philosophers developed bioethics they had a choice. On the one hand, they could affirm the ideal of care within a tradition of medicine that reached from Hippocrates to Benjamin Rush to William Osler. They could argue against patient objectification in research and insist, Hippocratically, on care as a communally grounded, social and ethical goal. On the other hand, they could ignore the history of abuse and excess and instead form arguments whose result, whether anticipated or not, was the promotion of state economics and the knowledge industry over the life and care of this or that fragile person. It is my argument that almost without exception bioethicists have always chosen the second alternative.

1950s Polio

Opposed to this sorry history of abuse and patient abandonment is another in which medicine and the society that supports it saw things differently. In the years 1951 to 1953 the most severe of a series of poliomyelitis pandemics swept the world.[63] From Copenhagen to San Francisco, local medical teams mounted an unprecedented effort to sustain the lives of patients, primarily young people, attacked by the virus. During a severe post-World War II recession more than sixty thousand cases were diagnosed in the United States alone, approximately twenty-one thousand of them resulting in either paralysis of the limbs or, more seriously, the respiratory muscles.[64]

In many cities school gymnasiums were turned into wards, cots installed from wall to wall. Nursing and medical students were pressed into service to help maintain those whose respiratory paralysis could only be countered, in the short term, by manual ventilation following a tracheostomy.[65] Negative-pressure ventilation machines, iron lungs encasing patients from foot to chin, and then more efficient positive-pressure respirators with volume regulation, were brought into service (see figure 2.9). There was no expectation those saved by these technologies would be returned to normalcy. Indeed, the assumption was that survivors would require ventilator assistance and personal care for the rest of their lives. Still: "The salvation of thousands of mostly young adults through a cumbersome process of mechanical ventilation was seen as a major triumph in both medical circles and the society-at-large."[66] For those with

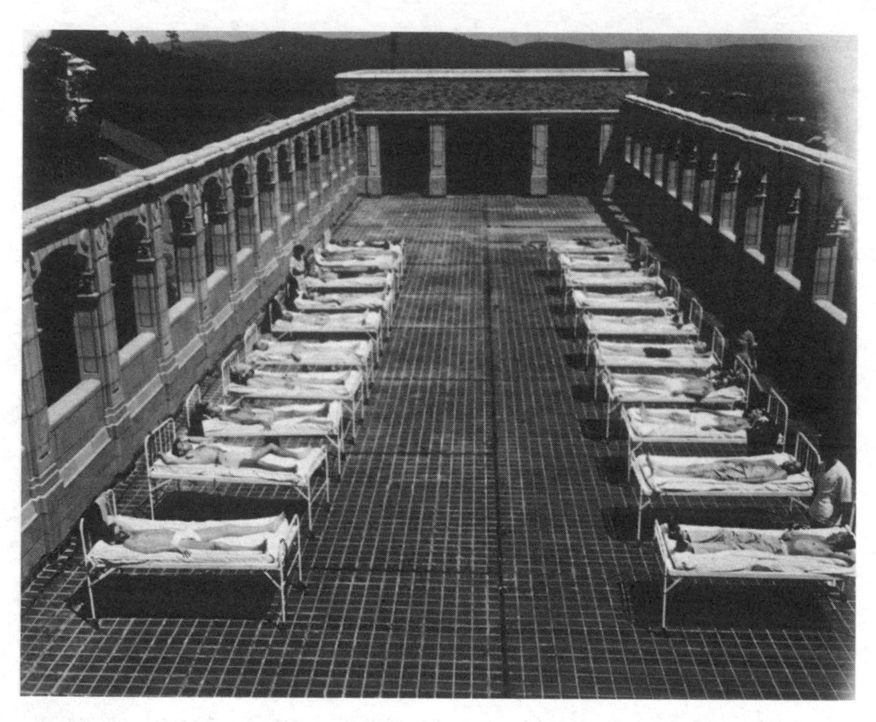

Figure 2.9
In the 1950s the last, devastating poliomyelitis epidemic required the treatment of thousands of patients, many through the use of the "iron lung" and others with extensive bed care and rehabilitation. *Source*: National Library of Medicine, Bethesda, MD.

permanently reduced limb function, "Crippled Children's Hospitals" were opened throughout the United States, and in other countries, to promote rehabilitation.

Nobody asked about the cost of the new technologies that permitted patient survival. No one warned that the continuing care and rehabilitation for those left with withered limbs would be economically unsustainable. Nobody suggested that the folk saved by these extraordinary interventions would be a social burden whose public cost of care could never be recovered. Nor did anyone whisper that the long-term severity of even the best-anticipated outcomes would leave the afflicted with a "quality of life" so intolerable that, as Binding and Hoche might have said, they would be better off dead. Medical and social ethics demanded society and its physicians do all that was possible to save and, after saving, to help rehabilitate polio's fragile survivors. Cost was not an issue because to *not* spend the monies, to *not* save the poliomyelitis patient, was unthinkable.

Futures

Bioethics was born, it is said, in the rush of technological advances in the mid-twentieth century, and publicly reported excesses—Tuskegee is an example—that raised questions about the nature of medical ethics and its ability to protect the fragile. By the mid-1970s the result was, Edmund Pellegrino writes, "the subjection of the entire corpus of medical ethics to serious philosophical inquiry."[67] This is at best only half true. Certainly a history of research abuses and excesses raised public questions about medical research as exploitative and inimical to the goals of society and of traditional medical ethics. But the idea that new technologies "highlighted tensions between old and new medical theories and practices, as physicians, scientists, and the lay public debated the increasing authority of scientific medicine" is at best incomplete and misleading.[68]

Technology and the medical methods of its application generally were celebrated for their life-preserving or at least life-prolonging potential. In the 1950s the iron lung was a popular symbol of medicine's commitment to care and the power of medical technologies to save those who previously would have died. With the development of the polio vaccine, scientific medicine was promoted as empowering an old ethic of care that was seen as bringing humankind to the threshold of a great new day. It was hoped that the broad community of physicians who cared for us as individual patients could together bring under control the congress of diseases that threatened us all.

The tensions that existed, and which grew into bioethical resolution, were less medical than social. Was the state first and foremost a protector of its citizens, irrespective of their individual capacities, or the guarantor of a future-oriented, economic vision? How one answered that question would largely determine the manner in which medical ethics would be constructed. In attempting to address the ethics of medicine bioethics necessarily had to weigh in on this divide. If, on the one hand, it promoted the earlier ideal it would condemn research excesses, advance the ideal of patient care and with that the community's commitment to each person in need irrespective of cost. If, on the other hand, it promoted the economic state as its principal focus, and of research as a priority generating jobs and income as well as saleable technologies, its arguments would lead in another direction.

Bioethics' answer was formulated from the start on the basis of what was advanced as a growing scarcity of resources that demanded the devaluation of some for the potential benefit of others, and of future states. The idea of scarcity became the defining idea that led bioethics away from the old Hippocratic ethic of community and care down the path to what it has become today. It didn't have to be this way. It's just the way it was.

3

Something Newer: Supply-Side Ethics

In the 1960s, a group of medical amateurs trained in a specific tradition of moral philosophy joined as citizens a national discussion on how best to allocate a scarce medical resource in the United States. Debate began in neither medical writings nor philosophical tracts but in the November 1962 issue of *Life Magazine*. Reporter Shana Alexander's story described the deliberations of a Seattle committee whose task it was to select a few from among the many patients seeking entry into what was then a new kidney dialysis program in that city. Just as poliomyelitis patients in the early 1950s had been saved from certain death by the introduction of the iron lung, patients in late-stage renal failure were offered a similar reprieve through dialysis. Dr. Belding Scribner's invention of the arterio-venous shunt and cannula permitted what had been a necessarily terminal condition to be transformed into one that was chronic and manageable. And again, salvation required a reliance on the continuing use of a physically limiting technology.

The problem was that few hospitals provided dialysis and the ones that did could not accommodate all those who needed treatment. The question therefore was how to choose the few who would be treated with available resources from the many who would die without. Alexander's story, "They Decide Who Lives, Who Dies," described the workings of the committee whose task it was to make this choice among Seattle-area patients.[1] Famously dubbed the "God Committee," it was an ecumenical mix of medical and legal professionals, of clergy and laypersons who together reviewed applications to the dialysis program. The label was brilliantly evocative at many levels. In a god-like fashion, the committee's judgments had the power of life and death for those seeking medically supported survival. Because the identities of the committee members were not revealed, the committee possessed an anonymity that made its judgments seem deistic, out of reach.

The medical reality for all potential patients was identical: dialysis meant survival but with physical restrictions requiring ongoing treatment. The lack of dialysis meant a relatively rapid death. For medical practitioners the problem was that the choice of care, and thus survival, was out of their hands because the care renal patients required could not be given either in the patient's home or the doctor's office. Physicians did not own the dialysis equipment; nor could they afford its purchase. It was not, as Rothman argued, that "physicians, in unprecedented fashion, turned over to a lay committee life-or-death decisions prospectively and on a case-by-case basis."[2] Physician did not turn over anything. Control over this life-saving (or at least life-prolonging) treatment was never theirs to dispense. Decisions on access to hospital-based dialysis programs were administrative and impersonal from the start. Their assignment was beyond the physician's control and thus beyond the physician's sphere of responsible action.

In the public debate that followed publication of Alexander's story the questions were threefold. First, people asked about the nature of the committee, about those who were making these life-and-death decisions about other human belings. Second, if a choice had to be made, what criteria should an ethical society employ? Third, some people questioned the very notion of scarcity as a rationale for treatment decisions. The very idea that a scarcity of medical resources required their rationing seemed, somehow, un-American. How could the greatest nation in the world be unable to afford life-saving treatments for its sickest citizens? Hadn't the poliomyelitis patients in the 1951–1953 window been saved by another wonderful if expensive medical advance? And *that* was in a period of severe economic recession, whereas November 1962, when the "God Committee" went to work was still the era of President John F. Kennedy's "Camelot," when all things seemed possible and . . . why not? The United States had emerged economically preeminent among nations following World War II, a country with seemingly infinite potential in both industry and political will.

In 1962 the United States had a sense of itself as a just nation in which, when problems were identified, solutions were quickly found. It is true that on Thanksgiving Day in 1960 Edward R. Murrow broadcast an exposé of poverty in the United States;[3] *Harvest of Shame* rocked the nation. But in the Great Society promised by President Kennedy, and then President Lyndon B. Johnson, poverty was a problem all agreed could and would be resolved. And yes, there was the festering issue of civil rights, but it, too, surely would be answered. For a nation whose leader promised to put human beings on the moon, the very idea of intransigent medical scarcity resulting in the preventable death of thousands of citizens seemed unpatriotic, almost seditious. As Harry W. Pearson argued in 1957, the "natural fact of limited means" is not natural at all but the result of clearly defined social choices based upon specific social objectives.[4] Thus if people who might otherwise be saved died because of a lack of dialysis services, there was a social responsibility for that fact. While all knew that markets function under conditions of relative scarcity—prices are bid up or down on the basis of supply—absolute, intransigent, natural scarcity costing lives seemed both unreasonable and antithetical to the nation's sense of self and self-esteem.

It is thus little wonder that many date the birth of bioethics with the national debate over dialysis in a context of scarcity.[5] The new sign of the times was the needy dialysis patient signifying a problem whose subject was not medical but ethical and economic. It is easy to be generous when there is more than enough for everyone. It is when choices must be made that the ethics of a people are tested. The idea of relative worth as a basis of selective treatment among supposedly equal citizens seemed an anathema to Americans who prided themselves on egalitarian policies promoted in a culture of productive abundance. At stake was the very idea of the American community in which opportunity existed, at least in theory, equally and for all. If choices had to be made, however, who better to ask than the moral philosophers for whom such problems were assumed to be a specialty?

Organ Transplantation

And, yet, scarcity became a legitimizing key that opened the door of medical practice to nonmedical philosopher-ethicists—first as commentators and then as players. In 1967 South African physician Christian Barnard introduced the heart of a dead black woman into the body of a living white male. That medical triumph, the first heart transplant, took place in an apartheid nation where blacks were subject to the whims of white citizens and where, had donor and recipient met when both were alive, they could not have ridden together on a bus, or sat together in a restaurant. Did the donor or her family have a choice in her donation? Was the heart taken without regard to the wishes of its source while living?[6] And how could *any* choice be free in a society where one race was so subjugated to another?

The question of the ethical legitimacy of the operation, and by extension of future organ transplantation programs, quickly took on a Kantian cast. In the most famous of Kant's categorical imperatives, the "supreme practical principle" of his philosophy was for all to "act so that you treat humanity, whether in your person or in that of another, always as an end and never as a means only:[7] To treat a person as a means was to deny his or her humanity, reducing the person to a utilitarian object. This in turn objectified humanity at large as merely a collection of instrumental beings, not moral ends in themselves. In the 1960s the referent of people as a means and not an end was the use of prisoners by Nazi physicians interested in experimentation on human subjects. To transplant the heart of a subjugated woman into the chest cavity of a member of the subjugating class seemed, at least potentially, to be similar ethically and thus similarly odious.

Organ Supply and Brain Death

It was with Barnard's first heart transplant that the issue of organ donation, and the criteria by which a donor could be defined, became publicly and practically urgent. Obviously, it would violate the Hippocratic Oath ("First, do no harm") to remove a donor's organ when he or she was still living. And yet, by the mid-1970s the need for donor organs was exigent. The question was how to secure a continuing supply of scarce, transplantable organs. That lead to this question: When did the dying become sufficiently dead to permit an organ to be removed? Because a person's organs begin to degrade immediately following the cessation of cardiopulmonary function, the window of opportunity for a successful transplant is limited by the ischemic rate of the organ (and it differs for each), in other words, the speed of its degradation. The ideal candidate is the person who expires on the operating table with the person needing the transplant prepared on another operating table in the same room, ready to receive the heart as soon as it can be removed from the donor's chest cavity.

Within a month of Barnard's first successful transplant, Henry K Beecher, who had earlier written the landmark paper identifying the inappropriate use of human subjects in U.S. medical research, petitioned the dean of Harvard Medical school to "create a committee to consider the use of patients in irreversible coma as potential donors."[8] The traditional definition of death—and thus of when a person's body could be used for its parts—depended on the irreversible and irremediable cessation of circulatory and respiratory function. The Ad Hoc Committee of the Harvard Medical School, headed by Beecher, distinguished a set of criteria to create a new category: "brain death."[9] Even if circulation and respiration continued, a person who failed neurological tests of brain activity would be defined as dead, and thus not coincidentally, available to serve as an organ donor.

It is correct but insufficient to say the Harvard committee "reviewed" clinical standards on which death might be pronounced.[10] This was more about ethics and law than clinical science. "A determination of death is a legal determination that a collection of living cells is no longer entitled to the rights granted to human beings, rather than a scientific or medical determination that all biologic life has ended. Reasonable people agree that human tissue loses its status as a person before there is complete cellular lysis but may disagree on whether 'humanness' legally disappears when brain function ceases, cardiopulmonary function ceases, or some other criterion is met. The question is, at its core, not a medical question but a moral or religious one."[11]

A motive goal of the Ad Hoc Committee, as Beecher and Dorr described it in an article frequently cited and often disputed, was "to increase the flow of organs for transplantation," and thus "secure the life-saving potential of transplantation."[12] While some argue this was an outcome rather than a primary goal,[13] it is the obvious implication of the Ad Hoc Committee's statement that "obsolete criteria for the definition of death can lead to controversy in obtaining organs for transplantation," which the Harvard committee's definition of brain death hoped to resolve.

This is not to suggest the whole was simply a charade to resolve a supply problem for materials required by the evolving industry of organ transplantation. New technologies permitted the maintenance of persons in a range of fragile states who would a decade earlier have died. These were seen as neither clinically nor ethically problematic, however, until the issue of graft organ supply arose in transplantation. As a result of both the new technology but also the perceived shortage of donor organs, a clinical set of definition was enacted by the Ad Hoc Committee as ethical and appropriate. The goal was humanitarian—saving the lives of some—and economic. From the start transplantation was extremely expensive (for the patient) and lucrative (for the professional). Epstein put this baldly and inelegantly but not incorrectly: "The need to change the definition of death became even more urgent when additional economic interests appeared on the scene—interests in retrieving organs for transplantation."[14] Those interests included, in a partial list, health insurers paying for dialysis for kidney patients (transplantation was more cost effective), hospitals charging for surgery and aftercare (a new revenue stream), surgeons who would perform the very remunerative surgery, and researchers interested in advancing transplantation as a general technology.

Death was defined, as a result, as occurring in the absence of observed neurological activity even in those whose noncognitive bodily functions continued. This new definition permitted a person's body parts to be excised and then deployed in service of others even while cardiopulmonary function continued. The argument was not that the persons in noncognitive states were better dead, only that they weren't *really* alive.

Bioethics and Brain Death

"The Ad Hoc Committee," Robert Veatch wrote in 1993, "was actually the first exercise in bioethics of differentiating facts and values. Early discussions with the Harvard Committee focused on whether calling someone dead was a matter of biological fact or a normative philosophical judgment about when to treat a person as dead."[15] The result was less a differentiation of facts and values, however, than an interpretation of facts through the lens of a value set including the improvement of graft organ supply as a general good.

The value that the Ad Hoc Committee laid upon its clinical facts carried more than a whiff of Immanuel Kant's philosophical perspective, and a full dose of his rigorous argument. Kant's whole metaphysic was based on the ideal of "human reason" and the human capacity to reason: "Every rational being exists as an end in himself."[16] It was that rational capacity that permitted the radical freedom that in Kant's philosophy made each person real; activating the will with which people independently could perceive moral law.[17] From this it seemed to follow that reason, and the will to reason, were what made each individual uniquely important. Where the faculty of reason (*Willkur*) was no longer biologically possible, where the person was clinically judged incapable of practical reason (*Willie*), the person could be dismissed as a body existing outside the Kantian sphere. Such a patient was a nonperson, dead in all but physical function that the new criteria deemed to be irrelevant. Life without a certain level of clinically identifiable cognitive activity was defined as no life at all and the cessation of care or active termination (withdrawing life support) was therefore deemed ethically acceptable.

More generally, organ transplantation was presented ethically as a beneficent,[18] communal good. That, in turn, rested conceptually on the potential for reciprocity, that we all may give or receive. Without that potential the idea of community was meaningless and the donor became merely an object of someone else's need. What troubled North Americans about the South African case was that policies of apartheid made a mockery of the idea of an egalitarian community in which reciprocal opportunity could prevail. It was unfathomable that, in South Africa, a white heart (or kidney, or lung) would be put into a black recipient's body. The whole was thus ethically problematic from the start.

This was an old debate transposed into a new frame. Binding and Hoche raised similar issues when in 1920 they defined as worthy of termination persons "who, through some event like a very severe, doubtlessly fatal wound, have become unconscious" and who might, they lamented, "endure so long" without conscious activity or purpose as to be the very definition of familiar and social burdens.[19] And, too as we saw, in *Buck v. Bell* (and the cases of Tuskegee, Willowbrook, and so on) the needs of the restricted individual counted little when weighed against those of the state.

What was new here was neither scarcity nor the broader question of the worth of restricted individuals, but rather the introduction of philosophical analysis as a means of evaluation or, depending on one's point of view, rationalization. Certainly, the moral philosophers engaged by the

Ad Hoc Committee were selective in the philosophy they applied. After all, Kant categorically opposed the transplantation that in his day involved implanting the teeth of the poor in the mouths of the rich on the basis that it objectified some for the benefit of others. Some have taken Kant's argument as suggesting that we, too, should reject organ donation even where the donor seeks participation on purely altruistic grounds.[20] Others have argued that a strict application of Kant's argument is inappropriate today.[21] Our society is more egalitarian and the potential for the economic objectification of the organ supplier therefore is less.

While the Harvard committee did not reference Hoche (it would have been politically unwise), what its members proposed was something similar to what he had advocated: the categorization of the persistently unconscious, and by extension fragile others, as nonpersons. The result was a normative philosophical judgment in service of a practical conclusion satisfying not Kant's humanitarian concerns but instead pedestrian supply goals.[22]

The values advanced by the Ad Hoc Committee demanded of physicians an abrogation of the traditional medical ethic that did not distinguish between those with capacity and those without. In that tradition the physician's job was to do the best he or she could for a patient without doing harm, irrespective of the patient's capacity or social abilities. Certainly using a body for its parts while the heart still beats was, in this old view of things, a harm. With the need for donor organs as a motive force behind the Ad Hoc Committee's mandate, however, clinical observations describing an individual's neurological status were transformed into a criteria set that "defined" death (some would say, today, "constructed") as occurring irrespective of continuing bodily function. The patient rendered dead by this definition was thus safely objectified as a resource object, a graft organ supplier. This was done through a kind of half-Kantian rational blush in which the abstraction of high philosophy was employed in the fashioning of a pragmatic supply ethic that restricted protected life as a defining clinical value.

Death: A Critique

Implicit in this new death were a number of assumptions that members of the Ad Hoc Committee did not consider. Central among them was that neurological science was capable of identifying rational cognition as a demonstrable neurological reality whose presence (or absence) could be accurately tested. If the science was accurate, then the "brain dead" were no longer and would never again be self-conscious, rational persons. Because they were not thinking persons they could be used as supply vessels without violating Kant's third categorical imperative prohibiting the objectification of others as means rather than ends to themselves. As had happened before, however (and as will happen again), the science was incomplete where not simply inaccurate.

In the 1990s, neurological reviews of patients previously diagnosed as being in "vegetative states" revealed as many as 43 percent had been misdiagnosed.[23] Stories of those like Terry Wallis—who recovered with fluent speech from a nineteen-year coma—became increasingly reported in academic and popular literatures.[24] To this was added data provided by newer imaging technologies which made it clear that assumptions on which "brain death" had been defined in the 1960s were at the very best inadequate.[25]

This created a potential problem for the ethicist-philosophers who for twenty years had embraced the Ad Hoc Committee's conclusions as well as the doctors who acted upon them. The question "of brain death wasn't as simple as most had assumed.[26] "The uncomfortable conclusion to be drawn from this literature," as Truog and Miller admitted in 2008, "is that although it may be perfectly ethical to remove vital organs for transplantation from patients who satisfy the diagnostic criteria of brain death, the reason it is ethical cannot be that we are convinced they are really dead."[27]

But if "some patients will [and have] die [died] who might otherwise have lived"[28] how can this be ethical? Certainly it violates the Hippocratic oath's promise to do no harm. The legal statutes and medical guidelines that advanced this type of "justified killing," as Miller and Truog called it, were based on the conclusions of the Ad Hoc Committee that were later proved incorrect. Thus the medical ethicist was faced with a choice. One response would be to uncouple the link first forged in the 1960s between the now disputed "fact" of brain death and the use of the unconscious as organ supply vessels. Doing this would affirm a traditional ethic of care irrespective of the living individual capacity or circumstance. That would likely decrease the availability of donor organs, however.

Another option would be to shrug away these new facts in the name of a pragmatic, utilitarian good: graft organ supply. And here we see the general rule of scarcity as it has been consistently employed in law and medical ethics. Where scarcity is assumed to rule, the high values of ethical concern for the individual are discarded in favor of the low values of utilitarian pragmatism. The "justified killing" of a fragile person for the benefit of others violates a raft of moral (and legal) principles. To justify that killing for the procurement of organs violates ethical injunctions against the objectification of the person. But in extremes principles of care and protection are reflexively set aside in the name of a perceived necessity, in this case resource scarcity, and a greater good beyond that of the physician's obligation (and society's) to first, do no harm.

Scarcity as a Medical Condition

By the mid-1980s, scarcity was bioethics' reflexive entry to a range of issues. Famously, in March 1984, Colorado Governor Richard D. Lamm argued that the public cost of healthcare in the United States was or would soon be unsupportable and therefore the fragile, kept alive by medical intervention, had a duty to die to assure more healthcare went to productive citizens as well as to assure a financially solvent society in the future.[29] It is an argument Lamm has made ever since in a variety of publications[30] and a range of public venues.[31] In a 1993 *New York Times* article he stated his position this way: "We've got a duty to die and get out of the way with all of our machines and artificial hearts and everything else like that and let the other society, our kids, build a reasonable life."[32]

The duty he proclaimed to a future as yet unlived is at once administrative (what hospitals should allow), individual (what patients should do), medical (how physicians should care), and political (what the public purse should compensate). Lamm's focus was never the immediate health needs of citizens but the requirement of future generations whose well-being might be (but was not yet) endangered by the profligate cost of contemporary medical care expended on the unproductive fragile.[33] Lamm perceived the community as divided between young and productive and thus worthy workers who would serve the future and fragile, burdensome, superannuated, or simply fragile nonproductive workers in the present. It is worth breaking down his assumption set to see its relation to more formal bioethical and philosophical thinking.

First, like Binding and Hoche, Lamm blamed medical technology—"All our machines and artificial hearts and everything else"—for keeping alive people who should otherwise have been left to die. Second, the ethical problem he perceived was not the provision of care for the needy but its cost in a society whose resources are or in the future will be so restricted that allocation choices will have to be made. Thus those deemed unaffordable—as Carrie Bell once was seen—could be dismissed as candidates for aggressive care, irrespective of their wishes. Third, implicit in all this was the insistence that citizens have a duty to future generations above a duty to themselves or their neighbors.

Lamm's scarcity argument was (and remains at this writing) that modern society faces a necessary choice of *either* saving a few today and thus sacrificing many in the future, or alternately, of saving the future many by sacrificing a few today. For Lamm, unproductive seniors were the sine quo non of those whose present needs could only be answered at the price of the future and its restricted economy. And after all, hadn't they been kept alive overlong by the expensive new medical technologies whose expense he saw as unsustainable? The result was not ageist, Lamm insisted, but humanitarian and philosophical: "I was essentially raising a general statement about the human condition," he told the *New York Times* in 1993, "not beating up on the elderly."[34]

We can infer Lamm's understanding of humanness from his argument. The virtuous, he believed, act not for themselves but for others, and especially for future generations. Human nature is or should be for Lamm selflessly utilitarian, perceiving the "greatest good" as superior to the needs of the individual at any time. That good is defined economically because society is at base an economic system whose accountancies are the single measure of good and worth. Where selfish individuals do not bow to the greater economic realities, society has the right (and perhaps the duty) to impose its limits on the individual's care (irrespective of medical benefit) for the greater good. Lamm thus argued at least implicitly—as had Oliver Wendell Holmes in the 1920s—that the primary goal of medicine should not be the care of the patient but the productive future state. Here was the modern neoliberal, one in which humanity is defined materially, the individual and his or her needs disappearing except as a cipher in some impersonal economic analysis. "Is it not the case that the truly new, and disorienting character of modernity is its seemingly being driven by merely material, statistical, tangential 'economic' constructions . . . in which all previous notions of belief and sociability have been scrambled?"[35]

Daniel Callahan

Richard Lamm was a politician and, to many, a bit of a crank. To transform his political argument into a social platform guiding medical choices required a philosopher-ethicist who might offer this view in a prettier package. That task fell to Daniel Callahan, founder of the most prestigious bioethics think tank in the United States, The Hastings Center (figure 3.1). From 1969 to 1996 Callahan served as its president and in that role was perhaps the best known and most influential of the moral philosophers who came to call themselves bioethicists. In 1987 Callahan advanced an argument very similar to Lamm's in *Setting Limits: Medical Goals in an Aging Society*.

Medical decision making could be considered a private affair between physicians and patients, Callahan argued, as long as the social cost was minimal and medicine's ability to sustain the fragile limited. Things

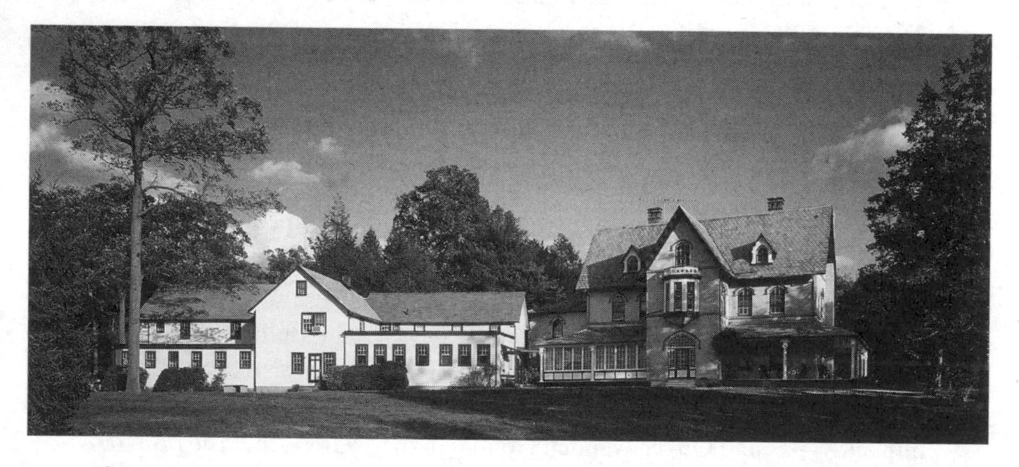

Figure 3.1
For more than twenty-five years, Daniel Callahan served as director of The Hastings Center, among the earliest and still among the most prestigious centers for bioethics in the world. *Source*: Photo, The Hastings Center.

changed, however, first with the introduction of new technologies and more effective treatment, and second when "a public commitment was made to provide at least minimal if not necessarily adequate healthcare for the elderly and the poor."[36] The result was Lamm's double whammy: new technologies kept people alive at a cost that was an intolerable strain on the public purse in a manner threatening future generations. In this argument economies and generations are synonymous.

Callahan blamed two programs enshrined in The Social Security Act of 1965 as the problem: Medicare supporting medical care for seniors and Medicaid's compensation of treatment for the poor. These acts created the world of Lamm's apocalyptic beggaring, primarily through the salvation of the socially superfluous, especially seniors. "The old can remain economically and socially productive . . . they cannot, however, remain socially indispensable in the way that children and young adults are for a society."[37] Where scarcity reigns, it is the duty of the socially dispensable to get out of the way, selflessly abjuring their own care to assure resources would be available for the "substantial pool of [young] people able to work well and hard, physically and mentally."[38]

Callahan advanced this argument in his 1990 book, *The Limits of Medical Progress*, as a kind of communitarian ethic (there are several) (figure 3.2).[39] It was, in effect, simple utilitarianism with a happy face,[40] an insistence that economic limits required the sacrifice of some for the benefit of the future many. Callahan knew this would seem to some immoral. But for him, as for Lamm, the problem was with that old morality that argued the worth of the individual irrespective of his or her productive and social capacity. "We have found our mortality wanting and have tried to modernize it. What have we learned? At the least we know that it can be an extraordinarily expensive economic venture, consuming resources at a rapid and growing rate."[41] The point of his ethic thus was economic. Medicine's goal, as he defined it, was or should be the maintenance of economically valuable workers.

The villain in this tale was medicine and its traditional, Hippocratic insistence upon patient care as a social and communal good irrespective of economic concerns. "The corrective cannot come from within the domain of health, which has no intrinsic limits. It can only come from a coherent perspective on the general perspective of society as a whole and of the individuals who compose it. . . . The best medicine is that

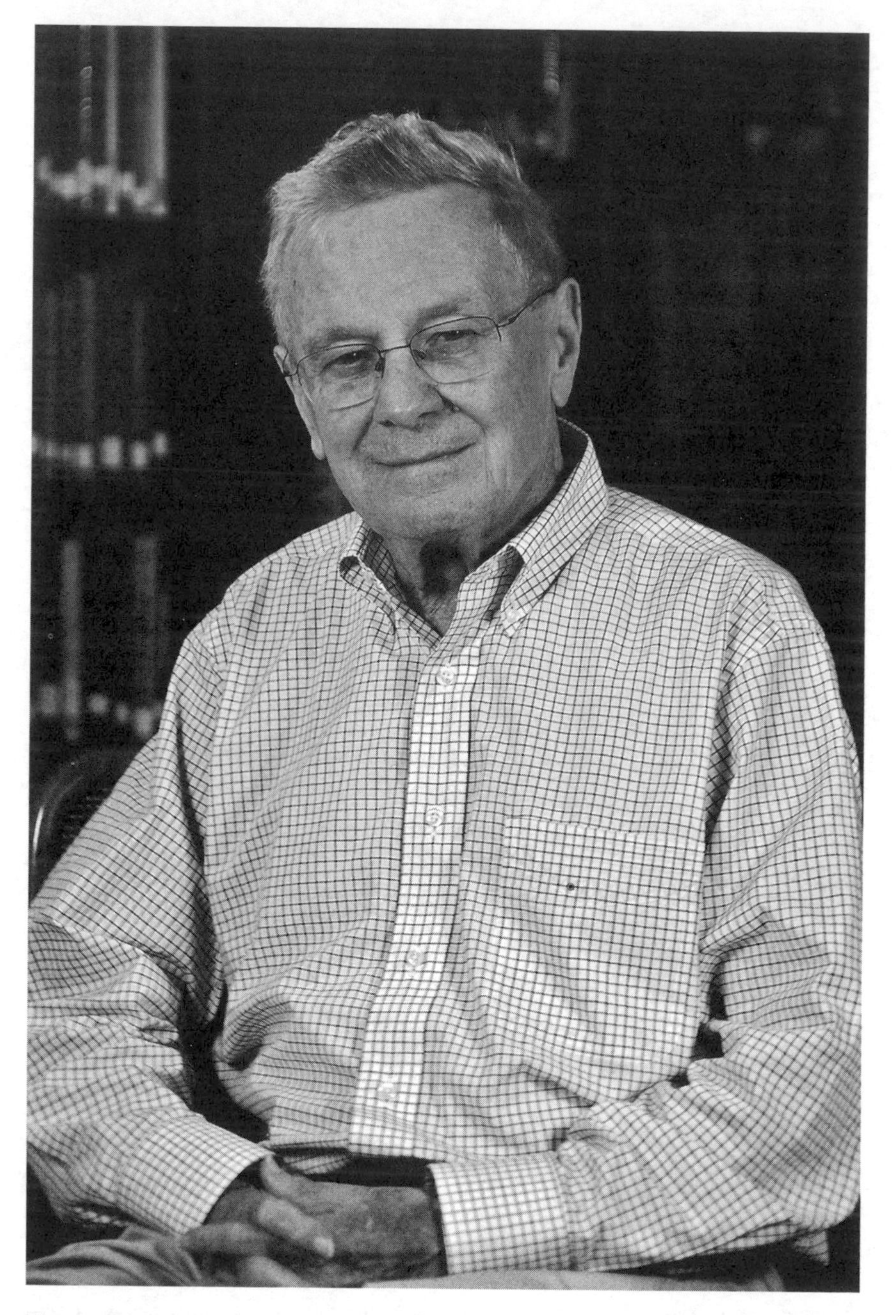

Figure 3.2
Now a septuagenarian, Daniel Callahan remains affiliated with The Hastings Center and continues to argue that scarcity demands that curative care for some seniors be sacrificed for the good of other, younger persons. *Source*: Photo, The Hastings Center.

which contributes to the health that makes society run well, to achieve its appropriate ends."[42] Medicine should therefore serve not the individual patient's need ("Into whatever house . . .") but instead first and foremost the needs of the state.[43]

This was a shocking proposition from the head of the foremost institute of bioethics in the United States. The traditional goal of medicine, to treat each patient to the best of the physician's ability—and the public ethos that had always embraced that ethic—were to be exchanged for another focused not on patient care but on economic stewardship. Instead of "physician, know thy self,"[44] a popular riff on Ben Franklin's "Physician, heal thyself," the motto was become: "physician, know thy place."

The mythology of bioethics asserts that in the 1980s the nascent ethic was advanced as the champion of patient autonomy and choice. It was this that in part distinguished bioethics from the old Hippocratic ethic that was, the new philosopher-ethicists asserted, unacceptably paternalistic. And yet in the late 1980s here was Callahan, the doyen of American bioethics, arguing patient choice (at least the choice of those who were elderly or poor) was or should be irrelevant in the face of futurist state economic concerns. The historic commitment of physicians to the needs of patients as persons and as community members was transformed into an unaffordable liability. Structurally, the resulting argument was the same as that of Holmes's 1927 decision in *Buck v. Bell*, and earlier, Hoche's concern over the costly maintenance of "idiots" and other "incurables."

Not surprisingly, perhaps, governments embraced Callahan's argument as a license to restrict health budgets and redirect services without thinking about system reform. In England, for example, physicians in a group practice facing the problem of insufficient state financing developed a policy statement by which they would assign care to persons on a relative scale of worth. The Asbury draft policy on ethical use of resources was described, and praised, in the *British Medical Journal.*[45] In it the elderly senior was disadvantaged, as were the unemployed, those without dependents, and so on. Loyola University philosopher and bioethicist Dave Thomasma, another doyen of the early days of bioethical formation, approved of this on the grounds that rationing of medical resources to favor the most productive and thus most worthy was, well, "rational" in a world of limits caused by intransigent scarcities.[46]

Greedy Geezers

A minor industry sprang up among gerontologists and sociologists who attacked Callahan's and Lamm's targeting of seniors as a superfluous class of superannuated citizens who were probably tired of life and in some cases maintained beyond all reason.[47] With Lamm and Callahan most accepted the idea of a natural resource scarcity requiring limits on healthcare. The problem, Callahan's and Lamm's critics said, was that they underestimated the continuing contributions of seniors as a class.[48] Callahan and Lam were promoting, the critics lamented, an "intergenerational war" pitting those popularly dubbed "greedy geezers" against the needs of potentially productive youth. [49] Greedy geezers were defined as seniors with money they spent selfishly on themselves rather than their adult children, either as a bequest after death or a gift in the present.[50]

The whole became an unseemly tangle over who had resources and who needed them. "At one and the same time they [the elderly] are characterized as a financially secure, healthy, homogeneous, powerful interest group, and as a massive, dependent burden on welfare, health programs, and the tax base generated by the currently shrinking workforce. In either case, they are seen as taking a disproportionate share of society's resources and disrupting intergenerational relations in the process."[51] Few doubted that society's resources were limited or that the limitations were both absolute and intransigent. Nobody disagreed that the care of some would have to be sacrificed for the good of all. The question was merely over who should be disenfranchised so that others might receive a full share of whatever was available.

For their part, politicians generally welcomed the announcement of a parasitic class of seniors they could blame for budget overruns, service provision failures, and tax increases.[52] They embraced as well Callahan's presentation of recalcitrant, spendthrift physicians as profligate healthcare villains, easy targets put in the bull's-eye by a bioethicist of real renown. The result was to focus the attention of officials and the public on the cost of care to the senior and the poor rather than the more general issues of public health.[53] Instead of a discussion of the ethics of national health coverage, or the potential inefficiencies of the healthcare system, the focus became the insupportable cost of care for the superannuated and by extension all those who were judged unproductive.

Reaganomics

It is not the least of ironies that much of this played out during the reign of the fortieth president of the United States, Ronald Reagan, who took office in 1980 at the age of seventy. That was already five years past the point where, in 1987, Callahan argued for only palliative but not curative treatments for unproductive seniors. For his part, Reagan energetically (one wants to say "youthfully") promoted a vision of government whose principal focus was the promotion of corporate and personal wealth.

Famously, he enacted tax breaks for the rich and tax incentives for corporations whose result, he promised, would eventually "trickle down" to the future benefit of society at large. Cutting back federal spending on social programs and deregulating the private sector would, in what came to be called Reaganomics, promote business health; cutting costs in socially mandated medical programs would, somehow, sooner or later build a better future (figure 3.3). The Callahan-Lamm argument fit perfectly with this vision.

The age at which curative care should be denied has always been something of a moving target that changed as Callahan himself aged. In 2010, by then a septuagenarian, Callahan continued to defend his argument: "I doggedly believe we will one way or the other have to set limits on health care for the elderly, even if a specific age limit will not do."[54] *Setting limits* is ethical, he continued, because "a good society ought to help young people become old people, but is under no obligation to help the old become indefinitely older." He is in good company. As Bill Bytheway put it in a 2010 review, the pertinent questions seemed to have become: "what do we do with all these old people?" and "how do we pay for them all?"[55] That was the only question of relevance. That years of social participation and service might deserve care, or the fact of continuing contributions by many, was deemed irrelevant.

The Malthusian Fallacy

Central to the Callahan-Lamm thesis—like that of Hoche and Binding before them—was the assertion that the source of the problem was new medicine technologies that kept alive those who would otherwise have died. On the one hand, new life-saving technologies held great potential for the medical care of sick people (Hurrah!). Scientific advances led to

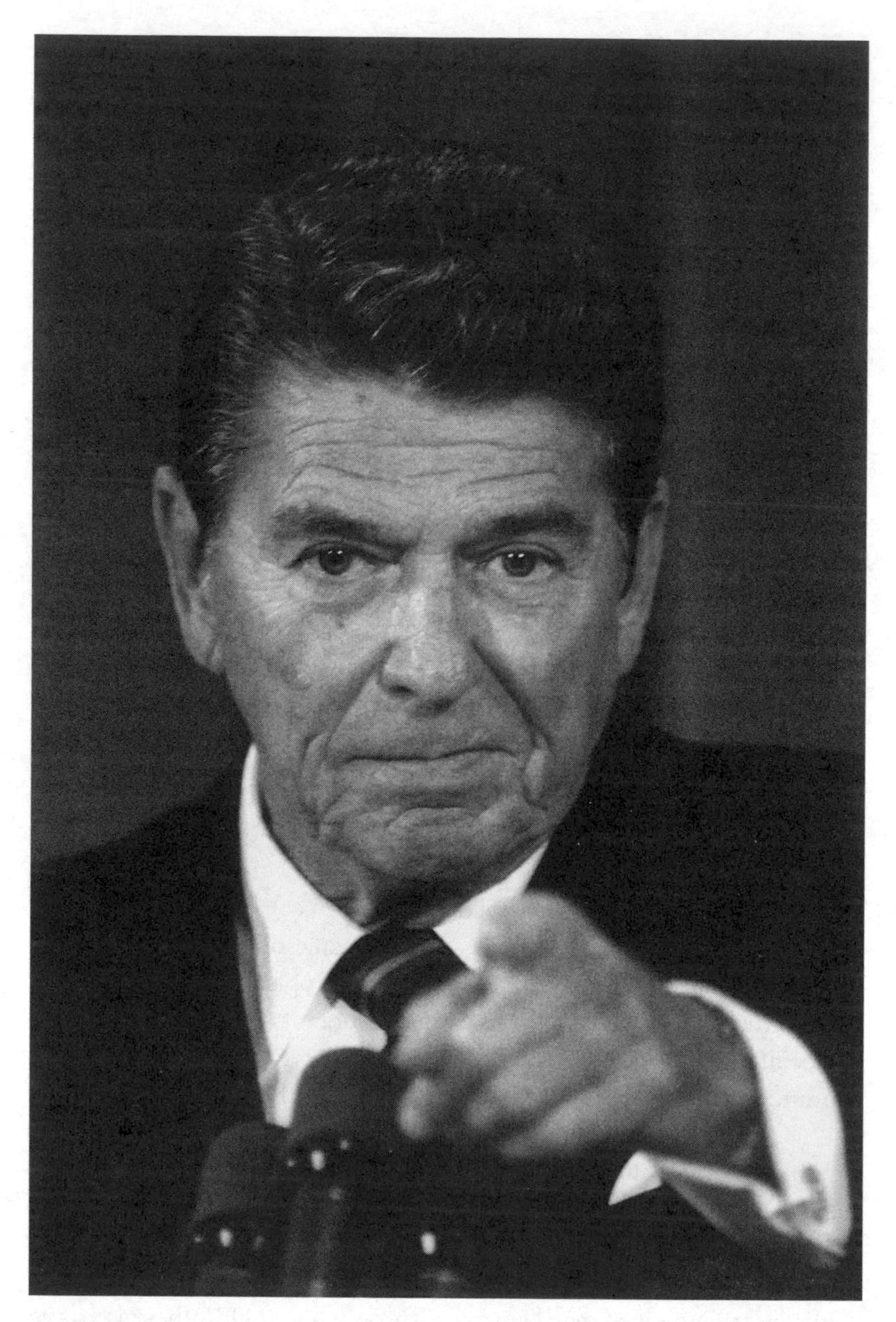

Figure 3.3
President Ronald Reagan, who took office at the age of seventy, oversaw a campaign to reduce health care costs through "managed care." These programs shifted responsibility for decisions regarding patient care from physicians to insurers.

new technology industries that contributed to public revenue streams at every level (Yay!). The resulting industries of medicine and its technologies employed tens of thousands of peoples who could be taxed, raising state revenues (Even Better!). But . . . new products were expensive (Oops?). Worse, they were often supported by public monies in the maintenance of unproductive, parasitic classes of people who were economic liabilities (Boo!). Bioethics offered itself as an evaluative consultant who could order this apparent conflict of good and bad in favor of economic priorities (Whew!).

At the heart of the argument, and more generally of bioethics' scarcity-based arguments today, is the Malthusian fallacy. Eighteenth-century Thomas Malthus assumed that "the power of population is indefinitely greater than the power in the earth to produce subsistence for man."[56] Population inevitably increased until a necessarily limited food supply became inadequate, resulting in "misery and famine." This was God's will, Malthus believed, a theistic enforcing of temperance and virtuous behavior upon an intemperate and sinful population. Bioethicists like Callahan, arguing from scarcity, have been substituting medical care for Malthus's grain supply-based limit in a structurally identical argument.

Malthus was half right. He observed a necessary relationship between population and its critical resource base: "In every State in which man has existed, or does now exist that the increase of population is necessarily limited by the means of subsistence."[57] But his assumption that supply is necessarily inflexible, and thus limited in relation to expanding demand was wrong. As the world's population expanded beyond Malthus's imagining so, too, did the supply of food and other necessities. Malthus—a demographer and Anglican theologian—did not perceive the possibility that both sides of the supply-demand equation are equally flexible and that both are dynamically related.

"Humans belong to the only species that continues to prosper even as we become more populous."[58] It has been the human genius to advance both agricultural productivity and animal husbandry to serve an ever-greater population base. It is not inevitable that demand will outpace over time a largely stagnant supply of this or that good. That Malthus was in error has not stopped neo-Malthusians from arguing similarly that population pressures will necessarily outstrip economic resources.[59] Here we can see, using medical care and its technologies as an example, the inadequacy of the assumptions on which supply-side formalists from Malthus to Callahan have based their arguments.

This is not to say there are no limits. But to say resources are not infinite is not to say they are necessarily scarce and must be rationed. We may choose to limit service to the elderly, the immigrants, or the poor on the basis of scarcity, but what we're really saying is that we'd rather spend our resources on other things, or people. In embracing scarcity as a natural condition, we permit the empowerment of the wealthy through lower tax rates rather than insisting upon tax programs that assure monies for care of the elderly and the poor. In embracing scarcity and the lifeboat, we ignore the needs of the lifeboat in favor of ship owners. It is a choice, not a natural necessity, and the failure to recognize that is a failure of ethics.

Medical Technologies: The Economic Case

New medical technologies will not necessarily bankrupt the state. It is not simply that healthier people are more productive, and thus are able to pay more taxes that support the public purse that pays for Medicaid and Medicare in the United States. It is also that new technologies require more workers to make the new products, and more doctors, nurses, and technicians to use them in diagnosis and treatment. That means increased employment at better-paying jobs, which translates into more tax revenues. Yes, medical care can be costly. But if state revenues are the problem then the promotion of new life-saving medical technologies is not the problem but the solution.

In 2000, for example, the U.S. biotechnology industry generated approximately $47 billion in revenue, $20 billion for the companies themselves and approximately $27 billion in revenues for their suppliers.[60] The industry and its suppliers paid a cumulative tax bill of approximately $10 billion. The biotechnology industry was also responsible for the creation of 437,400 jobs for workers whose incomes were taxable and thus contributed to the general economy. In the way of these things, that jobs creation led to jobs for millions of other, taxable workers. This is called the multiplier effect, by which each worker generates other jobs through his or her taxes and spending habits. Over the first decade of the twenty-first century these numbers increased markedly. A similar story can be told of the medical technologies industry providing CAT (computerized axial tomography) and PET (positron emission tomography) scans, MRIs, and other technologies. From 1997 to 2002, the market for diagnostic and other medical devices grew in the United States, from $57.7 billion to $75 billion dollars.[61] The U.S. share of the world market in these technologies, worth approximately $420.3 billion, was 42 percent. Again, this generated more jobs, the sale of more raw materials, and at each step vast increases in public revenues.

The same story of economic growth and increasing employment applies generally to the "Life Sciences Industry," and indeed, across all areas of medical technology and service. There we might include the colleges and universities where medical personnel are trained (doctors, nurses, lab technicians, physiotherapists, and so on) by an industry of tax-paying teachers supported by an army of income tax-paying support workers ranging from well-paid university deans to far less well-paid building janitors. Then there are the clinics that employ the professionals, each paying a range of state and federal taxes, as do the hospitals and private nursing homes that similarly employ more hundreds of thousands of taxable people.

The state's revenues are not simply stretched by healthcare but in a real way are very much indebted to it. The argument for necessary triage on the basis of cost alone fails unless one assumes it acceptable to promote industries but to deny their deployment to those whose taxes support the state. And in the event the use of the technology is restricted, demand for it is lessened and related jobs contract as a result. The argument thus fails, economically as well as ethically, unless one assumes the needs of the individual are irrelevant except to the degree that person performs (as consumer or producer) in a manner that serves the needs of the economy and an imagined and hoped-for future state of general economic prosperity.

Scarcity

The reflexive embrace of Malthusian limits served as a rationale for the abandonment of persons (the old, the feeble, the impaired) whose care was assumed by practitioners of the older medical ethic. In this perspective, bioethicists (and economists, and policy mavens who read both bioethics and economics) denied the personal for the impersonal and economic, obscuring rather than illuminating the questions bioethicists arguing from scarcity might otherwise have asked. Do we place the possible needs of a half-imagined future above the exigent needs of the person who is ill today? Is economic productivity to be the measure of human worth, and of patienthood in medicine? Is cost accountancy the measure by which treatment of the infant with polio, the senior with congestive heart disease, or the woman with breast cancer, is to be assessed (figure 3.4)? Is the practice of medicine a vocation dedicated to the care of the patient or is the practitioner merely a functionary of the state and its economic agenda?

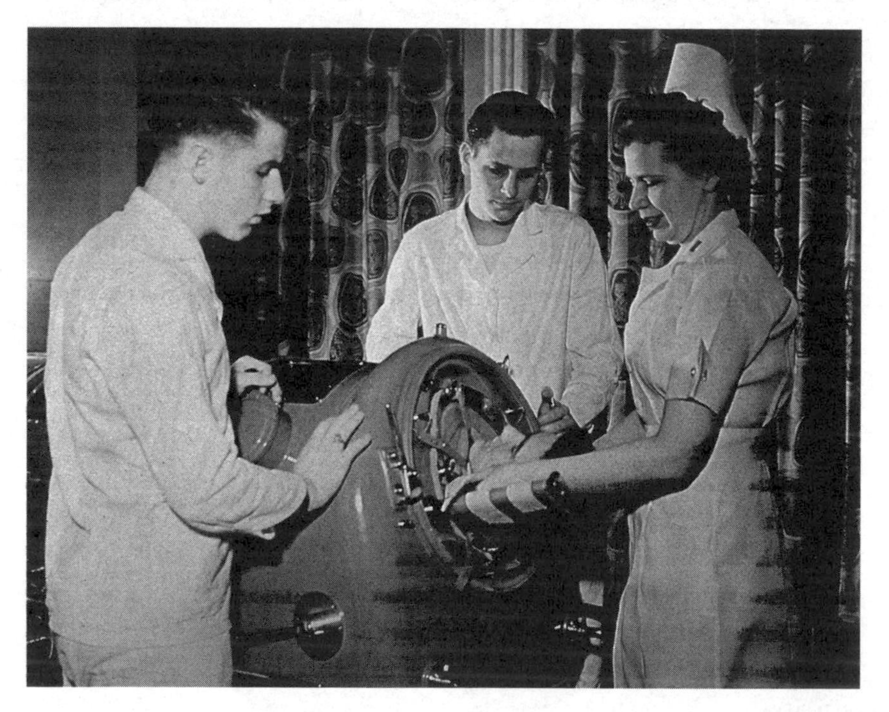

Figure 3.4
In this undated photograph, a nurse and two attendants care for a polio patient in an iron lung in the early 1950s. From Copenhagen to San Francisco, thousands of individuals were kept alive through the use of these expensive, cumbersome, labor-intensive machines. *Source*: National Library of Medicine, Bethesda, MD.

Lifeboat Ethics

By 1991 the argument from scarcity had become a generally accepted, bioethical and social truth referred to by the metaphor of "lifeboat ethics." In 1991, for example, Boston University's dean of medicine, Dr. Louis Lasagna, analogized the intransigent limits of health resources with those of the original overloaded lifeboat made famous in legal and social history in the landmark case *United States v. Holmes*.[62] The story Lasagna told in *Science Magazine* was this: A well-maintained American sailing ship, the *William Brown*, struck an iceberg in the North Atlantic in the spring of 1841. Half the passengers drowned when the ship sank; half were saved and brought aboard its single longboat. Overloaded, the longboat was in danger of capsizing. As a result, the crew threw sixteen passengers overboard in a desperate attempt to assure the survival of at least a few of the remaining passengers, and of course, themselves. One of those sailors, Alexander William Holmes, was later tried and convicted in the United States on the charge of manslaughter on the high seas.

Born in the longboat of the *William Brown*, lifeboat ethics has come to describe a class of ethical problems in which presumably inflexible resource limits are assumed to create special circumstances in which otherwise sacrosanct ethical principles can be relaxed if not wholly held in abeyance. The metaphor perfectly captured the argument of Lamm, Callahan, and the expanding community of bioethicists who accepted the role of, in effect, scarcity consultants. "The medical system in the United States today finds itself in an analogous predicament [to the passengers of the longboat]," Lasagna wrote. "The cost of health care has soared at a rate roughly twice that of general inflation, partly because of the proliferation of technological procedures—kidney dialysis, organ and bone-marrow transplants—that can quickly bankrupt a family."[63]

The editors of the *Cambridge Quarterly of Healthcare Ethics* used the lifeboat metaphor, substituting the story of the *Titanic* for that of the earlier *William Brown*. "The award-winning film *Titanic* released in 1997 once again brought to our attention the problems associated with the lifeboat ethic," they wrote. "One analogue in healthcare to the *Titanic* is the form of transplantation ethics and [more general] social policy."[64]

In modernity's lifeboat the ethical question is assumed reflexively to be not how to save everyone but how best to choose among the equally needy, some of whom must be die if any are to survive.[65] "Which patients should get the last available bed in the intensive care, or the single available donated heart, or the only remaining respirator?"[66] Perhaps, as John F. Kilner argued, we should seek a formula that offers a rule of maximum social utility irrespective of individual necessity based upon the resources society possesses at any moment.[67]

The metaphor became the reality, one whose narrative elements were taken as unquestionably real and generally exigent. Medical care was the lifeboat overfilled with the needy and the sick. The sea was the financial cost to the nation; its rough waters threatened to swamp the boat. Some had to be forsaken if some were to survive. Ethically and practically, all that was left was to ask, as did a Senate Special Committee: "Who Lives? Who Dies? Who Decides?"[68] In the ethos of scarcity no other questions were possible.

Two Ethics of the Lifeboat

The metaphor's limit is the ethic's failure. It assumes the limits of the lifeboat are exigent and unavoidable. This is, after all, what metaphors do: they structure the way a thing is perceived, distinguishing foreground from background. In the case of lifeboat ethics it focuses on the exigencies of the overcrowded boat in stormy seas, thus ignoring all the elements that brought a group of ship passengers to this extreme. In the metaphor's many venues of application its structure assures we do not question what brought so many people to the point of disaster. Hidden in the tale is the idea of causation, of avoidable disaster and its attendant responsibilities.[69]

In the lifeboat no good choices remain. One can only ask who is the weakest, the least likely to survive, the least able to contribute to the survival of others. Where all are equal and some must die the issue becomes at best one of grace in the face of dire necessity: the lottery, the drawing of straws, or, if a revolver is handy, a game of Russian roulette. That is ethics *in* the lifeboat where no good choices exist. Some *must* die, or be abandoned, so that others may live.

There is, however, another ethic one can apply, an ethics *of* the lifeboat whose focus is the complex of prior decisions that brought the lifeboat's occupants to the sorry contemplation of murder for salvation's sake. Using the index case as an example, the questions become: What was the *William Brown* doing under full sail at night in the spring of the year in waters known by all to be populated with icebergs? Why was there only one leaky longboat aboard a ship carrying more than eighty persons? And why was only one able-bodied seaman, Holmes, charged when more than a score of seamen answered the direct order of the first mate, Francis Rhodes, to "lighten the boat" by throwing sixteen passengers overboard?

Just asking these questions impeaches the bioethical insistence that the problems we face are unprecedented rather than old dilemmas transposed into a new form. The analogous questions are instantly clear: A physician might have to choose between three equally needy patients in an ER where he or she is the only surgeon on duty. That is a question of ethics *in* the lifeboat. Similarly, the doctor may have to choose between three patients who all need ventilation in a hospital with only one ventilator available. But why was only one surgeon on duty, or one machine in service when the ER's daily volume of patients made the necessity for more doctors and more resources inevitable? Who gets wheeled in first is a question of lifeboat ethics. An ethics *of* the lifeboat asks: Why was only one surgeon on call in a hospital with one ventilator, a hospital that is, perhaps the principal trauma center for a large community?

A second perspective arises in arguing an ethics of the lifeboat rather than the lifeboat ethics of intransigent scarcity—one that bioethicists have not rejected so much as never considered. To see this nothing serves quite as well as a close consideration of the index case that gave the metaphor its name, the nineteenth-century story of the *William Brown* and the court case that gave it standing in law and the popular literature.

4

Lifeboat Ethics: Scarcity as an Unnatural State

On the evening of April 19, 1841, an American sailing ship, the *William Brown*, was making ten knots under full sail when, shortly after nine o'clock at night, it struck an iceberg several hundred miles off the Newfoundland coast. Ten minutes later it struck another. After the second collision, the holds filling inexorably with water, Captain George L. Harris gave the order to abandon ship. Almost half of the sixty-five immigrant passengers and all seventeen crew members were saved in two auxiliary boats quickly provisioned with several days' rations of food and water. The captain and seven others went into the small jollyboat, the first mate and all other survivors into the open longboat. Just before midnight those who survived watched from astern as the *William Brown* sank with thirty-four passengers, Irish immigrants bound for America, still aboard.

The next day, Captain Harris steered the smaller jollyboat northwest toward Newfoundland after giving command of the larger longboat to his first mate, Francis L. Rhodes. "I also told the crew to obey all the mate's orders, and to do nothing without his consent," Harris would later testify. "They promised me they would do so—I bid them goodbye." The captain did not mention in his testimony that his mate told him that, "We cannot all live. Some of us must die, the boat is so leaky."

Designed not for the open ocean but for harbor use, the 22.5-foot longboat was overloaded and ungainly, its rudder barely operable. The first night of Rhodes's command, as the seas deepened and swells increased, he ordered his crew to jettison fourteen men and two women to lighten the vessel to increase its buoyancy and maneuverability. Sailing slowly through the ice the next morning the *Crescent*, an American ship outward bound for Le Havre, spied the longboat and took the remaining passengers and crew aboard. Several days later, a French fishing lugger rescued Captain Harris and his companions near the French Island of St. Pierre off the Newfoundland coast.

In 1912 another ship carrying immigrants from England to North America, and wealthy persons as well, was sailing at top speed at night in the same waters and at the same time of year. It, too, struck an iceberg. It, too, sank as a result. And like the *William Brown*, a significant percentage of its human cargo would go down with the ship because there were insufficient lifeboats for the salvation of all who had paid for passage. That ship was the *Titanic*.

In the 1840s, shipwrecks and marine disasters were almost as common as automobile pile-ups are today. De-mastings, wrecks, and maritime misadventures were a near-daily feature of the newspapers in coastal American cities. Where today we have a collection of police-blotter stories, the *Boston Post* of the 1840s ran a section with notices of marine wrecks and disasters. Despite society's familiarity with the dangers of transatlantic voyaging, however, the deliberate drowning of those saved to the *William Brown*'s longboat made this a special case.

The story of the *William Brown*'s longboat was shared between newspapers from Boston to Paris. A May 15 account in the *London Times*, for example, was a reprint of a story published two days earlier in the Paris-based *Galignami's Messenger*. Another story was published independently in London's *Morning Post* based on the narratives of the surviving passengers: "The tales which the survivors relate are piteous—horrifying," the story proclaimed. On May 18, the *London Times* published a joint statement by British and U.S. consuls in Le Havre, who together took depositions from the survivors and found that "throughout the affair we have not discovered any fact capable of drawing down blame upon anyone whatever." Everyone knew that sailing the Atlantic was perilous at the best of times. Ships sank, the officials said, especially in the early spring when icebergs populated the North Atlantic. Hard decisions had to be made and the wonder was anyone survived at all.

However, the story of the *William Brown* did not die with the official declaration that no fault could be assigned to the ship's crew or owners. The problem was, as a *Times* writer put it in an early article: "We have emigrant ships sailing every week, and if it held as law that 'might is right,' it had better be declared so, that the crew are justified under extremities in throwing overboard whom, and as many, as they think right, without casting lots or making any choices than their will." Here was a problem that was economic, ethical, legal, moral, and philosophical at once: *If* might makes right, *then* all those who sailed on commercial ships were at potential risk. Passengers could be drowned at the discretion of crew members. The Victorian question was, simply, whether might makes right.

At stake was the immigrant trade, a lucrative element of the economies of both the United States and Great Britain. Ships from the Americas carried raw goods to Great Britain that shipped finished goods in return. Immigrants from Great Britain were needed in the United States as laborers and as paying cargo to fill out the manifest of returning ships (bales of cotton were more bulky than finished fabric and fashionable dresses). Industrialization and enclosure acts had created a large class of former agriculturalists unemployable in British cities. They were seen as both a drain on the economy and a threat to civil order. Their emigration was thus an economic and a political necessity. But when travel was perceived as either too costly or too perilous, when the number of reported deaths at sea seemed particularly high, the volume of travelers declined as a result. And in 1841, the threats of death not only from the dangerous seas, but also at the hands of crewmen of a ship sunk by an iceberg, were seen by a growing number as one threat too many. Public reports of the *William Brown*'s sinking, and the subsequent drownings in its longboat, thus directly endangered the emigrant trade integral to economies on both sides of the Atlantic.

The people of *Le Havre* took up a collection to pay the fares to the United States of the crew and the survivors of the *William Brown*. When they arrived in Philadelphia in April 1842 one of those survivors, a Swedish seaman, was arrested and tried nine months later on the charge of "manslaughter on the high seas." Alexander William Holmes was accused of "throwing overboard from the longboat several of the passengers, among who was Francis Askins, the person whom the defendant is charged in this indictment with killing." Askins was a convenient name pulled from the list of those drowned by Rhodes and his crew; almost any of those saved from the sinking ship only to be drowned in the longboat would have served equally at law as victims.

All accepted the general facts of the case, reported in newspapers and later recited at trial by a number of survivors. The ship sank after striking an iceberg and half its passengers went down with the ship. Half of those saved to the ship's longboat were thrown overboard the following night. Holmes was one of the seamen who participated in the murder of the emigrant passengers saved from the sinking *William Brown* only to be drowned the following night. American newspapers promoted the trial as an experiment in moral philosophy to be played out in a federal courtroom in Philadelphia. What are the obligations of persons in power—in this case, seamen—when circumstances demand the sacrifice of some to save others? Is there a defense of necessity that might permit such actions when resources are so limited that some must be let die, or be killed, to give even the chance of life to others? Wasn't this just a case of human nature, the natural desire to live even at the expense of others in a Hobbesian world? If that were the case could one in fact prosecute someone for, well, being human?

True Lies

This is how lifeboat ethics got its name. It's a metaphor that rests, as most do, upon a set of incomplete facts carefully selected to construct a story that does little justice to the complex of events that occurred. Everything important is avoided in the telling, all the interesting questions are unasked. Yes, the *William Brown* sank in the springtime of the North Atlantic after being hulled by an iceberg. But . . . what idiot sails full tilt at night in waters that everybody knows to be littered with icebergs? Yes, more than half the passengers went down with the ship. But why was there only one lifesaving craft aboard a ship carrying a full complement of passengers from Great Britain to the United States? Yes, half the passengers saved to the longboat were later drowned to lighten its load in heavy seas. But who made the decision and who, if anybody, protested? And finally, yes, Holmes was one of the crewmen who helped jettison the passengers from the overloaded longboat. Why, however, was he the only one charged with the crime? Whose orders was he following and who, if anyone, opposed this apparently heinous act?

The answers to most of these questions, the secrets of the *William Brown* and its lifeboat ethics, lie in London's Public Records Office in

Kew Gardens. There reside the depositions of most but not all of the survivors of the *William Brown*, sworn statements recorded in the careful penmanship of a secretary to the British counsel to Le Havre, young Gilbert Gordon. There, too, is the correspondence between Gordon and his boss, Britain's foreign secretary Henry John Temple, Third Viscount Palmerston, KG, GCB, PC. An aggressive interventionist who asserted British legitimacy and rule everywhere, including on the high seas, Lord Palmerston (figure 4.1) had wanted a trial of the surviving crew members to take place in London, not in Philadelphia where it ended up. How he and his young counsel got snookered is a critical part of the way in which the idea of lifeboat ethics, and its view of human nature, was created.

Sailings

The *William Brown* and later the *Titanic* were at their map coordinates in the North Atlantic at the time of their destruction because they were sailing a great circle route, one that looks curved on the map, between their respective British ports of origin and their North American ports of destination. It was because they had not drifted far from that well-traveled route that the longboat and its survivors were found the morning after its crew drowned sixteen of their number. The great circle route was so popular because it described the fastest course between England and the United States, and the necessity of speed was dictated by the old equation that time equals money. Speed, not caution, ruled the nineteenth-century shipping trade.

Some, like the captain of the *Crescent*, sailed slowly among the litter of icebergs in the North Atlantic spring. Others like Captain Rhodes, and later the captain of the *Titanic*, Edward J. Smith, rushed across their likely field, trusting to chance and perhaps a lookout or two on board. There was no reward for the cautious captain who arrived late at port with ship and cargo intact. Bonuses might be paid, however, to the captain who came to port on or ahead of time. The faster the passage the quicker the ship could be unloaded, reloaded, and turned out to sea again. It was for maximum speed to generate the greatest potential financial return that Captain Francis Rhodes had his sailors bend on all sails on the night he sank the *William Brown;* in the 1820s the ship had

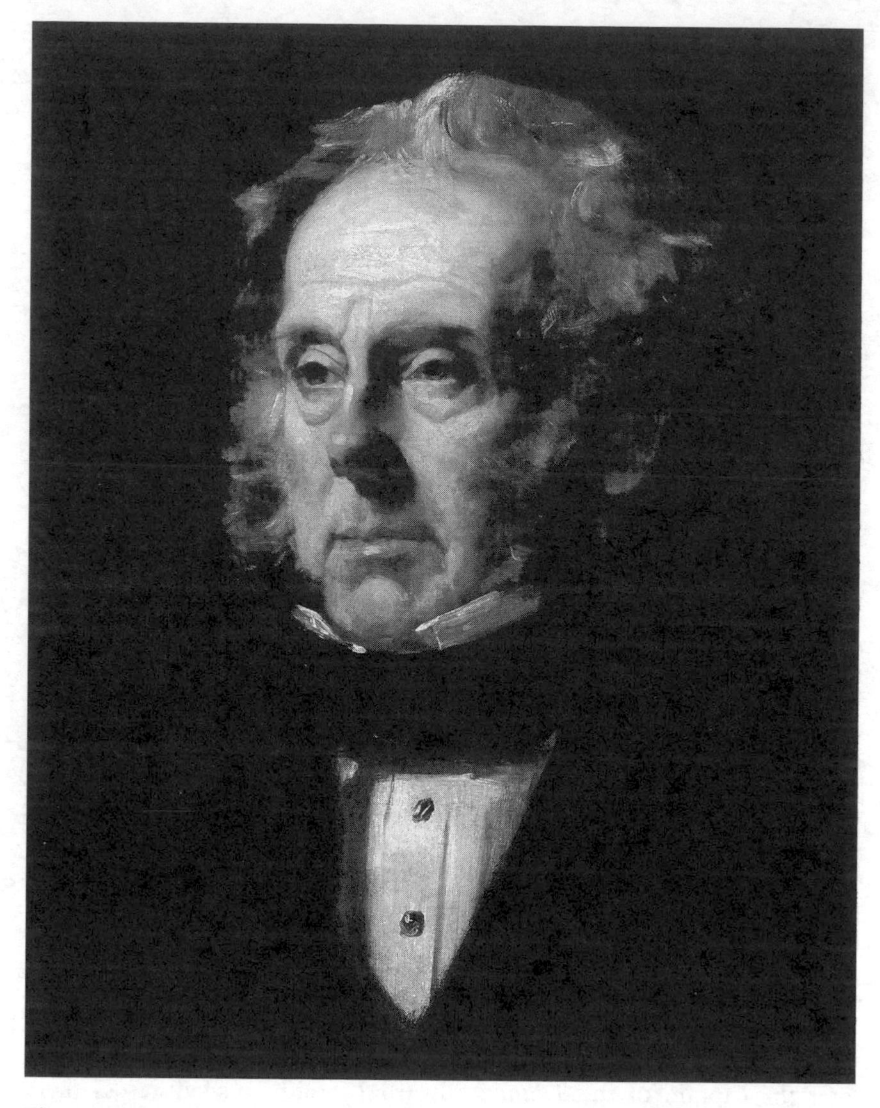

Figure 4.1
This 1855 official portrait gives the sense of Lord Palmerston in his maturity. A defender of British sovereignty everywhere, including at sea, he had sought to have the crew of the *William Brown* returned to England for trial. Painter: Francis Cruikshank, 1855. *Source*: National Portrait Gallery, London.

set a record for the speed of its Atlantic crossing. In 1912 it was the desire for speed, and the bragging rights of a record crossing, that placed the *Titanic* at full speed in the same waters in the same time of the year.

It was common knowledge that icebergs menaced the North Atlantic sailing route. Year after year, ships collided with icebergs and were sunk in the spring months; the few lucky survivors were generally found in leaky longboats and jollyboats by more cautious or just more fortunate ships (figure 4.2). Nineteenth-century weeklies on both sides of the Atlantic regularly reported iceberg sightings; captains meeting at sea would warn each other of the dangers they had seen in their respective passages. Brian Hill of the Institute of Marine Dynamics in St. John's, Newfoundland, has recorded the latitude and longitude of hundreds of North Atlantic iceberg collisions resulting in shipwrecks over the centuries.

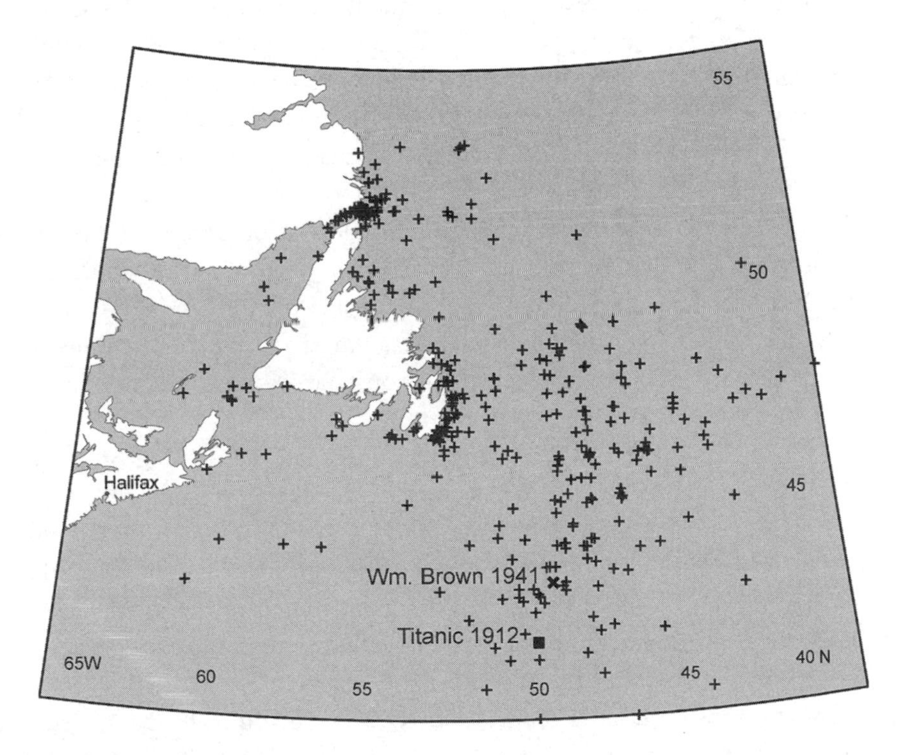

Figure 4.2
Hundreds of ships sunk through collision with icebergs were reported in the North Atlantic in the spring of each year from at least 1700 until 1920, when new international safety regulations were instituted. *Source*: Map by author.

Ship owners did not like losing ships but accepted the occasional loss of this or that vessel as a cost of business as long as profits accrued at a sufficient rate from the remaining vessels in an owner's fleet. The loss of human life typically was seen as a perhaps unfortunate but not truly lamentable cost of business. There were always seamen looking for a berth, always emigrants looking for passage. Nobody but the families of the drowned cared overmuch if members of either group were lost at sea. One nineteenth-century newspaper report gave the tenor of the age when it chronicled the loss of "twenty souls and 240 emigrants." While the former were lamented the latter were, well, just emigrants.

Ship owners adamantly opposed occasional calls for standards requiring a full complement of lifesaving craft on all vessels as an unnecessary and potentially ruinous expense. When the issue was raised in the newspapers of the day (or in the U.S. Congress, or the British Parliament) after this or that sinking, ship owners would warn that requiring all ships to carry enough lifesaving vessels for all on board would require they raise the fares for both cargo and for passengers. This, they insisted, would not only be inflationary (and thus bad for the economy) but would also damage the emigrant trade, making it less affordable to the poor. Nobody wanted that, neither the Americans in need of cheap labor nor the British seeking to rid themselves of surplus populations. The word "lifeboat" didn't enter the English language until the middle of the nineteenth century when it referred not to on-board vessels but to shore-based boats to be used in coastal rescue.

All this explains the *William Brown's* speed on the evening of April 19, 1841, in the iceberg-strewn waters of the North Atlantic. All this contributed to not simply its sinking but also the inevitable drowning of half its passengers because there were not enough lifesaving craft for all aboard the ship. And, of course, all this contributed to the dilemma of the leaking, overloaded lifeboat that carried more than thirty persons in heavy seas the day after the *William Brown* sank.

Every deposition, news report, and the trial record itself made clear that the decision to throw sixteen passengers from the *William Brown*'s longboat was the first mate's, Francis Rhodes. He was in command; Captain Harris had made each seaman swear to follow his first mate's orders. There is no more democracy in a lifeboat than there is aboard a naval ship. The decisions are the captain's, or in his absence the first mate's or whoever is the highest-ranking officer. To disobey a lawful command is insurrection (when done by a single individual) if not mutiny (when a group disobeys), and sailors were trained—in those days by the lash, and the threat of hanging—to follow orders.

Lifeboat Choices

Several survivors later testified that when given command of the longboat, Rhodes warned Captain Harris it was so overloaded that all in it could not survive. At trial survivors would eventually testify that, the morning after the *William Brown* sank, just before Captain Harris sailed his jollyboat toward safety, Rhodes broached the idea of a lottery that might determine who among his passengers would need to be drowned. Captain Harris refused to discuss the matter: "The mate then distinctly said, 'We must cast lots—we all cannot live—some of us must die.' The captain again remonstrated with the mate," one passenger testified in court. In response to Rhodes's concerns, "The captain replied, 'say no more about it, I know what you will have to do.'"

All agreed that while Rhodes had raised the idea of a lottery with his captain he brooked no discussion of drawing lots as the longboat wallowed the following night, the first night of his command. Instead he ordered the seaman to begin to dispatch the male passengers, one by one (figure 4.3). At least one sailor, Joseph Jack Stetson of Thomaston, Maine, made a point of this in his deposition and later, much later, in interviews given to U.S. newspapers.

For the nineteenth-century American, and Victorians generally, the failure to create a lottery of some kind was a potential sticking point that transformed common tragedy into malfeasance. In dire straits, drawing lots in a survival situation was a long-established custom of the sea. The most famous case of its kind in the nineteenth century was the wreck of the *Essex,* a whaling ship sunk in the mid-Pacific after being struck by a whale.[1] After his ship's destruction, that captain sailed with his surviving crew, parceled into small open whaling boats, caring for them as much as he could. One by one, survivors died of dehydration or starvation as their supply of fresh water and food ran out. Famously, the captain instituted a lottery among the survivors, one in which he was

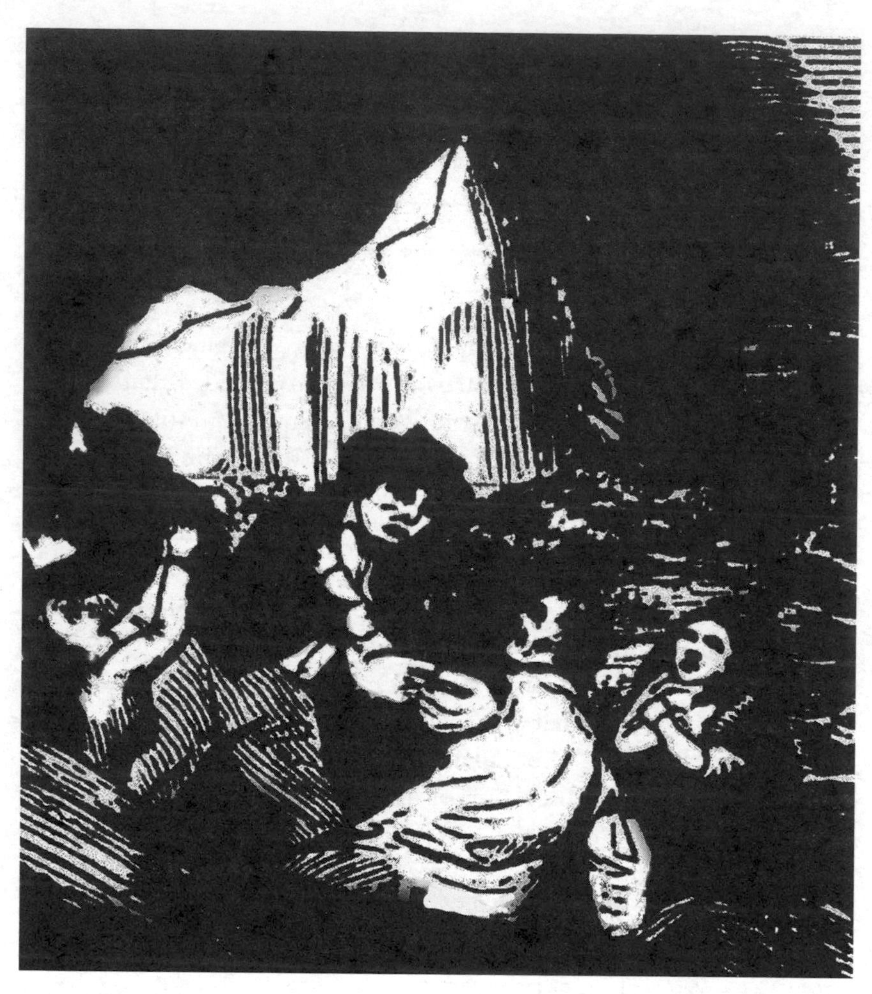

Figure 4.3
This 1845 woodblock by H. K. Brooke depicts the drowning of the *William Brown*'s longboat passengers by its crew in a popular telling of the disaster.

included, as the only honorable way of preserving the last of their meager resources to the seemingly inevitable end.

The sinking of the *Essex* was a unique event caused by an occurrence never before reported and thus impossible to foresee: a whale attacked the ship that carried its attackers, the men hunting it with harpoons, while they were adrift in their open boats. The sinking of a ship like the *William Brown*, however, was a predictable event. Ships sank every spring when some of those sailing the great circle route collided with icebergs in the North Atlantic. Were it not this ship, therefore, it would have been another. Still, for Victorians, and especially for Americans of the day, the memory of the *Essex* and the grace of its captain was a much admired, well-known model. It was therefore at least potentially an indictment of the crew members of the *William Brown* who simply chucked passengers into the sea at their first mate's order rather than more civilly and democratically drawing straws to decide who would be drowned. Thus, for many people living in the mid-nineteenth century, the story of the *William Brown* was at best ignoble if not necessarily actionable.

Depositions

The day after their arrival in Le Havre the survivors of the *William Brown*, both passengers and crew members, were brought before the American and British counsels to be deposed. The first to appear was Rhodes who, not surprisingly, cast his tale as one of inevitability in a boat that was difficult to steer, leaking, and overloaded. It was on the basis of these depositions that British counsel Gilbert Gordon and his more experienced counterpart, U.S. Counsel Rubin Beasley, released separate private statements to their governments as well as a joint public statement to the press. While the British Counsel's public and official reports were similar, U.S. Counsel Beasley's private report to his superiors was distinct from his agreed position in the joint statement.

The reason for this is clear. Beasley knew things that Gordon did not. The night before the official inquiry, Beasley had privately interviewed two dissident seamen, one of whom was John Messier, who had protested Rhodes's order and then refused to participate in the drowning. After deposing the two seamen Beasley dismissed them without telling Gordon, who therefore had no knowledge of their testimony. We know this from statements Messier would later make to newspapers in the United States after he was repatriated.

Messier told Beasley, and later American readers, that he had called for a lottery, one in which all including Rhodes would participate. Not only did the first mate reject his demand, but also, when Messier then refused to help in the drowning of the longboat's passengers, Rhodes ordered other sailors to dispatch Messier. Drawing his knife, he sat the rest of that long night waiting for one of his crewmates to approach. When the *Crescent* was sighted the next morning, Messier remembered, Rhodes called him a lucky fellow saved by the longboat's fortuitous rescue. The implication was that, sooner or later, Messier would have let down his guard, fallen asleep, and then been drowned at Rhodes's order. The blame for what happened, Messier said, was Rhodes's and his alone.

If damning in its portrayal of the first mate, Messier's statement was dangerous personally as well. After all, he had sworn to his captain he would follow Rhodes's order and he had violated that oath and in those days an oath was not to be lightly discarded. And, legally, the refusal of the mate's order could have been construed as at least insubordination if not a more serious offense. In his statement to U.S. Counsel Beasley, and later to American newspaper reporters, Messier admitted to mutinous insurrection in his challenge of Rhodes's order and his failure to answer the first mate's command. At the very least, a sailor who spoke in so scathing a matter of his superior, and who drew a knife against his fellow seamen, irrespective of the reason, would not soon find another ship.

Beasley knew that were Gordon to hear Messier's testimony, the British consul would insist upon bringing the first mate to trial in England. That was something that the American official did not want. If Lord Palmerston sought to assert British dominance at sea, Beasley knew that his superiors in Washington, D.C., were equally interested in the primacy of U.S. control over shipping in international waters. Yes, the passengers were British (or at least Irish) but the *William Brown* was an American ship and any legal or political review therefore should happen, Beasley believed, in the United States. To forestall any complications, he therefore ordered Messier and a shipmate telling a similar story released before

Gordon could hear their testimony. The British consul heard only what the American counsel wanted him to hear. Gordon was therefore more than willing to release the survivors after receiving the depositions of the Rhodes, the nonmutinous crew members, and the surviving passengers of the *William Brown.*

Even without reading Messier's testimony Lord Palmerston was dissatisfied with the official version of events. After receiving Gordon's initial report Lord Palmerston wrote to his consul ordering both crew and passengers returned to London. There, he said, the *William Brown*'s crew would be charged with the murder of British citizens, even if they were only Irish emigrants. But Lord Palmerton's order arrived after the survivors had left Le Havre, sailing once again to America. Most were on a ship bound for Philadelphia although Messier sailed separately, and earlier, to Boston. "Calamitous," Lord Palmerston called it in a note that survives in the archives. The case had passed beyond England and nothing more could be done about it (figure 4.4).

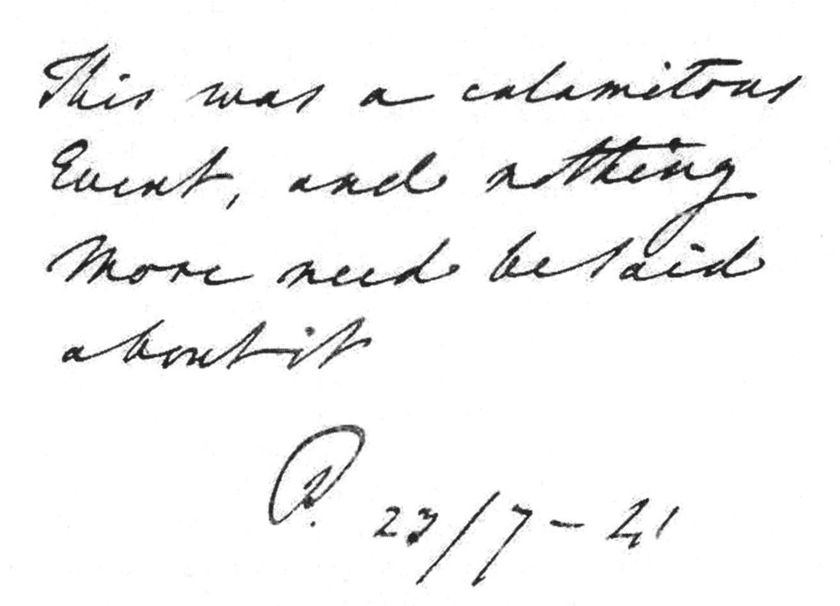
This was a calamitous
Event, and nothing
More need be said
about it

P. 23/7-41

Figure 4.4
When the survivors of the *William Brown* returned to the United States, they went beyond the potential jurisdiction of Lord Palmerston and British justice. The last note in the ministry's file was this dismissal of the affair.

Alexander William Holmes

In June 1841, when the bulk of the survivors of the *William Brown* arrived in Philadelphia, one seaman, Alexander William Holmes, was arrested on the capital charge of murder. When a grand jury refused to indict him on that charge, "ignoramused" in the language of the day, it was changed to "manslaughter on the high seas" under an 1890 statute, one never before or since used in a murder trial, giving U.S. officials jurisdiction over American ships anywhere in the maritime world. Why charge Holmes who, a Swedish sailor, was not even a U.S. citizen? There were, after all, American seamen on board who participated in the drowning. Why charge that seaman and not, say, Rhodes who gave the order to drown the passengers in the longboat?

Prosecutors might also have indicted the captain for sailing full speed at night in waters known to be rife with icebergs. That might have been construed as reckless endangerment and a willful disregard for the life and safety of others, the very definition of second-degree murder. Or, had they wished, U.S. federal prosecutors might have held the ship's owners responsible for the failure to provide lifesaving crafts sufficient to include all the passengers of the *William Brown*. Why *not* charge the ship owners (Americans out of Boston) for negligent homicide? They knew the risks of sailing the North Atlantic route when icebergs populated the winter sea.

None of these other options would answer the political realities of the day, however. What was needed was a judgment that would reassure passengers on oceangoing vessels in a fashion that neither indicted nor alienated American shipping interests. To indict the first mate would at the least reveal his captain's refusal to listen to Rhodes's concerns. Indeed, it may have resulted in a charge of abandonment against Captain Harris who, sailing away in his jollyboat, left the longboat's management to Rhodes's sole discretion. At the least, Captain Harris could have sailed the jollyboat in tandem with the longboat, keeping together his command. (That's what the captain of the *Essex* did with his whalers in their boats, people would have said.)

To indict Rhodes therefore would have been to indict the captain at one remove. That, however, would challenge the almost sovereign authority of ship captains in the days of sail, a difficult thing to do. It also would have upset both the shipping industry in which captains were prized as well as the congress of ships captains who together held considerable financial and political sway. Worse, a charge against the captain would have opened the door to other impertinent questions. Why was the *William Brown* under full sail at night in waters known to be densely populated with icebergs? And why did the *William Brown* carry only one longboat in ill repair? The answer to all of these questions, had they been asked, was simple. Ship owners demanded speed above all else and that was what Captain Rhodes gave them. They did not want the expense of extra longboats and it was not the captain's fault if they were not provided.

The United States therefore could not indict either the captain or the first mate without opening the shipping industry and its chain of command to scrutiny. Nor would it have been wise to indict a U.S. seaman who answered Rhodes's order to drown the passengers in the longboat. The merchant marine had a strong voice in U.S. political and maritime affairs and a strong sympathy among coastal peoples. Almost everyone knew someone who went to sea. And for every sailor there were eight or ten others who made their living either as maritime manufacturers, ship chandlers, builders and suppliers, or as innkeepers and lodging house managers for sailors in port.

To indict an American sailor therefore would have been to ask for political trouble from all quarters. But to indict a British sailor would have brought Lord Palmerston's interests into play. He might legitimately have called for the extradition of all for a trial in England. After all, it was *his* people who were drowned. At the very least he would have assured a strong British presence in the American courtroom, perhaps at the defendant's table. That, of course, would not have served U.S. interests, not at all. But Alexander William Holmes was neither American nor British but Swedish. There were therefore no special interests fighting hard in his corner except, perhaps, the Swedish consul and he was a minor figure on both the British and American political stages. Best of all, Holmes was the one hero of the whole sorry affair. He was the only crew member who, as the *William Brown* floundered, left the safety of the longboat to return to the ship to rescue a young girl who had been separated from her mother. As one cried to the other—the mother in the longboat and the child on deck—Holmes climbed back on board, grabbed the child, and brought her to her parent. This spoke, in the language of the day, to his "character" and would assure that when he was convicted (a foregone conclusion) his sentence would not be too harsh.

The Trial

The trial was reported in U.S. coastal cities and in England. Prior to its opening, U.S. newspapers promoted it as an experiment in moral philosophy and an exploration of human nature. "There will be many nice questions for settlement," the *New York Herald*'s correspondent in Philadelphia predicted. "Among others to be considered," the report continued, was "the determination of the law of self-preservation." This, newspapers promised, would be the issue of moral philosophy at the heart of the trial. Are humans selfless or selfish creatures? If the former, the drownings were an actionable moral wrong. But if humans are by nature selfish, reflexively driven to put their own lives first, then Holmes could not be prosecuted for "being human." More prosaically, the issue at law was a seaman's obligation to passengers: "whether they have a right to throw them [paying passengers] into the sea to save themselves or any others."

Holmes's lawyers, who never saw Messier's statement and did not know of its existence, argued two distinct but related defenses. First was the "law of necessity," one they insisted made blameless actions when they were the *only* actions possible to secure an individual's survival. This was akin to the principle of self-defense as a legal defense against the charge of murder. Second, they argued a defense of "human nature," insisting self-preservation was so deeply ingrained, so integral a part of the human psyche that a person cannot be faulted for acts of personal salvation even when they cost the lives of others. While unsuccessful—Holmes's conviction was a foregone conclusion—it is these arguments that have been cited in various cases over the last 180 years, including most recently the Canadian case *Regina v. Latimer* in 2001.

The maximum penalty under U.S. federal statute for manslaughter on the high seas was three years imprisonment and a fine of $1,000, a very significant sum for a seaman in 1842. But "in view of all the circumstances, and especially as the prisoner had been already confined in gaol several months," Holmes instead was sentenced by Mr. Justice Henry Baldwin to a fine of $20 and six months of hard labor in the Eastern Pennsylvania Penitentiary. The Seamen's Friend Society sought an appeal of Holmes's conviction as well as a presidential pardon. Neither was seriously considered.

The trial yielded the desired result. Captain Harris, who was asked no impolitic questions on the witness stand, was left with his reputation unimpeded and thus was free to command another ship. Captains were valuable commodities in the day and the loss of a captain direr than the loss of a ship's emigrant passengers. The first mate Francis Rhodes, conveniently at sea at the time of the trial and thus not available as a witness, was never censured and thus was free to serve on other ships, and perhaps, move up to a captaincy in time. The *William Brown*'s owners were free to collect from their insurers without worrying about compensation to the families of the drowned.

The trial's conclusion assured future immigrants that seamen did not have unilateral powers of life or death at sea. The head notes preceding the published report of *United States v. Holmes* gave the precedent officials on both sides of the Atlantic desired: "Seamen have no right, even in cases of extreme peril to their own lives, to sacrifice the lives of passengers for the sake of preserving their own."[2]

That safely obscured the important fact that nothing substantive changed. Ships were free to sail the great circle route at maximum speed in the spring of the year, guaranteeing some would sink without sufficient lifesaving craft to save their passengers. Ship owners were free to urge their captains to apply maximum speed in dangerous waters (maximizing ship usage as long as they survived) and first mates were left with no other responsibility than to heed a captain's command. Sailors were still beholden to their superior's orders, to be obeyed reflexively. They were put on notice, however, not to drown passengers when adrift in overloaded, leaking lifeboats. Order and the status quo were preserved.

The *Titanic*

The *William Brown* was remembered when other ships were sunk in collision with icebergs in the North Atlantic in the winter or early spring. In 1852 it was the *SS Arctic* and two years later the *City of Glasgow* went down with all hands, its demise so rapid that 480 passengers drowned en masse. In 1870 the *City of Boston* left Halifax in January of the year and was never heard from again, presumably wrecked and sunk with all hands and all passengers in the cold, iceberg-filled waters of the North Atlantic. Journalists recited all these and other ship names after the *Titanic* sank with horrendous loss of life in the spring of 1912. What the officials of the day lamented as a tragedy the newspapers described as one disaster too many. Everyone agreed something had to be done.

Commissions were struck and testimony was taken in both the United States and Great Britain to consider how something as dreadful as the death of a luxury ship ever could have occurred and how such disasters might be prevented. The answer was two-fold. First, all commercial ships were required by international agreement to carry a complement of lifeboats on board sufficient to ensure the safe placement of all passengers and crew in the event of a sinking. The repeated imbalance between supply (lifeboat seats) and demand (otherwise doomed passengers) that had resulted in thousands of deaths thus was eliminated.

Second, and no less significant, the North Atlantic sailing route was changed by international agreement during the critical months to keep ships out of the waters where icebergs were most frequently found in springtime. Bending the great circle route in this way added fewer than one hundred nautical miles to a trip of more than two thousand nautical miles from Liverpool to New York City. That added a little to all ships' sailing times but it kept them out of iceberg-filled waters. The result neither bankrupted ship owners nor forced huge increases in the cost of trade and travel on the North Atlantic. The new regulations did stop ships from colliding with icebergs and more generally prevented the drowning of passengers in maritime accidents when lifesaving craft were needed. Scarcity of these vessels disappeared and with it the metaphoric lifeboat dilemma it had created.

This is the problem with metaphor: "In allowing us to focus on one aspect of a concept, a metaphorical concept can keep us from focusing on other aspects of that concept that are inconsistent with that metaphor."[3] The story of the *William Brown* was constructed to argue the problem of ethics *in* the lifeboat as if its exigencies were natural and thus inevitable. Lifeboat ethics assumes the *only* question is who gets thrown overboard. It never asks whether anyone need be drowned at all.

The metaphor pretends to choice in that least democratic of environments: a commercial sailing ship in which the chain of command is clear and more or less absolute. The choice is the captain's, or in his absence, his designee's. He (or she) might choose to poll the passengers or the crew, but the responsibility is not theirs, not ever. And really, it matters little if the person in charge chooses an egalitarian lottery or the draconian murder of some for the good of the rest. The stark fact is that no good choices exist and some must die if any are to be saved. By the time lifeboat ethics is engaged all good solutions are gone. The "moral philosophy" that the situation was to engage was empty from the start of anything that might bear on the human condition, "human flourishing," or even simple justice.

With equal facility the metaphor of the lifeboat might be transposed from a story of irremediable scarcity into a cautionary tale about what happens when profits are put ahead of lives. In this ethics *of* the lifeboat the focus would be on the predicate acts whose consequence is the avoidable imposition of impossible choices. Sortal predicates are creatures of logic and philosophy, qualifying the resulting acts or elements that they modify.[4] In law, predicates acts are the "proximate cause" of consequential injuries that are the direct result of acts or events without which an event or injury would not have occurred.[5] The best-known application in U.S. law is in the U.S. Racketeer Influenced and Corrupt Organizations Act (RICO).[6]

It was precisely this type of thinking that neither U.S. nor British officials wished a jury to consider in 1842. If ships were likely to encounter icebergs in the North Atlantic in the spring of the year, then sailing at full speed at night was a predicate act directly leading to the sinking of the *William Brown* and the drowning of half its passengers. If company policy required captains to sail at all speed without respect to consequence, then the ship owners were responsible, their policies a proximate cause of the disaster. If ships frequently sank, as was clearly the case in the North Atlantic in the late winter and spring of the year, then the choice of route was, similarly, a predicate cause of any single ship's destruction. The owners were similarly responsible for failing to assure a sufficient number of lifesaving craft to protect all passengers, those who went down with the ship and later those in the leaky longboat. They might have argued "common practice" as a legal defense but that would only have shifted blame to those practices and the need for their alteration.

Similarly, blame for the longboat disaster necessarily should have accrued to the ship officers whose responsibility it was to assure the longboat and jollyboat were maintained in good order. Their failure was certainly a contributing cause of the lifeboat ethics' construction. Its rudder was defective and the boat leaked, together making its maintenance in rising seas difficult. If it had been in better shape it might not have wallowed so badly and Rhodes might have delayed the drowning of his passengers, all of whom might then have been saved by the *Crescent*'s arrival. In the metaphor of the lifeboat, however, none of this is considered. The lives of those passengers who went down with the ship because there was only the one longboat are irrelevant. The only concern is the choice made in the overloaded lifeboat. The whole of *United States v. Holmes* was thus a sleight of hand that slipped responsibility from the ship owners and officers to the seaman Holmes, obliged by maritime law to follow his superior's orders.

Bioethics and the Lifeboat

Bioethicists are very fond of lifeboat ethics and its assumption that some must be sacrificed that others may survive because there is not enough for all. They rarely ask "what ought we to do?" to avoid such disasters in the future. Their only question is "who do we sacrifice?" when artificial scarcities reign. A 2009 paper by Persad, Wertheimer, and Emmanuel in the *Lancet* presented, for example, a set of "principles of allocation of scarce medical interventions."[7] Their answer to the "persistent ethical challenge" of scarcity, after Callahan, "prioritizes younger people who have not yet lived a complete life." With Callahan and Lamm, Persal and his coauthors assume those to be thrown overboard from the medical lifeboat of care should include the old and infirm so the young and strong can be continued. It is called by some the "fair innings" argument and assumes we all have so many innings coming to us and any more than that is gravy. The young have yet to be given their time at bat and fairness thus demands the primacy of their care. How young is young, how many innings are "fair," as Daniel Callahan discovered, is a matter of perspective.

Norman Daniels talks about "society's normal opportunity range," generally dismissing care of those who fall outside it (those with chronic impairments, for example), as just and natural.[8] Here the ageist Lamm-Callahan argument becomes a more general thesis in which all those with what appear to be limiting characteristics are to be pitied, perhaps, but not helped. Just as ageism, defined in 1975 by Butler, permitted younger people to see the elderly as different and thus perhaps less worthy, now *all* persons of difference could be stereotyped as distinct and less worthy of care.[9] The argument expands the ageist argument to all who may have needs that society can choose not to meet because the basis of that need is not "normal." It is not that Daniels would not care for others if there were sufficient resources but because he assumes there are not—that scarcity reigns—then only those who exist within this normal range (those who, not coincidentally, are presumably most "productive") are entitled to society's caring concern.

Scarcity Unbound

All this makes of scarcity a "tragic discourse," in which intransigent natural and thus inevitable limits make hard choices and the attendant sacrifice of some unavoidable.[10] To transpose the metaphor to medical ethics it is only necessary to make doctors and nurses analogous to the lifeboat's crew, patients analogous to the ship's passengers. Bioethicists become, in effect, the apologists who argue the case for ship owners and the prosecutors, crafting their arguments within the lifeboat's confines. In this argument from scarcity they, like those engaged in the trial of Holmes, make a critical error: Scarcity is rarely natural. For every unforeseen and unexpected disaster, every *Essex* with its bull-headed whale, there are thousands of predictable, avoidable disasters like that of the *William Brown*. In the realm of human affairs limits are rarely immutable givens but instead the predictable consequence of economic choices and political decisions made with full knowledge of the dire consequences that inevitably will result.

The argument from scarcity serves primarily as an excuse for the failure to provide necessary resources. The dilemmas that result are real and exigent but not inevitable or intransigent. As David Harvey argued in the 1970s, "It is often erroneously accepted that scarcity is something inherent in nature, when its definition is inextricably social and cultural in orientation."[11] Whether the subject is medical service or petroleum reserves scarcity is, except in the very short term, typically a self-consciously created, avoidable result that is not inevitable even if, in economics, it is a necessity required for pricing mechanisms to function.[12]

To insist otherwise is not only bad ethics (putting blame where it doesn't belong) and worse philosophy (a misapprehension of the nature of the world we inhabit) but also demonstrably wrongheaded. After all, ships still sail the North Atlantic. They avoid by general agreement the iceberg-filled waters of late winter and spring, sailing a nautical degree lower than the great circle route. If by happenstance they are wrecked, all carry sufficient lifesaving boats to assure survival until someone can rescue the survivors. To do otherwise today is simply to participate in what all would acknowledge as unethical, actionable, criminal behavior. In this way the problem of ethics *in* the lifeboat disappeared after the *Titanic* when an ethics *of* the lifeboat and its predicate causes was instituted.

That shift in ethical focus, and the subsequent relief of scarcity, is not rare. Remember the problem dialysis presented in the early 1960s when *Life Magazine* reporter Shana Alexander was observing the deliberations of Seattle's God Committee. Here was a new lifeboat in which some had to die because scarcity ruled. There was no avoiding the necessity of choosing a few from among the many who needed treatment to survive. After some years of debate, however, the U.S. Congress changed the equation in 1972, voting to fund dialysis treatment for all those in need irrespective of their financial standing or social position. Scarcity disappeared as a result.

Some worried about the cost of such an entitlement just as nineteenth-century ship owners worried about the cost of providing lifeboats aboard their ships. The nation, they said, could not afford this new entitlement. In debate over the bill, however, Indiana Senator Vance Hartke told his colleagues that a nation able to afford billions of dollars annually on cosmetics and deodorants could "set our national priorities through a national effort to bring kidney disease treatment within reach of all those in need."[13] Senator Hartke remembered, as did others in Congress, the short-term failure of supply that occurred in the early years of the 1951–1953 poliomyelitis pandemic. The iron lung had been invented, it would save lives, but it was not immediately available. In the interim, gymnasiums of patients in respiratory failure were kept alive by nursing and medical students who hand ventilated patients while they waited for the life-saving iron lungs.[14] The rapid production and deployment of these machines was an expensive task most industrialized nations (Canada, Denmark, Holland, Sweden, the United States, and so on) reflexively chose to meet. In the United States their national distribution was assisted by members of the U.S. Army Medical Corps where needed (see figure 4.5).

To argue an ethics *of* the lifeboat is to insist the right-hand side of scarcity's equation is not an inflexible limit. That supply is not

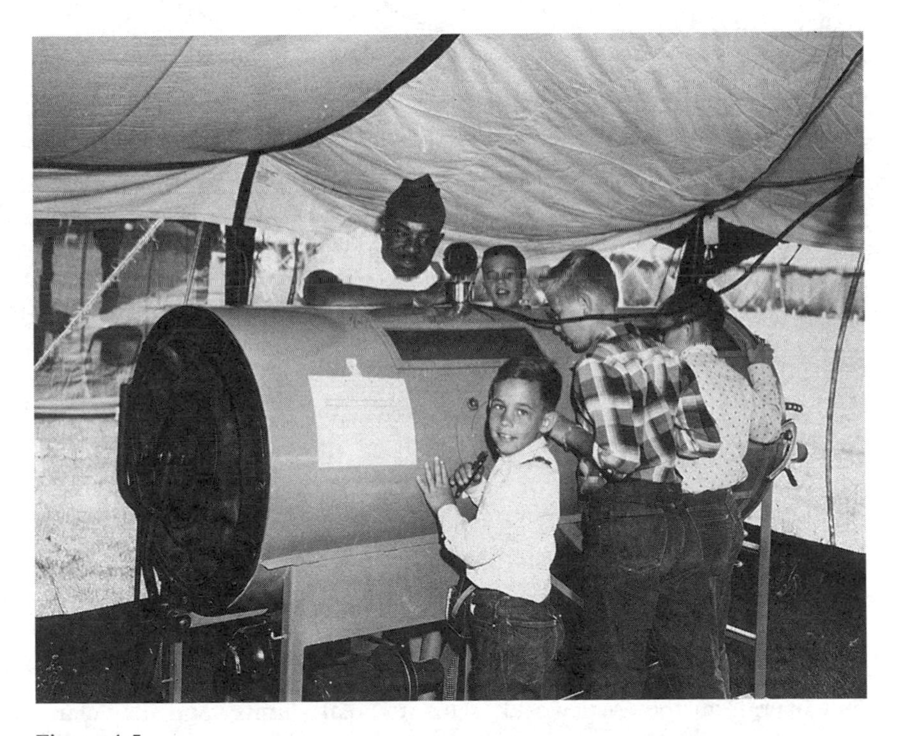

Figure 4.5
U.S. Army Sgt. Clarence Stewart demonstrates the use of an iron lung on Armed Forces Day in Denver, Colorado, in 1960. *Source*: Courtesy NLM: A01503.

necessarily an unchanging limit—instead it responds to our efforts—is the continuing lesson of the Malthusian threat that has never materialized. In history's eye we see this idea in the medicine of eighteenth-century physicians like Benjamin Rush and colleagues like Noah Webster who insisted that to fulfill their Hippocratic oath physicians must address the determinants of disease and not only treat those sickened when an epidemic struck. Some therefore joined the legislature and others local health boards to argue not only for preventive measures, like urban sanitation, but also more generally for the care of the ill irrespective of their economic or social status. Here, too, we see the medical ethics of nineteenth-century physicians like John Snow and Rudolph Virchow, and nurses like Florence Nightingale, who in different countries and facing different epidemics argued the antecedent causes of disease as the necessary focus of medicine's ethical duty.

Rebalanced Equations

Were bioethicists concerned with an ethics *of* the lifeboat, then bioethics might indeed be about what Brody called, in chapter 1's citation, "speaking truth to power." That focus would certainly expand the "moral space," and its attendant dialogue Andre proposed as the operational theater of the ethicist-philosopher. From bioethics' inception, however, bioethicists treated resource scarcities as a natural inevitability rather than the result of prior choices whose results were horrendous and anything but inevitable.[15] This failure of vision has, in a real sense, defined the bioethical role. The bioethicist is the triage specialist whose training in philosophy, but not typically in either economics or medicine, somehow allows him or her to assert, in the lifeboat of medical decision making, the criteria by which the protocols of noncare are to be arranged. As professionals they have a stake in the problem and none in its structural solution.

Bioethicists do not necessarily defend the status quo that gives us recurrent lifeboat dilemmas. Rather, they say (or at least have said to me) they operate in the "real world" with its "real" limits" and they claim my argument while perhaps in theory interesting is "impractical" in its application. They may be unhappy with the choices they help others make but there are, after all, only two ventilators and three patients who require ventilation to live. All this makes of bioethics a kind of short-term risk management science whose experts are uninterested in the nature of the problems they confront, only in their piecemeal confrontation. That response fails twice over.

First, assuming it impractical to identify and then fight to eliminate the proximate causes of lifeboat making, and the consequential necessity of life taking, is to insist what is obviously changeable is somehow immutable. This is the modern equivalent of the nineteenth-century ship owners' argument that changing the route of sailing ships in the North Atlantic was unworldly and that requiring all commercial ships have a sufficient complement of lifeboats both impractical and unreasonable. It is to say, with those who opposed physicians like Benjamin Rush, that urban sanitation and public sewer lines are too costly for the state to provide. That the result of doing nothing is typhoid fever and yellow fever is just the way it is. It is to agree retrospectively with those who argued, as did some of Senator Hartke's congressional opponents in the 1970s, that a federal entitlement for kidney patients requiring dialysis would be the ruination of the nation's economy.

Second, some bioethicists have argued to me they have no brief to consider the context of a lifeboat dilemma, only the dilemma itself. And within the confine of their job descriptions this may be true. But as ethicists their charge is to consider the appropriateness of actions through a method of analysis that is grounded in a philosophy that carefully considers not what is expedient or politically acceptable but instead what is right and good. In their failure to consider the structural cause of the problems they attempt to address they become mere apologists for the status quo—public relations consultants brought out to justify avoidable inequities.

Justice? In the lifeboat there will be no justice whether the charge is against an Alexander William Holmes (manslaughter on the high seas), a Frances Rhodes (incompetence, murder, whatever), or a John Messier (mutiny, insubordination, etc.). Any decision is bad because, simply, there are no good choices in an indefensible situation, only some that may appear worse, in retrospect, than others. If it is to be more than just an empty word, justice and the ethic that promotes it demand consideration of antecedent conditions; fairness requires a broader definition than exigent but avoidable necessity.

The failure is even more severe when we remember philosopher-ethicists are citizens first and professionals second. As Hippocrates knew, we all ply our trades within a community that sanctions our efforts and assigns us duties as both citizens and as experts. It is not enough, we learned at Nuremberg, to say, "That's the way it was," "those were my orders," or "I didn't know anything else." As citizens we are obliged to knowledge and to combat the violations of ethical conduct when they appear in our communities. For ethicist-philosophers presumably schooled in clear analytic thinking the duty is or should be even greater. And really, what is the good of an ethics that never asks what we ought to do to prevent disaster and sees as entire the pragmatics of triage in disastrous but avoidable situations? Why embrace an ethic that stops where the real work would presumably begin?

Scarcity Redux

In the previous chapter I argued that implicit in the scarcity that bioethicists have assumed is natural lies a Malthusian fallacy that can and should be challenged. Supply may indeed increase as fast as or faster than demand. In this same line of thinking an ethics *of* the lifeboat assumes the question of short-term cost is not the correct metric to apply to problems of resource scarcity. If a necessary, lifesaving system's expense seems insupportable the problem lies not in the number of persons who need that service but rather the system of thinking that restricts the equation's left-hand side—demand—without attention to the potential flexibility of the right-hand side—supply. Consider, for example, the assumption of scarcity in health resources in the United States. The U.S. healthcare system is certainly expensive and at present fails to cover more than 46 million citizens, those left out of the lifeboat of healthcare. The U.S. system of healthcare provision is widely recognized as the most expensive (at least in relation to gross domestic production [GDP]), least efficient, least equitable healthcare system among all the industrialized nations of the world. It is the national program without universal care even though its patchworked entitlements—Medicare and Medicaid, veteran affairs—cover a substantial portion of the population.

The problem of scarcity in U.S. healthcare is not the inevitable result of a plethora of new and expensive technologies that have saved lives we must, perhaps regrettably, triage away. Rather, at least in part it results at a structural level from a private, for-profit delivery system that builds profit seeking into the system at every stage, creating levels of onerous expense that would be unacceptable anywhere else. Since 1968, for example, Canada has spent a third less per capita than the United States on the health of its citizens without leaving—as the United States does at this writing—millions of citizens without comprehensive healthcare coverage. A principle source of this disparity is the "bloated overhead and bureaucracy among U.S. insurance companies and government" that in 2009 cost the U.S. healthcare system approximately $1 trillion dollars annually.[16]

Nor can one legitimately argue, as do many, that the costs of medical care and its new technologies have increased necessarily in real terms as a percentage of the GNP. At least in Canada, where private insurers are a relatively minor part of the healthcare equation, there has been a remarkable stability in the relation between health costs and the national income.[17] The exception occurred in years of severe recession, for example 1991–1992, where employment and production and therefore national revenues diminished while health costs did not. The short-term imbalance was rectified, however, when the recession ended. If healthcare is a priority and the method of its organization a root cause of costly inefficiency, then ethically and logically ("rationally," the bioethicist might say) the argument is for structural change. Certainly one cannot in good faith insist that resulting dilemmas of scarcity are necessary and inevitable. One can only say they are so in the system of health economics we have created.

Ignored in bioethics' ethics of scarcity are myriad ways to structure a U.S healthcare system to reduce costs and increase efficiency. Should one choose not to embrace any of those alternatives, then government revenues can be increased through programs of personal and corporate taxation. At least since the birth of "Reaganomics" in the 1970s, however, it has been a tenet of neoliberal faith that lower taxes inevitably are better. It may be that one cannot avoid the healthcare (or education, or infrastructure, etc.) lifeboat if the tax base is reduced to ensure the increase in corporate and personal wealth. But the preservation of rich corporations and individuals at the expense of the fragile is not a necessity but a choice, one that creates the problems bioethicists argue can best be resolved only with their expertise.

A Kantian Perspective

The issues of ethics that arise in this context are problems, as Harvard anthropologist and physician Paul Farmer argues, with Nicole Campos, of social structure and personal and social agency.[18] These structures are not natural in the sense that a people's geography is natural (you live by the sea, you live on a mountain) but instead are cultural responses that are by definition mutable. We can, as citizens or as experts (anthropologists, ethicists, physicians, and so on) consider the method by which social institutions and programs are structurally enabling or inhibiting, ethical or unethical, beneficial or problematic, defining them as enabling or inhibiting, as beneficial or problematic. One may debate their wisdom or villainy. What we can *not* do in good faith is ignore them or pretend they are inevitable and somehow, natural. Agency and its inaction occur within the social structures we create, not outside them. It is there the ethicist must focus if he or she is to be worthy of our trust.

Given the ways Immanuel Kant's works have been read, or more properly misread, by many ethicist-philosophers, it is tempting to suspect the source of bioethics' failures lies in the arena of Kant's philosophical writings. After all, it is the philosophical method he represents, and the broad paradigm he created, that lie at the philosophical heart of most bioethics today. Were this not true then the bioethicists' training in philosophy would be of little import and the reason for their consultation would disappear. By this reading, Kant is a good place to look for a rationale for the intransigent refusal of many—if not most—bioethicists to consider predicate causes and the logical consequences of their arguments from the standpoint of scarcity.

In his *Foundations of the Metaphysics of Morals*, Kant distinguished from the start what he called "practical anthropology" from the conceptual and moral imagining that was his principal subject.[19] His goal was not the consideration of practical dilemmas but the crafting of an argument about the nature of individual moral freedom, in which he proposed the autonomy of the rational individual reigned supreme. Will and its enabling reason were posited as distinct from the concrete cause-and-effect world and its clear chain of "if this, then that" events. Kant self-consciously avoided, in the main, the consideration of choices in a complex, problematic world. His subject was man as a being *with* choice, not the nitty-gritty *of* choices arising from social problems resulting from governmental policies. Kant thus largely set to the side the concrete and practical in his struggle to create an abstract metaphysic. His was a frame around which choice was enabled, not typically the practical choices that are made. "The problem of Kant's criterion of rationality," writes Charles Taylor, "is that it has purchased radical autonomy at the price of [practical] emptiness."[20]

It is empty because it is about rationality as a quality rather than its application to complex daily problems, or the emotions that often necessarily attend to their worldly consideration. Kant's question was not "what should I do?" or "what policy is better?" but "how do I define us, and the nature of choice?" The result was vacuous because it was a shell others might fill with the practical and political and social realities within which things like medicine are practiced *between* people. Taylor is one in a long line of critics who have seen this as a problem. As Peter Singer notes, in *Philosophy of Right* Hegel wrote that Kantian "theory can yield only the bare, universal form of the moral law; it cannot tell us what our specific duties are."[21]

This is not to suggest that Kant denied politics or practical matters. It is to say that at least in his *Critique of Practical Reason* and his *Groundwork of the Metaphysic of Morals* he did not focus on them. Still, he is relevant. Because he believed in humanity and the dignity of species members we can suppose he would have opposed political and social structures that systematically denied care to people on the basis of general economic advance. He certainly would have criticized programs whose inevitable result was the death of hundreds or thousands. The failure to consider predicate decisions favoring productive ends and profit over human lives is, he might have said, the false redefinition of *Homo sapiens* as a protected species, its members worthy of care, into individually dispensable members of *homo economicus*.

The assumption that because scarcity is profitable and entrenched it must be maintained reduces us all to ciphers whose right to existence is contingent upon this or that corporate or governmental balance sheet.

That assumption Kant would have despised utterly as the provenance of what he famously called a Kingdom of Means. In a "systematic union of different rational beings under common laws," Kant wrote in his *Groundwork*, "Each of them should treat himself and all others, never merely as a means, but always at the same time as an end in himself."[22]

In arguing the efficient sacrifice of those who might otherwise be helped on the grounds of alterable scarcity, bioethics promotes a Kingdom of (economic) Means over Kant's humanist Kingdom of Ends. In so doing it rejects the humanity of all that Kant, like Rousseau and most others, perceived as the essential good.[23] From this belief followed the importance of each rational being. It is in the sense of human good as a good that the Hippocratic injunction to care and not to harm can be read as a defining ethical imperative. It redefines medicine's goals, and those of the science in which it practices, as merely economic. By ignoring the ethical importance of structural causes of remediable scarcity (the rare case of the *Essex* aside) bioethics promotes as necessary a reality in which few choices are freely available and fewer are good. Kant, I suspect, would have opposed the result with every fiber of his being.

5

Biopolitics, Biophilosophies, and Bioethics

The oft-repeated phrase "politics is applied ethics" at once implies way too much and yet not near enough.[1] Politics is the dress that philosophy wears when it seeks to be seen as useful, its subject something that is practical and real, and thus important. Philosophy is the dress that politics wears to insist upon its truth and the rectitude of its programs. The two are like a reversible coat of two colors. Philosophy is the general form within which ideas of "good" and "bad," "right" and "wrong" are located as ethics. Politics is the manner in which the ethic of those ideas is enacted—"applied"—to critique the acts of some and justify those of others. There is almost always a political bias to philosophy's applicable order, a philosophical scent to the political odor.

"Societies, in order to endure, have to go on believing in themselves, in their vision of well-being, and imaging of the future [and thus of their past]. They have to pretend to be moral."[2] Philosophy and politics share the burden of defining and enacting the morals with which societies promote that self-belief. "Pretend" is perhaps too strong, a verb suggesting a self-conscious duplicity that masquerades as morality. It may be more a matter of naiveté; of assuming a morality that is real, distinct, and value-free (as if there were such a thing) that could be discovered and pronounced rather than self-consciously constructed and then carefully promoted as not only real but also "natural" and thus necessarily correct.

When Oliver Wendell Holmes rendered his opinion in *Buck v. Bell* he was articulating a political and social philosophy, a set of values that could be enacted legally. In doing so he argued an ethic that diminished the rights of the individual in favor of the future economies of the state.

When Senator Vance Hartke argued in the U.S. Congress for dialysis as a national entitlement he advanced an ethic of care in which the needs of the fragile citizen took precedence over the potential cost of that care. Philosophically this advanced a belief in the inherent worth of the individual, even (and perhaps especially) those fragile and unable to serve the nation productively. Those who contested with Hartke did not dispute the ethical importance of the individual. Instead they argued the primacy of the cost of their care to the future balance sheet of the state. Implicit in this argument was the assumption that future economic well-being was a good distinct from and more important than the welfare of individual citizens.

Daniel Callahan argued that rapid acceptance of bioethics resulted because it "dovetailed very nicely with the reigning political liberalism of the educated classes in America."[3] It was not liberalism's focus on the worth of the individual, however, but neoliberalism's cost accountancies that dovetailed so nicely. The willingness to assume scarcity as a natural limit and economic projections as the assessor of care decisions was what earned bioethics a place at the table. Ethicists-cum-philosophers like Callahan, for example, denied the primacy of personal choice on the basis of the state's future economic needs. The patient who was elderly, or by extension simply fragile, was a burdensome expense and thus could be abandoned—whatever he or she might wish—in the name of state economic futures.

It did not have to be this way. Early philosopher-cum-medical ethicists might have insisted upon the liberal importance of the individual irrespective of his or her age or characteristics. They might have argued with Senator Hartke the moral primacy of the individual citizen over the economic projections of state officials. Had they done this, then the logical conclusion would have been an advocacy for the fragile individual at all levels of concern. As analytic thinkers, moral philosopher-cum-ethicists at least might have parsed the idea of intransigent limit rather than embrace it as a naturally restricting truth. Instead, most comfortably accepted the general framework of Callahan's argument from scarcity, and his promotion of cost accountancies as the metric of ethical choice. The result denied in all but name the liberal promotion of the person and his or her freedom to choose.

In this way, I argue, bioethics gave up the ethical game from the start.

Biopower

Strangely, at least to me, bioethics is typically presented as if politics, political systems and their economic manifestations are wholly irrelevant to the ethical and moral consideration of medical practice and research. It may be that the analytic methodology bioethicists advance as their own is conducive to a logic that is not simply supportive of but also conducive, in application, to this perspective. Yes, the philosophical tradition on which bioethics is built emphasizes the rational individual. And, yes, bioethics has promoted itself as a champion of the liberal ideal of freedom and choice. But what we learn from the history of philosophy is the distance separating the conceptual framework from the messy practicalities of practical interpretation and social implementation. The divide between theories—in Kant, in Hegel, in Marx—and application is vast. Bioethics focused the "murderous splendor" of an economic divisor for ethical divisions in a way that assured that, in practice, individual choice would matter less than general necessity. In rejecting as inadequate the traditional ethics of medicine bioethics abandoned a primary, practical commitment to the person in need.

Consider the history of the noun. Bioethics conjures a very Foucauldian sense of modern agency, of the politics and technologies that together create a biopower "that takes as its object life itself, the life of the human qua living being, that is, the life of the human insofar as it is a living being."[4] It is not that those lives are perceived as sacred or even equally precious, however, but instead that they are equally countable. Each is a cipher within a scientific and political order grounded in a system of official categorization. The importance and reality of those lives is determined not by individual worth, or relations (doctor-patient, sovereign-subject, parent-child), but more coarsely within a "biopolitic" of measurement (costs of care, rates of birth to deaths, rates of reproduction) that has nothing to do with the particular person and everything to do with systems of general assessment. In a fundamental sense the biopolitics of biopower is about administering societies in which the individual is anonymous and irrelevant except as an entry in the ledger of public accounts. "A power whose task is to take charge of life needs continuous regulatory mechanisms," wrote Foucault. "Such a power has to qualify, measure, appraise, and hierachize, rather than display itself in its murderous splendor. A normalizing society is the historical outcome of a technology of power centered on life."[5]

There is no indication that Foucault was reading the early bioethicists or that he had their works in mind while he and they were writing simultaneously from very different perspectives. Nor is there any hint that bioethicists in the 1970s or 1980s were very aware of Foucault and his works. But in both the politics of Foucault and the working of bioethicists what was at stake was the definition and valuation of human life either as a specifically valuable good, and thus the value of the individual person, or as simply an accountable cipher in a broadly bureaucratic context. Through its embrace of scarcity as a natural limit, and of economic projections as a basis for care decisions, bioethics created the context of Foucault's "murderous splendor" whose effect is to assume the inevitability of the lifeboat, marginalizing some and wholly disavowing others. In this way the best liberal sentiments of protected humans with choices was denied from the start.

Bioethics: The Eugenic Noun

It was Van Rensselaer Potter, a research oncologist at the University of Michigan, who coined the noun "bioethics" to describe the ethical focus of those who would help humankind to a self-conscious "participation in the processes of biological and cultural evolution."[6] "Bio" was to signify the biological system of the species and "ethics" the value systems that would fashion a vision of self-directed evolution for the eventual betterment of future humankind. Participation in the processes of evolution quickly came to mean embracing mechanisms of the species' biological self-direction. It has never meant (although it might have) either a close ethical engagement with the cultural and social determinants of health and disease or the needs of the individually fragile.

From the start bioethics was thus linked conceptually to Sir Francis Galton's nineteenth-century eugenic program whose focus was also the self-directed evolution of humankind in service of a more homogenous and productive future. This perspective lives today in the bioethics of those like British philosopher and ethicist John Harris, who makes "the ethical case for making better people" in a bioethics not of the individual in his or her need but the species at large as a focus.[7] Implicit in both

Galton's argument and this bioethic is the assumption that human defects can be precisely identified and then weeded out over time, person by person, to promote a homogenous population of healthy, productive, socially adjusted future workers. The specifics of contemporary eugenic bioethics are considered in chapter 8. Here the general relationship between the ideal of genetic improvement and the development of bioethics is briefly reviewed.

Evolution and Eugenics

Galton was captured by the Darwinian idea of evolution as a simple function of hereditary selection. The simplistic notion of the "survival of the fittest" fit well into an economic perspective in which "the best" would survive the reproductive battle and those who were not would wither and disappear. That the precise mechanics of this process of selection and transformation were obscure made no difference to Galton or his successors. The promise was the reality and that was enough. This kind of biopower-cum-bioethic fit nicely into the agenda of the industrializing nineteenth-century state in which people were classified as either productive workers or economic burdens. The goal of biological science was to be the fashioning of the former and the elimination of the latter.[8] The result was the eugenics of the early twentieth century.

Van Rensselaer Potter's bioethics built self-consciously upon Julian Huxley's 1942 reformation of Darwin (and Galton) in Huxley's *Evolution: The Modern Synthesis*. Huxley took the basics of Darwin's pioneering ideas, and the work that followed upon them, to create what admirers of the day called "the great generalization" of evolutionary biological theory.[9] In the 1970s, Potter advanced this simplistic Darwinian perspective, believing that then-emerging genetics would permit the eugenic dream of a self-directed species future. This was the time of the first real imagining of DNA and RNA as the carriers of inheritance and the things that make us biologically human (and of course, make chimpanzees chimpanzees, sparrows sparrows, and so on). If we could only understand genetics at this fundamental level then we humans at last would have the tools to create a future "us" whose members would be if not perfect perhaps perfectible. From this perspective early twentieth-century eugenics was not ethically wanting or morally distasteful. It was simply that the old science had been inadequate while the new science of DNA was (or soon would be) capable of fulfilling the old eugenic dream.

Looking back the whole was incredibly naive. It assumed a mechanistic model in which genes were assumed to produce instrumental characteristics that would wholly describe the resulting person.[10] Weeding out bad genes would remove defective persons, and thus undesirable characteristics in the citizenry, thereby permitting a society of better people to emerge. Today we know the relationship between these constituents is far more complex. Simply, "There are no genetic factors that can be studied independently of the environment" whose structure is dependent, in turn, on human action and agency.[11]

The complex of characteristics that together make up the individual—coordination, height, I.Q., weight, and so on, are the result of complex, toxicogenomic, gene-environment interactions.[12] Genes are the overture, not the symphony, a statement of general themes modified across the movements of the individual life. Noninherited influences on gene expression are called epigenetics,[13] whose complexities make hash of the old determinist genetics that early bioethicists believed would be the mechanism powering the simple, eugenic reformation of humankind.

To say past visions were simplistic is not to say they were not compelling. Andre Hellegers latched onto Potter's noun when asked in 1971 to head a new institute being created at Georgetown University, the Joseph and Rose Kennedy Institute for the Study of Human Reproduction and Bioethics. In putting bioethics in the institute's name Hellegers, a physician, assured the noun would be transformed into a verb describing an active process of ethical control, in applying a value system to human reproductive biology. At the Kennedy Institute and elsewhere "the study of human reproduction" implicitly if not explicitly was to be directed toward the development and assessment of clinical mechanisms in service of programs that would weed out undesirables and promote desirable persons in future generations.

At stake was the old philosophical ideal (Rousseau, Kant, Hegel, etc.) of humankind as a protected entity whose members deserve equal consideration, protection, and treatment irrespective of their individual attributes, characteristics, or social performance. This was as well the virtuous good underlying the old ethics of medicine in which each patient deserved care. Bioethics promised instead a biopower whose eugenic view was general rather than specific, one of a future species whose members had been selected if not eventually designed to conform to a homogenous template of acceptable characteristics. In such a program the individual never stands as critical, only the general good of programmatic change is important. By its name, in this read, bioethics gave up the promise of individual care and concern from the start.

Bioethical Assessors

In the 1970s bioethics' philosophical progenitors developed a set of characteristics defining both the role of the bioethicist and a specifically bioethical perspective. The ethicist might be a physician but medical training would not be a necessary element of his or her expertise. He or she might be a legalist but those engaged in this new ethics would not need to be well versed in the law. Nor would bioethicists require training in economics even though from the very start economic assumptions were an engine propelling bioethical agendas. Rather, the bioethicist was to be a philosophically trained expert adept in *valuation*, in defining worth and worthiness across the sciences that were the biology of humans in their frailties and strengths. This assumed the analytic approach of the philosopher would serve to answer the practical problems of medicine. "The focus of bioethics is not on moral activity or praxis in a broad sense," writes Bruce Jennings. "The moral agent envisioned by liberal bioethicists is a weigher of options, a balancer of conflicting values and interests . . . from outside the community within which the decisions are made and from outside the practices of decision making themselves."[14]

The Hastings Center

The philosopher-ethicist thus was to be an outsider: not a "guest in the house of medicine," as Mark Kuczewski argued in an earlier quotation, but rather like the realtor who comes to the house to gauge its worth. To accept the bioethical adjudicator one had to accept the moral folk theory introduced in chapter 1, and with it the premise that practical problems can be resolved through a specific analytic approach based on disinterested, dispassionate reason that ignores the complexities (emotional and practical) of contested events. Without that premise, bioethicists were just interested amateurs, pretenders in a world where they had no standing.

The argument for bioethics and its philosophically grounded approach needed a center from which it could be promoted. In 1969 the Hastings Center was created under the leadership of Daniel Callahan as an "independent, nonpartisan, and nonprofit bioethics research institute." Its mission was and remains, its website states, "to address fundamental ethical issues in the areas of health, medicine, and the environment as they affect individuals, communities, and societies." This was not a research institute that developed new medicines, new surgeries, or new approaches to them. Its first director and guiding force was not a biologist, economist, geneticist, or a physician, but a philosopher. The Hastings Center's members were and in the main remain academics steeped, like Callahan, in the philosophic traditions of Hegel, Heidegger, Kant, Mill, and so on. The center's raison d'être was valuation. The *Hastings Center Report*, first published in 1971, was to be the premier venue in which bioethicists argued their institutionally grounded, philosophically erudite points of view. It would be the model for a range of journals that proliferated as the demi-discipline grew.

Here we have one of those debates that academics so adore. In 2007 Baker and McCullough argued that the critical framework of bioethical practice was based upon the "appropriation" of Kantian philosophical methods and perspectives, which were then applied to issues of practice.[15] It was this insistence on a philosophical high ground that gave bioethics its legitimacy. Tom Beauchamp, a coauthor of *Principles of Bioethics*, and earlier, a principal author of *The Belmont Report*, dismissed this argument as at best out of date if not simply inaccurate.[16] It was not that Kantian wisdom did not have a continuing currency in bioethics, Beauchamp wrote, but that it did not and had never dominated the ethical framework of the field.

The scholar's question is whether medical ethicists "apply" Kantian methods and principles or merely "appropriate" snippets, "theory fragments," to create arguments with a veneer of philosophical insight.[17] Beauchamp insisted that if bioethics was ever about deducing the answers to contemporary problems through the close study of Kant's high philosophy, well . . . that went out with tie-dyed shirts.[18] In this he is correct. So, too, however, are Baker and McCullough. A sense of Kantian principle and method in relation to problems of medical practice and research is enunciated again and again in the bioethics literature. References to

Kant, especially his *Groundwork for the Metaphysics of Moral* but also his *Critique of Practical Reason*, are de rigueur constants in the books and journals that defined bioethics in its formative years. Even today, no university program in bioethics is complete without lectures, and usually whole courses, on Kant and the continuing relevance of his works to biomedical research and medical practice. How could it be otherwise? Bereft of any specific, practical knowledge relevant to medical dilemmas, it was only an expertise in the philosophical tradition and method Kant symbolizes that gave bioethics its sole set of credentials.

Raising Kant's banner, and that of philosophy generally, gave to bioethics a general veneer of historical power and the appearance of analytic rigor. The problem was, however, that asserting the methods of analytic moral philosophy as a basis for practical valuation crossed a firm line between the theoretical and practical in Kant's writings. As Hegel and other critics have continually pointed out, Kant never applied himself to the pedestrian problem. "This is not because Kant himself lacked interest in such practical questions," writes Peter Singer, "but because his entire theory insists that morality must be based on pure practical reasoning, free from any particular motives."[19] Kantian theory sketched broad parameters, never detailing the landscape of specific duties or responsibilities. Put another way, Kant was about the high and mighty and from this perspective remained necessarily distant from low-down, messy, practical realities.

But the issues that bioethics sought to address were messy and complex. One may talk about a society of the good, and if that good is defined economically then all valuations will take on the assumptions of the economic system of the day. Similarly, the ethicists may argue with Kant, the supremacy and sanctity of the individual person with the freedom to choose. But in the lifeboat—where some must die that others may live—that choice becomes devalued where not meaningless.

Almost from the start, bioethics opposed in practice, if not in theory, the older medical ethic whose moral center was the preservation of the individual patient irrespective of social cost. It did this not because the person was irrelevant but in the neoliberal economics of the day was too expensive. This, as we have seen, was inimical to the values of the older medical ethic in which care irrespective of cost was a priority. Callahan was right when he argued that society could not trust physicians to allocate medical resources in the care of patients because his concern was cost and their concern was care. The two ethics, one traditional and the other neoliberal, could not easily coexist. As it developed, the older ethic's ideal of individual care and social concern first was diluted and later generally ignored in service of a neoliberal accountancy in which the cost of care was the illness to be addressed.

Research: Subjects and Objects

The first institutional test of bioethics came in 1974 when the U.S. Congress created The National Commission for the Protection of Human Subjects of Biomedical and Behavioral Research.[20] Its task was to identify "basic ethical principles that should underlie the conduct of biomedical and behavioral research involving human subjects and to develop guidelines which should be followed to assure that such research is conducted in accordance with those principles."[21] The result would be a document called *The Belmont Report*.

It is easy to forget at this remove why Congress perceived a need for an official committee to review what was in fact old, familiar ground. As we have seen, Osler worried about this very subject—and the effect of research protocols on patient-physician relationships—in 1907. Throughout the twentieth century, U.S. politicians repeatedly proposed state or federal legislation to protect human subjects in research only to be beaten back each time by researchers who warned that regulations focusing on subject protection would impede the progress of the medical research industry. Like the nineteenth-century ship owners who argued successfully against changes to maritime procedures in the North Atlantic, twentieth-century medical researchers insisted that added costs for research subjects would be their financial undoing. But as happened in the nineteenth century in the North Atlantic, incidents occurred with sufficient frequency to represent an independent peril to business as usual.

The Problem

The question of human exploitation in the name of advancing medical knowledge was a critical concern—public and professional—following

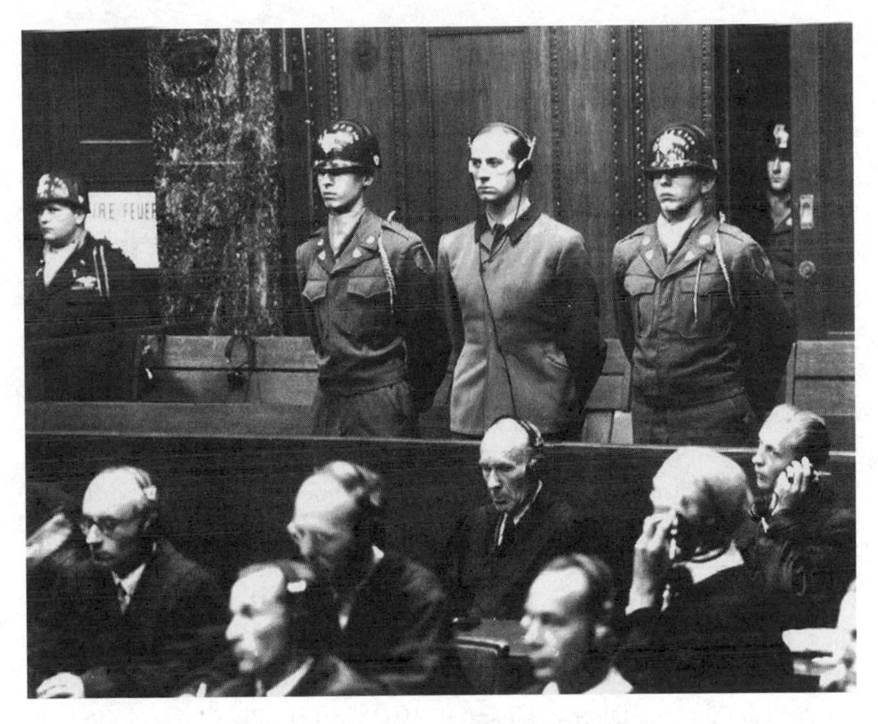

Figure 5.1
This famous photograph was taken in the Nuremberg courtroom. Standing flanked by two guards is Adolph Hitler's personal physician, Dr. Karl Brandt.

reports of Nazi physicians' experimentation on forced human subjects in Germany in World War II (see figure 5.1). The world was repulsed and the actions condemned in the Nuremberg Trials that generally condemned the advancement of knowledge over human safety and need. But in the 1960s, with the lessons of Nuremberg still fresh, a series of well-publicized reports described a pattern of patient exploitation and injury by U.S. researchers who argued the needs of science trumped those of the fragile. The National Commission was founded to address this problem in a manner that would facilitate rather than jeopardize the burgeoning and profitable industry of medical experimentation.

A 1960s court case considered the practice of New York physician Clarence Southam, who beginning in the 1950s routinely injected HeLa cervical cancer cells—named after the woman from whom they first were harvested without permission, Henrietta Lacks—into the arms of (mostly poor) patients to see if they would develop tumors at the injection site.

The chief of virology at Sloan-Kettering's Memorial Hospital, Southam later "began injecting them into every gynaecologic surgery patient" with the disingenuous explanation that he was "testing for cancer."[22] What he really wanted to know was whether these cells remained virulent across numerous cellular generations.

It was only in the 1940s that physicians began diagnosing cervical cancers in situ with a procedure that involved scraping the cervix to harvest cells that could be seen under a microscope. The procedure was common by the time a poor black woman, Henrietta Lacks, was examined and treated at Johns Hopkins University in Baltimore in 1951. Uniquely, the cervical cancer cells harvested in her examination were "immortal," able to divide continuously as long as they were in a proper medium. The discovery of an immortal cell line was exciting stuff, and Johns Hopkins researchers shared them—without Lacks's knowledge or permission—with colleagues around the nation and the world.

Southam wanted to know whether the cells while obviously alive—they still were dividing—were also actively virulent. In 1963 Southam made an arrangement with Dr. Emanuel Mandel, director of medicine at the Jewish Chronic Disease Hospital (JCD) in Brooklyn, to include JCD patients (mostly immigrants, many with minimal English) as research subjects. William Hyman, a member of JCD's board of directors, attempted to get these studies stopped after other doctors complained to him about the dangers. Unsuccessful at an in-house solution, he sued in a case that was broadly reported.[23]

Trial testimony made clear that unknowing patients were infected with cancer cells that resulted in localized tumors at the injection site, and in some cases, more serious cancers. This was not a case of individual researcher excess but rather a general research practice. Witnesses described as common the use of patients as research objects without their consent or, as in this case, without concern for their safety. "If the whole profession is doing it," asked Southam's lawyers, "how can you call it 'unprofessional conduct?'"[24] Following the court case, an investigation by the federal National Institutes of Health (NIH) revealed that only nine of more than fifty grantee institutions the NIH supported financially had any program at all that might protect the rights of research subjects.

Were all this not enough, in 1976 *Rolling Stone* magazine published a story about Henrietta Lacks, publicly describing for the first time the

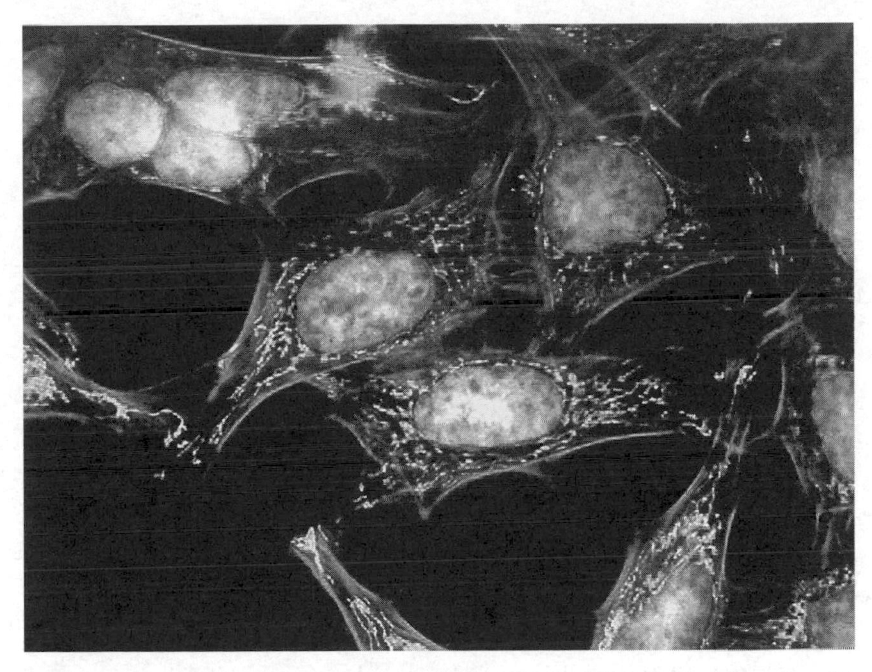

Figure 5.2
This is a micrograph of Henrietta Lacks's famous cervical cancer cells. They are stained to improve legibility. The cells have been stained to reveal their structure. *Source*: Dr. Gopal Murti, Science Photo Library, http://www.sciencephoto.com.

woman whose now famous cells had been harvested without her knowledge or consent (figure 5.2). Her family was never informed that her famously immortal HeLa cancer cells became the basis of cancer and genetic research for generations. Henrietta Lacks's use, or as some saw it her abuse, confirmed the fears of many African Americans who never believed Tuskegee or Willowbrook (discussed in chapter 2) were isolated incidents. The impression of uncaring researchers knowingly injuring patients, or at least putting patients in danger, endangered research itself. The appearance of exploitation of the poor in general and African American poor specifically was odious, and widespread. If patients were merely objects to be used by researchers, and the Southam trial made it clear this was a common sentiment, why would anyone choose to be a research subject?

Some argued that regulations enacted by the NIH in 1966 were sufficient to promote patient protection in human subjects–based research.

These included the idea of independent research review boards that in theory would assure at the least some form of oversight. And, of course, there was Osler's old idea of truly informed consent brought into the postwar era in a 1957 court case, *Salgo v. Leland*.[25] But from the perspective of the public whose members would be solicited as research subjects, the revelations of subject endangerment in popular reports of researcher excesses needed something more. The National Commission for the Protection of Human Subjects of Biomedical and Behavioral Research was formed to find a balance between the needs of the research community and the concerns of potential research subjects.

The Belmont Report

Commission members gathered at the Belmont Conference Center in Elkridge, Maryland, then a part of the Smithsonian Institution, to compile what has ever after been called *The Belmont Report* (*Belmont*). It distinguished from the start between medical practice, "interventions that are designed solely to enhance the well-being of an individual patient," and research designed to test a hypothesis in a way that developed "generalizable knowledge."[26] The Commission would consider only the latter and not the former, an ethical arena presumably best left to the old ethics of medicine.

The distinction between "patient" and "subject" was something of a cheat, however, creating two separate ethical contexts for what was, really, the same set of participants. The subjects required by medical research programs were typically patients like Henrietta Lacks, persons with diagnosed conditions. Studies of multiple sclerosis required MS patients; studies of cancer required cancer patients. By separating medical practice and research as if needed (and needy) research subjects were not also medical patients, *Belmont* presented, as James Anderson puts it, a "decontextualized picture of knowledge" promoting an ethical fiction of distinct classes for whom distinct ethics might be applicable.[27] Researchers were typically the physicians of record for these patients-cum-research subjects. Sloan-Kettering's Southam, for example, injected HeLa cells into patients he was treating as part of a research agenda that provided no benefit and resulted in harm to those patients; the Tuskegee farmers were patients who assumed incorrectly their syphilis was being treated; Willowbrook's children were under the care of physicians who infected them with hepatitis.

All this would or should have been broadly condemned under the old medical ethic whose sole moral focus was the care and protection of the patient. And certainly, *Belmont*'s authors could have endorsed this ethic as a signal guide in their deliberations. To do that would have argued, as well, the primacy of short-term care over the potential of long-term knowledge that might be gained in the draconian use of unknowing patients as research objects. That older ethic might have been advanced with reference to Kant's argument for humanity and its categorical prohibition of people as means rather than ends in themselves. *Belmont*'s authors didn't do that, however. In separating the medical patient from the research subject, and arguing a distinct ethics of research, they opened the door for a bioethical perspective in which the needs of the patient-cum-subject would ever after be secondary to those of the knowledge industry and its potential production of future benefit.

Belmont: Principles

The greater good argument was presented with a kind of philosophical gloss in which the individual was to be respected in a system guided by beneficence and justice for all. Its guiding principles would be, first, "respect for persons" as autonomous, rational human beings, and second, a "beneficence" that maximized the communal benefits of the research while minimizing potential risks to research subjects. The third principle, justice, was to ensure "reasonable, non-exploitative, and well-considered procedures" that would be fairly administered in a manner that assured an equitable distribution of benefits and burdens.

The result was to be an adroit balancing act whose high-minded philosophical stance assured that benefits accrued first and foremost to the knowledge industry and its researchers. The burdens were principally to be borne by the patient-cum-subject whose medical needs were secondary to the needs of the research program. Whatever the outcome, there were always real health risks for the patient-cum-subject. After all, the efficacy and safety of the drugs and therapies in trial were unknown.

The only justification here was the potential benefit to future patients, and to the research industry itself. Even if a research program was successful its benefits would likely come too late for the patient in the research trial.

Grievously absent in the justice ideal presented by *Belmont*'s authors was a rigorous principal of distributive justice that might have assured a real sharing of benefits, not simply the unequal distribution of burden. The authors might have argued for participation of the subjects (or, of their families if they died) in any profits that resulted from the tests in which they participated. At the very least the care of the subject as a medical patient might have been guaranteed over time irrespective of the efficacy of the drug or procedural trial. Where federal monies supported research programs (many and perhaps the majority under National Institutes of Medicine grants), *Belmont* authors might have argued for a public distribution of any benefits accruing from the work. That could mean either public ownership of resulting patents or at least payments from the research industry—one involving drug testing and producing companies—to the public based on profits that resulted from the research.

None of this happened, however. Because the patient and the research subject were defined as distinct there was no injunction to assure the patient's care. Nor was distributive justice a real concern. It was simply assumed that market mechanisms would answer all questions of the just distribution of the generalizable knowledge that resulted from human subjects–based research. Practically, that meant "justice" would be left to the marketplace.

Nor is this mere history. The *Belmont* authors' separation of patient from research subject, of medical care from medical research, continues today. The "theaputic orientation" and its ethics are assumed to be distinct from the "scientific orientation" and thus to answer a distinct bioethic.[28] The "traditional and decisively patient-centered account of physicians' obligations" can be discounted by all except for the nonresearching professional whose care begins and ends at the bedside.[29] And yet, nobody has demonstrated how to distinguish between the patient in care and the patient as research subject. It has thus been impossible to ensure patient care and protection as priorities within the broader regimes of research (figure 5.3).[30]

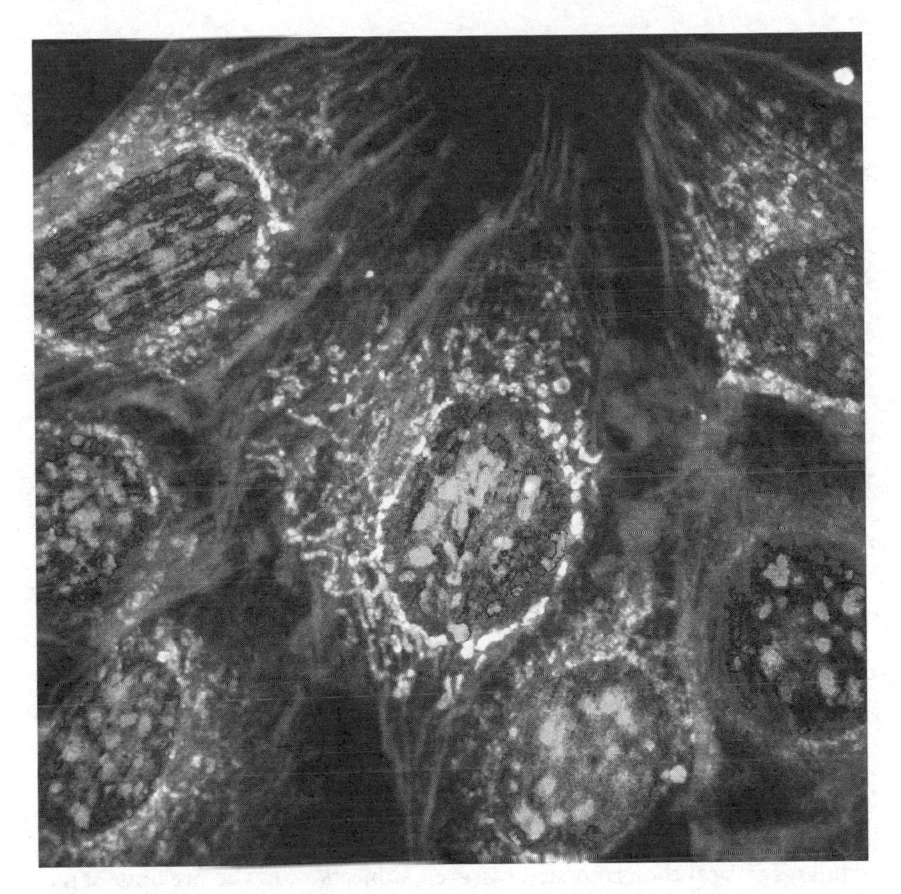

Figure 5.3
Here again are the HeLa cancer cells, identified with a different stain. They stand as a symbol that exemplifies the use and misuse of patients as patients as research objects. *Source*: Science Photo Library, http://www.sciencephoto.com.

Belmont's answer was one in which the potential for general knowledge and tomorrow's greater good took precedence over the immediacy of the sick person's needs. It was short on practical procedures of protection, long on high-minded principles whose methods of enaction were unclear. That served nicely to promote a patina of protection without hampering the research industry. It also served to reduce the efficacy of the old medical ethic, removing its injunctions from the world of the medical researcher. That perspective continues, I argue in chapter 9, today.

Risk and Consent

The general parameters for research proposed in *The Belmont Report* were enacted by federal regulations in 1981 under President Ronald Reagan and then extended in 1991 under his successor, George Bush. These presidencies were grounded in an ideology arguing that, first and foremost, the business of government was business and its promotion. They further believed as an article of faith that business and industry do best what government necessarily can't ever do well. Both championed the idea that decreasing federal supervision (but not federal funding) promoted business and research and thus was itself an instrumental good. *Belmont* fit nicely into the political spirit of the day, its principles constituting a general ideal rather than a pragmatic set of protective protocols. As such, and with minimal oversight, industry was left to build its bottom line.

Operationally, the Federal Drug Administration (FDA) was given the power to loosely supervise a four-step program by which new drugs are tested before being marketed, each requiring more and more human subjects.[31] The first phase requires a small number of healthy subjects to test the general safety of a new product; the second phase tests safety and efficacy of a product on a number of sick patients who, if the drug or procedure is successful, might be helped by it. The third phrase employs several thousand sick research subjects if, in the previous stage, reported side effects are not too severe. The final phase is a cost–benefit analysis in which the efficiency of the new drug is compared with that of other drugs with the same general treatment goal.

Informed Consent

Across this very complex series of trials involving thousands of people *Belmont* promoted "informed consent" as a bulwark against patient abuse. Its power was built on the moral folk theory's assumption of the rational, self-aware individual capable of making his or her own decisions. By informing them of procedures—potential risks and benefits—they are then free to either participate or not based on a full consideration of the program they are asked to join. There was nothing particularly new here. Osler championed an idea like this early in the twentieth century. And, too, the 1957 court case *Salgo v. Leland* appeared to insist upon patient disclosure as a necessary constituent of patient choice.

The result has been, as Wilson and Epstein succinctly put it, a set of "legally fictitious procedures which is not really capable of doing what it is primarily supposed to do: respect the patient's autonomy."[32] Patient disclosure and informed choice, they argue, are good ideas lost in the realities of the research paradigm. A patient with MS (or ALS, or HIV, etc.) is told there is a clinical trial for a new drug. On what basis will the patient make his or her choice? If it is a stage one or two trial they can't be told about the dangerous side effects because they're not yet known. They can't be told about the drug's real potential because it is not known. They are not told about the number of laboratory animals that have died in the testing. And if the patient asks, "What is the drug?" the answer will be largely meaningless unless he or she has studied both biochemistry and the nature of specific disease mechanisms the new drug is designed, at least in theory, to address.

Not surprisingly, the patient often assumes that participation in this or that drug trial, or to the application of a new experimental surgical procedure, will contribute to his or her care and treatment. This is politely called the problem of "therapeutic misconception": the mistaken assumption of research subjects that the research will somehow benefit their own situations.[33] But in many research contexts the goal has nothing to do with the care of the patient who is the research subject, only with gaining information about the drug or procedure for which he or she is a research object.

The patient must rely upon the physician for guidance. Yet increasingly, the physician acts simultaneously as a caregiver and a well-compensated recruiter for the research program needing test subjects. "The attraction for most physicians is that they can see that for each line item, the pharmaceutical companies are paying at least twice as much (and even up to five times as much) as an insurance company or government agent would for the same services. Each office visit . . . generates two to three times the revenue as does seeing patients as part of standard medical visits."[34]

The patient assumes his or her physician's primary ethical concern is the patient's care. But the primacy of that old ethical obligation is superseded contractually by the physician's obligations to the research program.

The result has been a series of medical misadventures and legal imbroglios. One of the best known, in recent years, occurred at The Hospital for Sick Children, in Toronto, Canada, where a physician-researcher, Dr. Nancy Fern Olivieri, faced legal action and official censure after attempting to stop a drug trial she believed injurious to hospital patients.[35]

The promise of "informed consent" and its premise of free choice are even more problematic in the United States where physician care for some of the more than 46 million persons without health insurance is sometimes predicated on participation in a research trial. That is, acceptance as a patient is dependent on a person's willingness to serve as a research subject in trials the physician-researcher is hired to recruit for and supervise. The idea of free and "informed choice" becomes meaningless where "choice" is reduced to either no care at all, or treatment within a research program whose efficacy is unknown and whose safety is uncertain.

As a final indignity, the system built upon *The Belmont Report* shifted the ethical onus for research safety to the research subject him or herself. If the person with a terrifying disease (AIDS, ALS, MS, etc.) is killed or injured in a research program—well, the subject signed a consent form. Obviously, he or she knew the risks.

Still, researchers and research-oriented physicians chafe at the necessity of consent as an impediment. Ian Roberts, for example, argues the very idea of consent is itself an unethical impediment to patient treatment with new drugs and procedures.[36] Consent, in this reading, violates the physician's duty to care while impeding the progress of research. Roberts and his colleagues favor abandoning the meaningless ritual of consent in favor of the reflexive imposition of research protocols on injured and ill patients. That the treatments being tested may not serve as well as older procedures and may carry new and unexpected risks is explained away as, simply, the way it is.

Review Boards

Nor are supposedly independent, institutional review boards—earlier instituted by the NIH and then advanced in *Belmont*—a bastion of patient protection. More typically the practice is a kind of "ethical imperialism"—Zachary Schrag's phrase—in which critical oversight typically is minimal and so, too, is the idea of rigorous subject protection.[37] Review board members are drawn from supervising institutions (a hospital or university) which have a strong interest in approving research as a way of raising needed monies. Those chosen for review boards, including bioethicists, often lack the knowledge in biochemistry, biostatistics, or medicine required to judge the safety of proposed research. As one nurse who participates in a university-based research program told me privately, "I ask about this and they say, 'it's complex. Trust us.' Nobody else seems to be concerned."

Osler, who understood the necessity of research, would have been appalled. As we have seen, he insisted that *if* Hippocratic medicine's primary principles of patient care and caution were to be protected *then* no experimentation on human subjects should be undertaken without the possibility of real benefit for the patient-cum-subject.[38] In the language of Kant we might say that when patient care became a secondary priority the research subject became no more than a research object, a cipher in the Kingdom of Means rather than a protected person in the Kingdom of Ends. Thus both traditional medical and later Kantian ethics would reject necessarily and unequivocally the paradigm that has followed on the ideas and ideals of *The Belmont Report*.

The Philosophical Flavor

What does "respect for persons" mean? Clearly, Kant's "deep and robust theory of autonomy"[39] is reduced from a theoretical shout to at best a practical whisper in the world that *Belmont* opened to researchers. As Lewis White Beck says in his introduction to Kant's *Foundations of the Metaphysics of Morals*, a perceived duty to protect persons in general, and especially those unable to protect themselves, reflected the essential good of a "common moral humanity" underpinning Kant's philosophy.[40] With *Belmont*'s research priorities that essential good was locked in the future benefits that may someday accrue to research. The immediate needs of fragile persons, of patients, were at best secondary.

There is something nicely Hippocratic in Kant's description of the protected and special nature of humanity. The moral physician does not only treat the smart and able but all who need medical attention, irrespective of their abilities. The goals of medicine were, in Kant's ethics, based on humanness and not performance categories. So, too, *The*

Belmont Report said, human subject research needs a similar sense of humanity as a good. "Some persons are in need of extensive protection, even to the point of excluding them from activities which may harm them."[41]

From the start, however, this sense of the protected human was subjugated by an allegiance to the writings of various utilitarians, especially John Stewart Mill.[42] One sees this in the *Belmont* authors' idea of "beneficence" as not an absolute injunction to do good (and thus nonmalfeasance, to do no harm) but instead a maximizing of benefits not for the patient but in terms of the "generalizable knowledge" research might produce. This reduced the primacy of individual care into a contingent good whose importance was outweighed by the promise of future benefits defined as potential knowledge. We find the same transposition of old values into new meanings in the redefinition of "justice" as not equality or equity among a citizenry but as an "equitable" sharing of burdens (to the patient) and benefits (to research).

The tensions that result, the impossible inconsistencies, cannot be reconciled. On the one hand, *Belmont* enjoined researchers against selecting subjects on the basis of "their easy availability, their compromised position, or their manipulability."[43] On the other hand, it is precisely the compromised patient (with cancer, multiple sclerosis, or some other disease) who is needed most as a research subject. And these patients, available through their physicians, are easy to manipulate. Similarly, "informed choice" is promoted as a protected good but has become either an empty ritual or an unforgivable impediment and inconvenience to research, depending on the author one seeks to quote. And of course there is this final indignity: even if a research project is successful and a new product is eventually brought to market (typically long after it might help the test subject) its cost may be so prohibitive that none but the wealthy can afford it.

Managing Medicine

It didn't have to be this way. *Belmont* might have begun with the Oslerian ideal of the primacy of patient care and protection, insisting it took precedence over the uncertain future good promised by research programs. It could have considered the composition of review boards, including perhaps citizen or patient representatives as necessary members. And, too, it could have insisted upon an absolute separation of physicians enjoined to treat (and protect) the fragile patient and researchers whose allegiance to patient care is necessarily at best secondary. But then it would have been a different report. As written, *Belmont* was successful in two different ways.

First, it appeared to provide a measure of protection for research subjects without unduly inhibiting the research industry. Second, *Belmont* was a proving ground for bioethics as a system of adjudication that could address issues of medical care and research in a way that did not impede the knowledge industry. Professorships were funded to support those who would teach bioethics, write papers about it, and serve as bioethical consultants to industry and government. Bioethicists would sit on institutional review boards. Political commissions sought the wisdom of moral philosophers who promoted themselves as medical ethicists. Many gained positions at well-funded institutions like the Hastings Center and the Joseph and Rose Kennedy Institute for the Study of Human Reproduction and Bioethics, later called simply the Kennedy Institute of Ethics. None of this was because, as Albert Jonsen put it, "health care had become a powerful institution, with powerful technologies."[44] That happened long before. Big Pharma did not emerge full-blown from the ether in the 1960s. Its modern incarnation had its origins in the lowly technology of the medical pill patented in 1884 by Henry Solomon Wellcome and Silas Mainville Burroughs. That permitted the profitable mass production of a standardized, easily distributable medical product.

Nor need we think that it was a bold new world of research newly requiring human subjects that called forth this new industry of ethical valuation. Rabinbach has the late nineteenth century chock-a-block full of what today we would call biomechanical engineers testing ways to increase the efficiency of industrial workers. Others, as we have seen, were similarly active—psychologists and physicians—identifying the "idiots," "morons," and other "defectives" who could be classified as nonproductive social burdens. Historically, therefore, there was nothing particularly "new" or "unprecedented" in the issues that, in the 1970s, gave rise to either *Belmont* or bioethics. In a real way we had seen it all before except that now it was wrapped in the high language of the principled philosopher.

The Physician: Stripped

What was new, perhaps, was the manner in which the non-research, treating physician was made the whipping boy of the new medicine. The steps by which this took place are very clear. First, President Reagan's administration announced a crisis in the cost of national healthcare. The answer, his officials argued, was to free capitalism and its entrepreneurs by slashing regulations that industry officials saw as costly while decreasing private and corporate taxes whose return, not coincidentally, paid for federal health and welfare programs. *If* research is an important industry, then it should be encouraged through tax breaks, flexible research protocols, and so on.

Because the costs of healthcare appeared to outstrip available revenues in the present, the costs of medicine therefore had to be restrained. Medicine was, in the language of the day "rationalized" into "managed care" under a system of cost–benefit analysis that served not the patient but the economies of care in general. "By assigning values and standards to clinical practice," as Jill Fisher put it, "medicine became less a social good [as it had been] and more a set of commodities to which individual patients have different degrees of access.[45] When *Belmont* separated the ethics of patient care from the ethics of patient use in research, it opened the door to a prioritizing of economic benefit over the needs of the fragile and the ill.

The result was to reduce fields of choice—for the patient and the physician—even as the bioethicist was proclaiming informed choice as a fundamental good. Patients were no longer free to choose a physician they found amenable but instead were assigned physicians from a pool approved by an insurer chosen by the patient's employer. Physicians with their patients were not free to choose the treatments that seemed best but instead were required to select from insurer-approved treatment options based on cost–benefit ratios rather then the sometimes-eccentric realities of patient circumstance. The patient became a consumer and the physician an employee contractually responsible to the insurer rather than the patient alone.

If the goal was to decrease the cost of care on a per capita basis the whole was a dismal failure. Year by year, those costs have increased in the United States. If the goal was an ethics of patient protection from research the results were similarly lamentable, as I argue in chapter 9. Worse, the one person ethically obliged to place the patient's care above all other considerations was in this process virtually removed from the equation as a decision maker. Medicine was emasculated as the physician's vocation was shrunk to a client roster approved by insurers who set the fee schedule and determined what drugs and procedures could be prescribed or performed (and thus compensated), what rehabilitation (if any) would be offered.

Bioethics was a part of this transformation. As moral philosophers bioethicists might have argued the primacy of care as a philosophical good. They might have joined this to the old Hippocratic ideal of medicine, as Osler did, in a relational ethic of caregiver and care receiver. They could have promoted a system in which research participation would guarantee patient care. They might have argued, in the name of patient autonomy, for a health system that permitted free choice of medical providers rather than choices limited to an insurers' pool of available doctors. Indeed, they might have argued the necessity of universal care itself as ethically necessary as well as cost efficient. *Belmont* and its successive authors might have promoted a stronger argument about the responsibilities that attend among needy patient, physician, and physician employer in society at large. Bioethicists did none of these things. Instead, they blamed the doctors.

Paternalism

Into the 1980s the ideal of the Hippocratic physician held real sway in both the popular imagination and the professional arena of medical societies. For the new ethic to take hold, the ideal of the Hippocratic physician whose primary duty is to the patient had to be disgraced. At the precise point in history when physician responsibility for patient care was being overridden by hospital administrators (with regard to dialysis) and insurers, just as Reagan's managed care reduced the scope of physician authority in the hospital, bioethicists were busy mythologizing (demonizing may be a better word) physicians as a class of arrogant, imperious twits in need of restraint. In this trope it was not medical insurers, pharmaceutical companies, or researchers who were out of control, but the damn doctors themselves.

The argument was called "paternalism" and it rapidly became a pillar of the bioethical argument. Not coincidentally, it promoted as a consequence the bioethicist as the patient's protector against the autocratic physician whose predilection for imperious treatment decisions needed restraint. The idea of paternalism, and of patient choice, is treated more fully here in chapter 9, but a brief introduction is useful at this point. A 1983 special issue of the journal *Theoretical Medicine*, edited and introduced by Laurence B. McCullough, is as good a locus of this transformation as any. A philosopher with a BA in art history, McCullough spent two years as a postdoctoral fellow at the Hastings Center (1975–1976) and then, after a brief stint at Texas A&M University (with appointments in medicine and philosophy), nine years (1979–1988) with a joint appointment at the Kennedy Institute of Ethics and Georgetown University. With that superior pedigree McCullough was the gold standard of the academic philosopher turned bioethicist. Here was the way he described paternalism in medicine:

> Medicine makes a distinctive claim, namely, that based on its objective (in the sense of transindividual) body of knowledge, skills, and experiment it knows what is in the best interests of the patient whose health care needs it seeks to serve. At the same time patients, based on their own subjective (in the sense of individual) values and beliefs, claim to know what is in their own interests. Paternalism—the interference with another's autonomy to prosecute or protect that individual's best interest—is the concept in moral philosophy that captures what is at stake in conflicts between medicine and patients over what is a patient's best interests.[46]

These three sentences are a model of the kind of axiomatic writing that permeates bioethics, permitting unsupported opinions to be presented as unquestionable conclusions. Medical expertise is reduced to a "claim" of knowledge. Patients have their own knowledge base, their own experience base that is assumed to be both equal to and stand in natural opposition to the physician's. The essential conflict is therefore between two equal and competing perspectives and their respective adherents. "Paternalism," for McCullough, was "the concept in moral philosophy" that captured what happens when these two equal knowledge bases—one personal and public, the other professional—were placed in opposition.

Historically, paternalism is not "the interference with another's autonomy," however, or anything else necessarily bad. But then as noun or adjective it was not born on the high plains of moral philosophy. The word is derived from the Latin word for father (*pater*), and meant, before its bioethical appropriation, "a policy or practice of treating or governing people in a fatherly manner." According to the *Oxford Online Etymology Dictionary*, paternalism was used in the late nineteenth century to describe responsible "government as by a father over his children." Across the first half of the twentieth century the word thus carried a sense of personal responsibility and caring, not arrogance and imposition.

Bioethicists redefined the word to serve very specific ends and then hung it all on the hook of a "moral philosophy." As used by bioethicists, paternalism became a byword for the imposition or withholding of treatment by physicians irrespective of the express wishes of a patient. Paternalistic medicine denied patient autonomy, and thus personal choice. Certainly there were—and are—arrogant physicians. There are also many shopkeepers, bureaucrats, bus drivers, lawyers, mayors, police constables, and not a few professors of philosophy who share the trait. Whether physicians were more prone to this trait than others is a question considered here in chapter 9.

What is clear is that, as it was argued, the whole was suspect. Physicians were on the one hand legally (and ethically) responsible for a patient's care. On the other hand, their practice was carried out in an environment of ever-scarcer resources (remember the Asbury draft policy mentioned in chapter 3) and ever-greater restrictions. Private insurers employing physicians imposed upon their treatment choices a range of controls and protocols whose sole purpose was to decrease cost. These became the parameters within which physicians could prescribe and treat. As a result the physicians' practical sphere of action was being reduced at the precise moment that bioethicists attacked them for treatment choices as if these were not being bounded by insurers and other cost-containment strategists.

There was another problem. The paternalism literature assumed physicians and patients shared a sufficiently equal knowledge base such that the preferences of neither group should dominate. The patient—an advertising executive in Toronto, Canada, a dockworker in New York City, a field hand in Texas, a cook in Minneapolis—was assumed, at least implicitly, to be able to make treatment decisions as informed as those of the imperious physician. That doctors might have knowledge this or that patient did not was a possibility the literature, written largely by ethicist-philosophers generally ignorant of medicine, politely ignored. But knowledge inequalities between physicians and patients have been, as Robert Bartz reminds us, a constant at least since the days of Socrates. "I have often, along with my brother and with other physicians, visited one of their patients who refused to drink his medicine or submit to the surgeon's knife or cautery," we read in *Gorgias*, "and when the doctor was unable to persuade them, I did so."[47]

We want physicians more expert in their vocation than are we, the patients. We want them to argue for our best chances even if we are concerned about the potential of those recommendations for havoc. That patients might be unrealistic in demands for procedures that may be injurious or impractical is a possibility bioethicists who rallied to fight paternalistic medicine never considered. That physicians were the ones charged—ethically and legally—with making allocation decisions in a context of scarcity was a fact largely unremarked. So, too, was the degree to which physicians were bounded by cost protocols that dictated the treatment decisions they made.

The litany of paternalistic physicians whose treatment caused harm is long: Jewish Hospital, Tuskegee, Willowbrook, and so on. The problem was rarely the Hippocratic physician treating the patient in need, however. Rather, the excesses that spurred bioethics forward were more typically the result of physician-researchers who had abandoned the primacy of patient care for the lucrative ideal of research as a future good.

In the end, arguments about paternalism had little to do with the realities of patient care and treatment by the average physician. Daniel Callahan had said physicians were the problem in a medicine whose costs were expansive. Here was a means by which they could be put in their place. As a reward for their service, bioethicists were permitted to promote themselves as patient champions in the new order. Where disagreements occurred they were the risk management specialists skilled in practical (I want to say colonial) and ethical decision making. In effect, the Hippocratic physician was demoted to a clerkship at the evolving big box superstore that was American-style consumer medicine.

Biopower became bioethics became bioconsumerism . . . all in a single gulp.

6

Principles of Biomedical Ethics

By the late 1970s bioethics had its agendas and the administrative nodes for their advancement. The Hastings Center and the Kennedy Institute of Ethics were principal foci of the valuators who assumed scarcity as a natural limit to healthcare and an impediment to research (not enough human subjects), and who more generally argued the failure of medicine's traditional ethics of care. What bioethics lacked was a manifesto that would formalize its arguments and serve as an instructional document for the courses in bioethics that moral philosophers turned practical medical ethicists were increasingly teaching. Tom Beauchamp and James Childress remedied this deficit with the 1979 publication of the first edition of their *Principles of Biomedical Ethics*.

Principles has been both singularly influential and uniquely successful. Its approach "has been the dominant orthodoxy in the application of ethics to medicine for a generation," in large part because it "lends itself so well to the checklist project, of reducing medical practice to algorithms."[1] That checklist, and the argument for its utility, "has served as groundwork for the training of countless students and professionals in medicine and biomedical ethics world-wide."[2] The whole works if, but only if, assumptions of the moral folk theory are accepted, however. Then, as Mark Johnson wrote in passage cited earlier, "moral reasoning is thus principally a matter of getting the correct description of a situation, determining which moral law pertains to it, and figuring out what action that moral law requires for the given situation."[3] *Principles* has sought, since its first edition, to argue its ethic on the basis of a philosophical method and perspective its authors believe permit the production of broadly acceptable if not in fact universal principles applicable to medical issues.

Principles has stood across its multiple editions as at once an argument for bioethics and a statement of what it is and should be. It has been sign *and* signifier, the modern advertiser's dream product that at once announces a commercial need (clean skin) and a product to service that need (Ivory soap). Indeed, it is sometimes praised in the form of advertising promotions in which both problem ("I experienced it") and solution ("I use it") are simultaneously advanced in a personal testimonial. British bioethicist Raanon Gillon, for example, wrote in 1996 that "as a standard basis for moral assessment in biomedical ethics that is compatible with a very wide variety of moral theories, I recommend and use the 'four principles plus scope' approach advocated by the Americans Beauchamp and Childress in their famous and standard text book, *Principles of Biomedical Ethics*.'"[4]

Modestly, Gillon went on to note that his own work, *Philosophical Medical Ethics*,[5] was a mere gloss on Beauchamp and Childress's great text. *Principles* advanced, and Gillon praised, the principled pillars of Beauchamp and Childress's work that include (1) respect for personal autonomy, (2) nonmalfeasance (the obligation not to harm), (3) beneficence (try and do good), and (4) justice, the obligation to treat competing claims fairly. Gillon is no sports personality enlisted to sell razors or shaving cream, no movie star whose image can be expected to sell a bottle of Scotch. He is a serious British bioethicist-physician and a central player in British medical ethics. Inadvertently, perhaps, his use of the endorsement form correctly treated *Principles of Biomedical Ethics* as a product seeking to create and simultaneously to fill a market niche among a class of medically engaged consumers. These included, and include today, the academic world in which *Principles* is taught (in applied ethics courses and in medical schools); the world of working ethicists, where it is a reference; and the legal world where questions of medical practice and its ethics are adjudicated.

One problem with discussing *Principles* is that it has changed across six editions spanning more than thirty years of continuous publication. Some of the changes have been trivial which others have been substantial and indeed fundamental. Some may see its decades of transformation, edition to edition, as a strength; a furthering of arguments that, solid and articulate in the beginning, have become better with age. Alternatively, more than thirty years of textual change may be seen as evidence that, for all its authoritative tone, *Principles* is anything but definitive in arguments whose foundations are contingent and uncertain.

A somewhat exasperated John Arras described *Principles* and its authors as analogous to the Borg species in the science fiction TV series *Star Trek: The Next Generation*. As a race, the Borg searches the galaxy (or at least its Alpha and Delta Quadrants) for other species whose qualities they might assimilate in the search for the perfection of their own. "Many of Beauchamp and Childress's critics know the feeling. No sooner do they launch a seemingly crippling broadside against the juggernaut of PBE [*Principles of Biomedical Ethics*] . . . than their critique is promptly welcomed with open arms, trimmed of its perceived excesses, and incorporated in the ever-expanding synthesis of the next edition."[6]

It's a very useful analogy. The central fact of the imaginary Borg is that no matter how many other species they assimilate, the Borg remain . . . Borg. They may add this or that characteristic to their shared consciousness (they are a "hive" species), but the nature of their society and its organization remain constant. Similarly, amid its many changes *Principles* has been constant in its fundamental argument. Edition to edition it has asserted a methodology and its applicability. The disinterested dispassionate thinker, usually a philosopher, may perceive a singular moral law whose constant, indeed universal values may be briefly summarized and generally applied by the careful thinker. Complexity is banished when correct values are correctly applied.

From the start, *Principles* sought to expand upon the essential vision of *The Belmont Report* in two ways. This is not surprising given that Tom Beauchamp, a principal participant in *Belmont* was to be a coauthor of *Principles*. But where *The Belmont Report* enunciated three general principles applicable to issues of human subject research, *Principles* expanded its set to four principles. These would be applied not simply to the arena of medical research but also to all questions of medical care and treatment. These principles were advanced as substantial in their utility, but also definitional, bounded not by a time, culture, or political perspective. They were argued as universal, constant, timeless, necessarily true and . . . real.

It is no surprise that the bioethics that results from *Belmont* and in *Principles* has a self-consciously Kantian flavor. It insists there is a path to moral knowledge. That path requires the application of a dispassionate, analytic, and rational methodology whose result reveals applicable truths irrespective of the vagaries of individual, clinical, political, or social circumstance. Once perceived, *Principles* insists, these can be applied to issues of medical practice and research.

Perhaps Beauchamp and Childress's greatest achievement has been to advance this general Kantian perspective (universal moral law, rationality, etc.), and the moral folk theory derived from it, as a methodology so broadly acceptable, so universal that even those who do not admire Kant will reflexively accept the general manner of the text's argument. From the start, therefore, *Principles* has been three things. First, it has been an argument for bioethics as a necessary successor to the older ethics of medicinal practice in society. Second, it has asserted a specific kind of thinking as the only appropriate means by which issues of medical practice and research can be ethically adjudicated. Third, it has argued that from the philosophical method come a small set of principles that are definitional and universal (they define what morality is in a way all right-thinking people will accept) and thus generally applicable.

Many others have criticized the work's principlist focus as inadequate. But the broader perspective of *Principles* remains foundational. It is taught generally and widely. And even where its principles are dismissed as too little, its general argument and broad perspective, outlined in this chapter, are generally accepted. Thus in addressing its limits the limits of the field it has helped to build are addressed as well.

The First 106 Words

All this is made clear in the first 106 words of the fifth edition of *Principles*, the most recent, at this writing, available to Kindle users:

> Medical ethics enjoyed a remarkable degree of continuity from the days of Hippocrates until the middle of the twentieth century. Developments in the biological and health sciences then led to critical reflection on conventional conceptions of the moral obligations of health professions and society in preventing disease and injury and meeting the needs of the sick and injured. Although major writings in ancient, medieval, and modern health care contain a rich storehouse of reflection on the relationship between the professional and the patient, these writings are inadequate for contemporary biomedical ethics. This historical record often neglects problems of truthfulness, privacy, justice, communal responsibility, and the like.

To avoid a similar narrowness, we begin with philosophical reflection on morality and ethics that is removed from the history of professional ethics. Such reflection affords some distance from assumptions still evident in the biomedical sciences and healthcare.[7]

There is no quibbling here, no, "We will attempt to show . . ." or perhaps, "we will argue . . ." common to science and social science writing. Like the writing of McCullough, cited earlier, the rhetoric brooks no debate. The magisterially declarative writing states opinion and surmise as unequivocal fact. And as in all good sales pitches, it asserts as evident and exigent a problem it is fashioned uniquely to resolve. Broken down, what results is a series of interlocking assumptions, building one upon another, whose proofs are never provided.

To begin, there is the problem statement: The ethics that had governed medicine for centuries will no longer serve for two reasons. First, it is dismissed as incapable of addressing "developments in the biological and health sciences." Second, the older ethic is more generally deficient in its promotion of virtues we today value and insist upon in our social relations: "truthfulness, privacy, justice, communal responsibility, and the like." Thus even if the older ethic was capable of assessing the issues arising from new sciences its judgment would be suspect because it lacked values we believe are necessary constituents of any ethical conclusion. The solution is a new ethic in which these values are clearly articulated, one based upon a system of "philosophical reflection" largely removed from but somehow relevant to the ethical practice of medicine the authors sought to inform.

Here the implied predicate presents what is, in the end, a kind of logic trap. The declarative form insists we accept reflexively the premises on which the conclusions depend. There is no "if" to the insistence that new sciences and technologies have created problems the older ethic is incapable of resolving. The opening of *Principles* permits no demand for proof that that older ethic was deficient in a range of virtues that make it generally inapplicable in a society that finds justice, individual worth, and truthfulness important. Because we are just and truthful we need bioethics, a new ethic that reflects our virtues in the face of unprecedented new sciences. Where do we find that new ethic? Where else, but in the field of thinking where ideas of worth, justice, truthfulness, and so on, are constructed: philosophy. Here is the problem and if there is a problem then here is the solution.

To buy into *Principles* does not require the reader buy into Kant. Accept the premise of the moral folk theory that insists upon dispassionate rationality as a way of discovering moral truths and you're hooked. Nor does the reader necessarily need to believe in the principles that *Principles* espouses as long as he or she accepts as important the virtues the old medical ethic is said to lack. In this way bioethics becomes inevitable, and a philosophical approach to issues of medical care and treatment a necessity.

But if the older ethic is redolent with truthfulness and an ideal of justice then a newer ethic may not be needed. If the older ethic is capable of assessing and valuing changes in medical science and practice then a new ethic is not required. Much of the material in the previous chapters has been included to permit the argument that *Principles* fails not simply because its checklist mentality is inadequate and simplistic but also because the conditional premises—the implied "ifs"—on which bioethics is argued as a necessity are simply untrue.

Traditional Ethics Critiqued

The opening lines of *Principles* imply that the older ethic was inflexible and unchanging and thus incapable of handling new science, new data. While the virtues underlying that ethic remained relatively stable across centuries the means of their application changed over time. After the early days of Hippocrates, for example, physicians were not required to teach for free the children of their instructors even though the idea of respect for senior practitioners and their knowledge remained intact. As Daniel Hall notes, this remains a principal tenet of the "Fellowship Pledge" for the American College of Surgeons whose members swear that: 'Upon my honor, I declare that I will advance my knowledge and skills, will respect my colleagues, and will seek their counsel when in doubt about my own abilities. In turn, I will willingly help my colleagues when requested.'"[8] The goal was the best care of the person through the skills of not simply the physician but the physician in association with all who swore the old allegiance in service of the individual in need. That service was communal and depended on a collegial commitment to care as a principal good.

Collegiality as a way of improving patient care through the application of the best of shared knowledge remained important even as the forms it took were transformed across the centuries. In the nineteenth century, for example, regional and national medical societies became the new mechanism within which physicians explored the changing face of science as well as their responsibilities to each other and to society at large. These professional associations were, in turn, recognized by individual states as the logical foci of medical opinion and professional supervision. To them were added the public health organizations and boards joined by physicians who saw in those public positions a method to improve the health of both their own patients and the community at large.

What remained constant into the middle of the twentieth century when bioethics decided the old ways would no longer serve was the principal Hippocratic injunction to care as an ethical responsibility of the practitioner: "I will follow that system of regimen which, according to my ability and judgment, I consider for the benefit of my patients, and abstain from whatever is deleterious and mischievous."[9] Nor were the principles of the old ethic restricted to the practitioner. They served as well as a motivating force behind much of the research that brought medicine into the late twentieth century. The Hippocratic ethic described nicely, for example, the ethics of Dr. Rudolf Virchow in the nineteenth century. That century's father of cell biology and social epidemiology was, as Sherwin Nuland put it, "a spokesman for the philosophy of the Hippocratic Coans. He recognized, as do all modern healers, the primacy of understanding pathophysiological processes if one is to cure disease."[10] Famously, Virchow understood these processes occurred within socioeconomic and political contexts that inhibited or promoted the occurrence of health or disease. The physician's obligation to promote patient health—and thus the health of the societies in which patient and physician together lived—required attention to social constructions contributing to disease events.

It is therefore hard to understand Beauchamp and Childress's magisterial rejection of the older ethic on any basis but their unsubstantiated charge that the older ethic lacked social virtues bioethics would, in its stead, promote. Nor is it clear why any would think that reformation, if needed, would best come "from outside the community within which the decisions are made and outside the practices of [clinical] decision making themselves."[11] Why choose as reformers those with neither practical experience nor detailed knowledge of the subject and its underlying science? "Curious," the student in his Bob Marley tee shirt might say. "What they proposed is a nonmedical ethic of medicine."

The Twentieth Century

If the authors of *Principles* sought to argue the inadequacy of the old ethic to serve patient needs, they might have chosen as a date the spectacular failure of U.S. physicians to condemn surgeon Harry J. Haiselden and his euthanasia of infants in Chicago in the second decade of the twentieth century (see chapter 2). There were clear violations of the physician's Hippocratic oath not only to preserve life but also to act solely for the benefit of the patient. At the least, the failure of the U.S. medical community to censure Haiselden might be advanced as a failure of ethical practitioners to ensure collegial conformity to traditional practice goals.

Or with equal justice and a better sense of history, the failure of the old ethic might be seen in the forced medical sterilization of women like Carrie Buck at the behest of the state (as discussed in chapter 2). Similarly, one might think of Tuskegee as a landmark of a failed ethic when, in the late 1940s penicillin provided a robust treatment that was never offered to the patients being studied. A detailed reading of these and other events—for example, the experimentation on human subjects by Nazi physicians—suggests not the limits of the traditional ethics of medicine, however, but instead the danger that occurs when that ethic is overshadowed by the perceived needs of the state. Where the allegiance of the physician is not to the patient but to an employer whose perspective is economic rather than humanitarian the virtues of the oath are easily ignored.

By the 1950s, and certainly the 1970s, the earlier excesses that might seem to argue the failure of the old ethic were publicly and professionally perceived as violations of both the ethics of medicine and society's broad ethic of human rights based upon a belief in the sanctity of the individual person. The two were mutually reinforcing. Thus the use of medical patients as forced medical research objects was condemned generally as at once clinical and social violations and thus criminal. This was evident in the Nuremberg trials and the general condemnation of medical researchers engaged in programs objectifying human subjects at Jewish Hospital, Tuskegee, Willowbrook, and so on. In the United States the state's right to forcibly sterilize women, already reduced in law in the 1940s, was withdrawn in 1972 by the U.S. Supreme Court decision *Roe v. Wade*.[12]

Thus with at least equal correctness and on the basis of better historical evidence the middle of the twentieth century might be seen as a time when the core values of the old medical ethics were being reaffirmed and rejuvenated. The failures that had occurred resulted from the cooption of physicians as instruments of economic policy rather than as champions of patient care. The traditional medical ethic was not outmoded but in the process of revitalization.

What are we to think about the physician whose professional allegiance is not to the patient but to an employer whose interest in the life of the patient is at best secondary? Here was a problem that needed attention. The older ethic assumed a preeminent caring relationship between the patient and the physician. Both were joined in a social compact that valued each citizen, in the old Greek way, as a member of society. The history of twentieth-century excesses occurred where the ethical obligation of the physician to the patient was overshadowed by either a research orientation in which the patient became a cipher, or where government priorities prevailed, an economic burden. Here was a messy area crying for ethical deliberation, one that placed the needs of the state, or of the corporation engaged in medical research, in conflict with those of the individual members of that state.

Alas, this is not a problem *Principles* would perceive, let alone consider. Nor was it a problem bioethicists would choose to engage.

New Technologies

Principles states that "developments in the biological and health sciences then led to critical reflection on conventional conceptions." What developments? The most expensive, radical new technology of the mid-twentieth century was the cumbersome and life-preserving iron lung that in the 1950s was the salvation of young poliomyelitis patients—saved

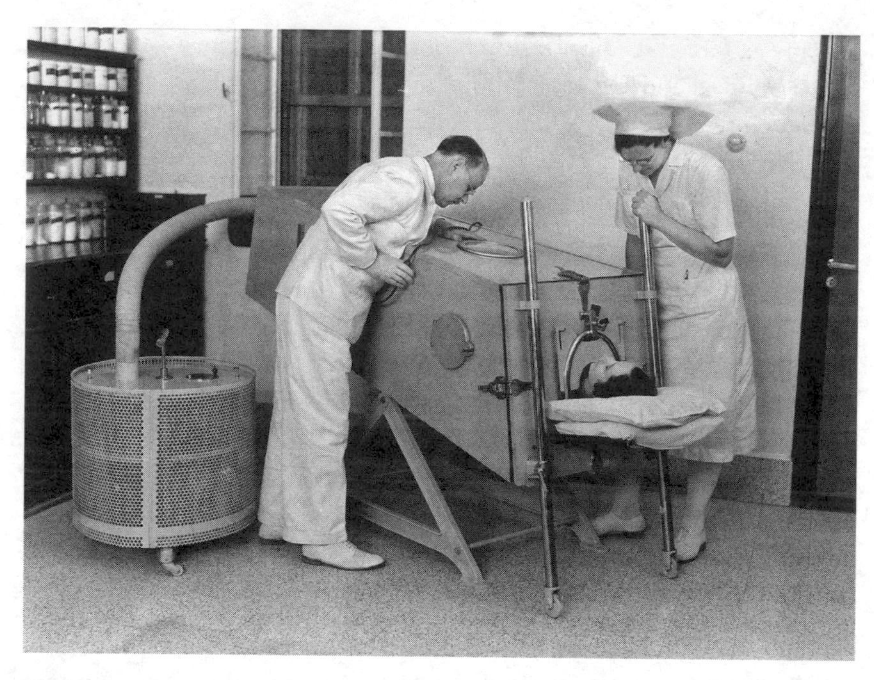

Figure 6.1
The iron lung was the most expensive and restrictive of new technologies introduced in the second half of the twentieth century. And yet its use raised no questions about either cost or "quality of life." It was—popularly and professionally—hailed as a technological triumph that saved lives. *Source*: Science Photo Library, http://www.sciencephoto.com/media/300097/enlarge.

for what all assumed would be a physically restricted life (figure 6.1). Its introduction raised no "critical reflection on conventional conceptions" of medicine and its technologies. Instead it was broadly perceived as a reason to celebrate the power of new technologies to promote the traditional ethical goal of medicine, saving lives that otherwise would be ended by disease. Nor was this seen as an intolerable burden to the state. Indeed, the state was fully engaged, as a photograph of U.S. military personnel showing off the technology demonstrates. No problem there.

In the 1950s and 1960s a host of other new devices and procedures (for example, bypass surgery for cardiac patients) was introduced, all permitting doctors to do what they had sworn to do: save lives and maximize the health of the patients they served. None of these innovations were perceived as ethically problematic. When dialysis was introduced in the 1960s, it presented no new ethical challenge for practitioners but did, at least for a few years, create a social challenge related to cost.

In the same vein, the needs of mid-century medical research programs did not create unprecedented new problems. As we saw, Osler worried about the objectification of patients as research subjects early in the twentieth century. And, earlier, the use of orphans and the poor as objects of medical research was a subject of public as well as professional concern well before Osler's 1907 writing. The sanctity of care and the needs of the patient as primary were ethical priorities in the Nuremberg trial judgments. If there was a challenge to the traditional ethics of medicine at mid century it lay not in the complexities of new science and technology but in the impatience of researchers and their employers who were less interested in patient care than in cost control and product development.

Genetics

Perhaps Beauchamp and Childress's "developments in the biological and health sciences" referred to the slow unraveling of the double helix and its constituents (DNA, RNA, enzymes, proteins, and so on) that began in the 1950s. While fundamental as science this did not throw medicine or its accompanying ethic into a tizzy. Indeed, it would be decades past mid century before the slow advance of this evolving knowledge base had any substantial effect on medical practice. While this subject is covered more thoroughly in chapter 8, it is worth noting here that few diagnostic and even fewer curative procedures were introduced as a result of this science.

To take one representative example: In 1960 Peter Nowell and Davie Hungerford published a paper demonstrating that chronic myelogenous leukemia (CML) was characterized by an aberration on chromosome 22.[13] A decade later another geneticist, Janet Rowley, showed this aberration resulted from a swapping between the ends of chromosomes 9 and 22 in a process whose mechanism was unclear. It was not until 2000 that these insights led to the creation of a treatment, the drug Gleevec, inhibiting the production of the abnormal protein that caused the problem. As a result, survival rates of CML patients rose from 30 to 90 percent. This advance, and others of a similar nature, evoked no ethical controversy among physicians. Hematologists and oncologists, general practitioners and nurses engaged in patient care all cheered a new treatment for this old killer. So, too, of course, did the patients and their families who together looked to medicine for care and treatment.

The issue raised by Gleevic's introduction was not one of medical ethics but economics—who pays? In 2010 in the United States the drug cost up to $100,000 a year per patient depending on dosage levels, patient location, health plan, and the profit margins of local pharmacies. In Ontario, Canada, the cost range was $12,500 to $32,000 a year. Physicians gladly prescribed the drug wherever it was available. Public and private health insurers, however, were reluctant to embrace Gleevic because of its cost. The drug's expense caused them problems, not the prescribing physicians. Similar issues arose, a decade earlier, over the cost of drugs required by HIV-positive patients. Doctors wanted to treat all who needed care but insurers were reluctant to pay the price.

"The emergence of bioethics at the inception of the 1970s coincided with medical and larger-than-medical developments taking place on the American scene."[14] Synchronicity does not prove causality, however, even if it may suggest it. Amid a wealth of technical advances improving the ethical physician's ability to save lives and care for patients it was the "larger-than-medical" developments—economic and social rather than clinical—that were the real issue. The question was the degree to which care of the person should take precedence over the costs of that care in a for-profit system of medical production and product delivery in which care providers and suppliers were free to charge whatever they thought the market might allow. Neither *Belmont* nor *Principles* sought to consider these issues, however.

Truthfulness, etc.

Perhaps the most preposterous assertion of *Principles'* opening paragraphs was that the old ethics was deficient in "truthfulness, privacy, justice, communal responsibility, and the like." The Hippocratic oath is very clear on the issue of privacy: "Whatever, in connection with my professional practice, or not in connection with it, I see or hear, in the life of men, which out not to be spoken of abroad, I will not divulge, as reckoning that all such should be kept secret." Similarly, the oath is clear in its declaration of communal obligation: "Into whatever houses I enter, I will go into them for the benefit of the sick, and will abstain from every voluntary act of mischief and corruption."

These service ideals, embedded in the old ethic, were not challenged by the new technologies and science. Nor were they discarded. In 2010 the oath of the American College of Surgeons, for example, affirmed for its members the "fellowship pledge" first pronounced in the old ethic's Hippocratic oath.[15] That pledge included a vow to practice surgery "with honesty" while affirming and supporting "the social contract of the surgical profession with my community and society." More than thirty years after the first edition of *Principles* first appeared, honesty, implicit in the traditional oath, was reaffirmed in this restatement of "the highest traditions of our ancient profession."

Implicit in the traditional oath was a justice principle: treat all individuals on the basis of their need irrespective of other criteria. It was this ideal of care as a social value that sent physicians into the homes of fifteenth-century plague victims, eighteenth-century yellow fever patients, and nineteenth-century cholera patients. It informed the work of social reformers such as Dr. Rudolf Virchow, Chicago's Dr. Alice Hamilton in the early twentieth century, and more recently, physicians like Harvard's Paul Farmer[16] and the neurologist Oliver Sacks.[17] The justice ideal implicit in the traditional medical ethic was engaged by the vocational ideal of duty invested in the physician as a member of his or her community. The Guild of Surgeons' fellowship pledge, for example, still has its members swear "to affirm and support the social contract of the surgical profession with my community and society." If truthfulness were a criterion it would seem that *Principles*, not the medical profession, fails its standard.

"Professional Ethics"

The heart of the matter resides in *Principles*' promise of a "morality and ethics that is removed from the history of professional ethics." Here, unnoticed, was a radical transposition accomplished with a few keystrokes on the computer keyboard. In describing medicine as a professional ethic whose elements were distinct from its practice, Beauchamp and Childress made of medicine just another profession—like accounting or advertising—without special duties or obligations. What Abraham Verghese has described as the "medical calling"[18] was transposed into a marketplace business like any other, one whose ethics would be that of any marketplace supplier. Medicine thus becomes, in *Principles*, simply one more commodity distributed by one more kind of professional. Physicians were no longer bound by a covenant of service but were service providers and, as such, professionals whose primary obligation was not to the "customer" but to the employer, the insurer, or the research institution. Remember Daniel Callahan's insistence that doctors are mere technicians who should be restricted to the administration of procedures, rather than their selection for the benefit of a patient? As professional technicians of medicine, he said, they should know their place. Bioethicists, *Principles* implies, would be the ones who will explain it to them.

"And the Like . . ."

It is in this spirit that the authors of *Principles* condescendingly (I want to say cavalierly) dismiss as inadequate the old ethic's "rich storehouse of wisdom." At the end of the first paragraph "and the like" was inserted to suggest the broadening field in which the authors' bioethics was to be applied in future unspecified ways. The implication was that not only would *Principles*' bioethics replace the older ethic, but also it would do so in ways too numerous to mention. What*ever* the problem, Beauchamp and Childress's biomedical ethic would be the solution. From this perspective the final sentence is ominous. It promises that proponents of the new bioethical order will avoid the "narrowness" of the traditional medical ethic. The obvious question is: what narrowness? Building line upon line of unfounded assertion leads to a conclusion that defines as exigent problems as yet unperceived but for which the authors' bioethics will be the inevitable answer.

All in all, the first 106 words of *Principles* is a masterpiece of its kind, building fact out of surmise in a seamless construction that makes conjecture real. Its mixture of condescension, error, and sheer authoritative chutzpah is simply brilliant. It insists on problems the older ethic cannot treat and then insists their treatment must be based on a philosophical perspective ignorant of the practical issues of medicine itself. There is no other reasonable response to the first page of *Principles* than to close the book and toss it against the wall. Frustration at this point is not simply understandable but laudable.

"The Philosophical Detour"

Principles' philosophical detour was doomed to fail because it was, to use a painterly analogy, all ground and no figure. It is useful to see *Principles* as an extension of *The Belmont Report,* transposing its research ethics, crafted in part by Tom Beauchamp into his and Childress's biomedical ethic in a one-two ethical punch.[19] *Principles* built upon *Belmont*'s three principles of medical research to create a set of mid-level norms presumably applicable to all issues arising in the governance of medicine in society. *Belmont* was focused on research and *Principles* on broader themes of general medical ethics. In both cases a philosophical method promised to provide essential values that could be translated into practical ethical guidelines in specific situations.

Only Isaac Asimov's famous three laws of robotics, first presented in his 1950 short story collection *I, Robot*, have been more succinct in the advance of a simplistic set of principles-as-laws whose activation requires a complex consideration of competing individual and social moral interests. The difference is that Asimov crafted his rules with full awareness of their practical limits. They were *in theory* a universal rule set capable of governing without amendment the action of thinking machines in relation to each other and their human creators. What made the stories so much fun was that what seemed logically (and philosophically) complete was revealed, in story after dramatic story, to be open to abuse, misinterpretation, and sheer confusion.

Broad laws and general principles, the stories said, are never capable of capturing the nuanced complexity of competent beings, even "thinking machines" with "positronic" brains. Thought of in this way, as a fictional device, the principles of biomedical ethics might have been an admirable pedagogic device. The smart student would be taught to ask, "How many ways does this fail in practice?" Alas, Beauchamp and Childress promoted their rules as principles as if they were complete, inclusive, infallibly serious, applicable truths.

Moral Folk Theory Redux

Invoking "philosophical reflection" served to promote the authority of *Principles*' authors, philosophers, and the methodology they brought from moral philosophy. The implication was that the power of philosophy and its reflective method would enable adepts to identify and then answer moral problems arising from the new science, conundrums the old medical ethic and its practitioners presumably were incapable of addressing. So irrespective of the principles proposed, *Principles* championed a methodology of problem definition and resolution. In service of this goal, its authors formalized the essential assumptions of the moral folk theory introduced in chapter 1: "Reason guides the will by giving it moral laws—laws that specify which acts are morally prohibited, which are required, and which are permissible. Universal reason not only is the source of all moral laws but also tells us how to apply these principles to concrete situations."[20]

Principles' authors did not quote Mark Johnson, of course. Rather, as Beauchamp has said, "the works of Kant were carefully consulted for the wisdom they offer."[21] But whether one quotes Kant or Johnson the result assumes there *is* a single set of moral laws discoverable by rational individuals willing to participate in a specific type of reasoned, unemotional reflection. Further, these rules stand apart from the circumstances of their application or the base needs of the person who seeks their wisdom. The result is something beyond culture and beyond the individual . . . a necessarily universal truth out there, waiting to be discovered. As Charles Taylor put it: "Rationality involves thinking in universal terms and thinking consistently. Hence the maxim underlying any proposed action must be such that we can universalize it without contradiction. If we cannot do this, then we cannot as rational wills [reasoning beings] conscientiously undertake this action."[22]

The whole thus depends on the moral philosopher's faith that dispassionate rational reflection will provide answers reflecting applicable, universal truths. Those answers will be singular and independent of context. Were it otherwise, the law would lose its purpose because every Tom, Dick, and Harry (and every Raul and Serafina) could rationally conjure a consistent set of laws that seemed right to him or her, if *only* to him or her. That would never serve because universal principles rationally derived from revealed moral law (and there was only one such law to be revealed) by definition do not brook eccentricity or multiple interpretations. Further, these laws must be such that they can be understood and then applied consistently in a practical way that leads to one and only one solution to a real world problem.

Kant had no problem in postulating this kind of unconditional. As a Christian he believed in God as the universal lawgiver and thus in moral laws that were absolute and real. It was every person's right and obligation to discover God's universal laws for him- or herself. Through Kant we learn, in other words, to seek the law, not the lawgiver.[23] This theology-at-one-remove underlay Kant's metaphysics even as he struggled to craft a philosophy that was independent of religious dictates. "The exciting kernel of this moral philosophy, which has been immensely influential," writes Taylor, "is the radial notion of freedom. In being determined by a purely formal law, binding on me solely qua rational will, I declare my independence, as it were, from all natural considerations and motives, and from the natural causality which rules them."[24] That is: all natural considerations and motives but one, a belief in the universal law and an allegiance to it.

This *is* thrilling. It makes each of us a rational will capable of independently discovering God's universal that is out there, somewhere, waiting for us to find it. Its perception occurs wholly apart from the natural desires and emotions that exist amid the interpersonal and social uncertainties that attend to real problems. Thinking about them would only impede us in this search, however, distracting us from the universal truths that are within our free, rational grasp if only we seek it purely. From this perspective the ignorance of moral philosophers about the realities of science or the practice of medicine becomes a virtue. Unlike patient or practitioner the analytic moral philosopher is unfettered by the ambiguities and complexities that attend upon the treatment of one person by another in a community.

Bioethicists become the law seekers, in this imagining, unencumbered by the messiness of the real. The problem is that the bioethics of *Principles* is agnostic, its arguments made without reference to a deity. And yet the assumption of a single moral truth is inherently theistic. Without that, laws are not discovered but crafted; they are not eternal and universal but tentative and specific to the culture in which they are produced. We are left with nothing but moral pluralism, a set of assumptions that each leads to a different outcome, a different practice depending on the context of first their construction and then their implementation. Logic and its methods of problem definition and resolution only go so far and rarely far enough. That's why Asimov's three laws of robotics were sufficient in theory but never in practice to order robot-human behavior in that fictional world. And that is why the principles Beauchamp and Childress proclaimed were never sufficient to resolve issues of medical care and research.

In the end, the authors of *Principles* found themselves in the same jam as Kant who, ultimately, could not present, as Taylor put it, "a new substantive vision of the polity in which it [his philosophy] is to be realized."[25] Kant's problem was there was no clear link between the ecclesiastical polity of his ethics and the polity of the state within which he lived. That is, the state of ethics derived from his vision of moral law could not be transposed into a system of popular morality in the political state of his day.

To argue an agnostic vision of applicable moral law *Principles* (and *Belmont*) would have had to define a state (in its widest sense) that answered to the virtues their ideals promoted (justice, beneficence, etc.). But at no point in its many versions do *Principles*' authors take on the nature of the state in which they seek to order the complexities of medical practice and research. They assume its benevolence. They assume its potential for justice. They assume the freedom of the individual is not only permitted but encouraged (by all but doctors) in the socioeconomic systems in place in the second half of the twentieth century. But, as we have seen, the idea of the individual in his or her freedom was decidedly secondary to the priorities of neoliberal cost accountancies advancing the future economics of the state over the immediate needs of the individual.

Humanness

Kant grounded his philosophical imaginings in a belief that humanity was special and therefore to be nurtured and protected. Humankind was God's work, after all, and His highest creation. Underlying his thinking therefore was not simply a respect for human dignity (*menuschliche Würde*) but the dignity of humanity at large (*Würde der Menschheit*).

"Kant finds the universal principle of morality in the feeling—and not in the idea—that 'human nature' is, as such, worthy of respect."[26] That is, the traces of the grand law he seeks to discover, and thus of God's handiwork, are lodged in the nature of humanity at large. "There was a time when . . . I despised the people, who know nothing. Rousseau corrected me in this. This binding prejudice disappeared. I learned to honor man."[27] It was in the humanness of personhood that each individual's potential for morally perfectibility resided. It was in the human ideal that individual moral freedom was situated. In both resided the hope for us as a moral, self-aware species seeking the good.

The purpose of Kant's *Groundwork for the Metaphysics of Morals* was "nothing more than the investigation and establishment of the *supreme principle of morality*" and thus the basis of ethical and moral reasoning.[28] That investigation was predicated on his belief in human worthiness and thus the inherent worth of individual human beings. Certainly, Kant was all for the "practical faculty of appraising" over the "theoretical in common human understanding."[29] That was why he distinguished between what bioethics conflates from the start, abstract ideas of human dignity and choice on the one hand, the practicalities of social action and interaction on the other. But practicality was not his goal. It was, however, the goal of *Principles*.

Had *Principles*' authors—and other bioethicists—taken seriously the philosophical grounding of bioethics, "the philosophical detour," there was a way out. They might have embraced Kant's sense of humanity as privileged and protected, and thus an organizing principle of the ethics they sought to create. The idea of humanity as a protected good might have served as an existential universal from which other values could be derived. But without that strong humanist core as a unifying concept, the result is frosting without any cake beneath it, pleasing perhaps but unsubstantial.

Physician-philosopher-cum-ethicist Tristram Engelhardt saw the problem early on. In *Belmont*'s deliberations he suggested a principle of "respect for humans as free moral agents, concern to support the best interests of human subjects in research, intent to assure that the use of human subjects of experimentation will on the sum redound to the benefit of society."[30] This would have made of humanity at large a largely protected category and "free moral agents" a subset of humanity at large. The emphasis for medical research would, as Osler had suggested, emphasize the care and protection of the human subject first and foremost.

If with Engelhardt we begin with the common and protected humanity of all persons, deriving from that universal the importance of each individual, we make of that commonality an absolute referent against which all ethics and morality are to be fashioned. It was this ideal that in the first half of the twentieth century was embedded in more than thirty-seven national constitutions, the United Nations Charter of 1945, the General Declaration of Human Rights of 1948, and later, a host of other conventions—including those supposedly governing research use of human subjects.[31] The dignity (and protection) that results is not based on individual characteristics or traits but communal species membership.

Belmont's authors chose instead to advance a more limited "respect for persons." *Principles* transformed respect for persons into respect for an abstract ideal, "autonomy." "Beauchamp and Childress did not identify respect for persons as their principle and foremost principle. Instead, in *Principles of Biomedical Ethics,* the principle of respect for persons became the principle of autonomy, or *respect* for *autonomy*," typically defined as a type of demonstrable rational capability.[32] To value autonomy meant drawing a circle around those having a set of identifiable, observable, contingent characteristics, permitting a kind of self-conscious cognition.

In this formulation those judged autonomously incapable, the Carrie Bucks of society, could easily be denied care or respect. Having been denied respect they could then be denied protection. Crudely put: bye-bye dummies, idiots, and morons. Bye-bye those who fail to meet some measure of demonstrable performance the ethicist-philosopher advances as worthy. The result cut away the heart of the arguments of Kant and his successors while still somehow insisting upon their "wisdom" as a basis for bioethics.

After both *Belmont* and *Principles* a vigorous cottage industry developed among ethicist-philosophers seeking to parse the line between autonomous and thus enabled persons and those who were more or less disposable except, perhaps, as research subjects or graft-organ repositories. Thomasma listed the essential attributes of the protected person of bioethics as consciousness, the ability to communicate, self-awareness, and the potential for growth and development.[33] The result, as he and Eric Loewy set out these criteria, were: "The major distinctions along the continuum of personhood are nonperson, preperson, person, and postperson with many gradations in between. Nonpersonal human life forms are those that do not possess the potentiality for personhood."[34]

Personhood as a function of cognitive and communicative performance became the principal criterion distinguishing the ethically protected from the morally expendable. The result divided humanity and its social members into categories of real people with choices and nonpersons without choices. These categories of worth were easily married to the idea of scarcity of resources. If Carrie Buck is an idiot she can't think, at least not as the philosopher defines thinking, and is therefore disposable. There is no injustice or inequity in her forced sterilization to inhibit her ability to produce more "idiots" who will be similarly useless burdens upon the state. If a stroke has destroyed a person's (call her Freida) communicative faculties, and affected her rational mind, then a decision for noncare or termination (withdrawing respiratory assistance, nutrition and hydration, etc.) is only logical. The cost of her maintenance argues for that choice.

The result is a thoroughly conflicted ethic. It proposes the autonomy of the person and his or her choice as sacred while permitting and perhaps encouraging the disavowal of individual choices (by the person or surrogate) in the absence of this or that contingent attribute. While asserting the value of the autonomous person it simultaneously permits that individual choices be dismissed (for example, the desire of the fragile senior for curative care) on the basis of communal necessity, defined economically. Chapters 7 and 8 will argue the inadequacy of almost all of the attribute categories that bioethicists use to parse the human condition into salvageable and disposable lots.

At the center of the bioethical construction—*Belmont* to *Principles* and into the present—is simple ignorance leavened by hubris. Bioethicists assumed that medical science was capable of assessing the characteristics of the person as an autonomous, cognitive being along the continuum described by Thomasma and Lowry. Hubris was engaged when, as philosophers, bioethicists did not deem it necessary to investigate the science that was and remains incapable of such determinations. To offer one example: In the mid-1990s studies of persons assumed to be in "persistent vegetative states"—and thus beyond the autonomous pall—found that between 15 and 34 percent were misdiagnosed. Many were in fact minimally conscious if not, in a few cases, wholly conscious, but were "locked in" without the capacity to speak or act independently.[35] By the first decade of the current century, new neurological evidence drew into question if not disrepute the assumptions of communicative and rational limits that into the mid-1990s seemed indisputable.[36] On the basis of the best of neurology one could not argue the abandonment of the person on the grounds of what were in retrospect coarse and inaccurate systems of cognitive assessment.

Simplicities

Great philosophy does not necessarily make great ethics. At best its argument is a first step in the mapping of our journey from here to there, from concrete problem to acceptable resolution. Ironically, in attempting to fashion a set of principles that were universal and law-like, Beauchamp and Childress gave us a principled set that was very much like those embedded in the old Hippocratic ethic it sought to replace and the Judeo-Christian ethic whose religiosity it sought to ignore. *Belmont*'s respect for the person was more or less the old Judeo-Christian virtue of "respect for others" that for Hippocrates meant care for the patient irrespective of his or her abilities. Beneficence, the injunction to do good wherever one can, was Hippocrates' "Into whatever house I go . . ." Nonmaleficence was in fact simply the Christian injunction to abjure evil or, in the Hippocratic argument, to "first, do no harm." Arguments for and from justice are not new. What was new here, however, was the transformation of these hoary ethical injunctions into a utilitarian balance of benefit and harm. To the extent that it advanced the "knowledge industry" over the person, social constraints over values of care, the result denied the best of old ethics bioethics attempted to restate and retain.

The Common Morality

"The world is independent of my will," wrote Wittgenstein (*Tractatus* 6.373). But the authors of *Principles* seem to suggest, "My will is independent of the world." In doing so they, and the majority of bioethicists today, assume the polity of the state, its organization and its ideals, are a given whose elements need not be considered. As Hippocrates knew, however, applied ethics is about individuals in relation to others coexisting within a community. Morality is always constructed within the shared boundaries of experience and circumstance. If one seeks to create an ethic of practice its attention must attend at least as much to the ethics environment of the community as it does to the moral imagining of the person.

Ethics is never an isolates' game. The question of "what should I do" is a convenient shorthand for a complex query about what can be done with and to and for another in a context that may either promote or inhibit his or her care. The context of choices is anchored at once in an external reality "out there," a philosophy of good and right; "down here" in the clinic with the resource available, and "over there" in a political conversation on economic order.[37] That complexity is what *Principles* ignored from the start.

The Common Morality

Given the preceding, it is not surprising that the principalist is a thoroughly endangered species except, perhaps, in bioethics. "I want simply to call attention to leading assumptions of principlism," wrote Charles Bosk in 1999, "namely, that the individual is the proper measure of all things ethical, that tools for measurement transcend culture, and that there is a single, correct solution for each ethical problem, which is largely independent of person, place, or time. At the time that this ethical universalism is gaining ascendance in the world of medicine, it is being rejected in virtually every other sphere of society."[38]

The problem was, and remains, that the philosophical groundwork on which specific principles can be argued in ways that are applicable and generally accepted has never been clear. Philosophy is an orientation, not a game plan. Perhaps accepting this, and the limits of their argument, by the end of the 1980s Beauchamp and Childress gave up on a philosophical groundwork for their ethics as a practical endeavor. "Beginning with the third edition of PBE [*Principles of Bioethics*], published in 1989, Beauchamp and Childress relocated the source of their bioethical principles from philosophical theory to what they came to call 'the common morality.'"[39]

Had Beauchamp and Childress begun their third edition by writing, "Wow, were we naive! All that fine philosophy stuff didn't work. We're going to switch gears, maybe try some anthropology," it would have been both admirable and (dare I say it?) honorable. To write that would have been to admit the failure of the enterprise at large, however. That would have raised questions about the legitimacy of a bioethics that promised answers based upon the philosophical methodology lodged deep in its foundational core. Instead, Beauchamp and Childress continued to insist on the philosophical as a necessary methodology; otherwise, why read them at all? Instead of the universal good they promoted in its place a "common morality." Forget philosophy. As for common wisdom? Call a pollster.

Positing a "set of norms shared by all persons committed to morality,"[40] the authors' definition of common wisdom implies that all those who disagree either with the norms' definition, or the bioethicist's interpretation of those norms, are not committed to morality. And because the judge here is to be the bioethicist whose job is to interpret and apply this morality, the norms are those things that the bioethicists accept as common and shared by right-thinking people. The result is exclusory; reducing the "moral space" Andre sought, as described in chapter 1, to one approved by the bioethicist.

The original goal of bioethics was to create a singular and broadly accepted "canonical content-full morality" that would serve across the landscape of medical practice and research.[41] That goal has failed spectacularly. Not only is there no single common morality, but also the idea of a conventional and generally accepted set of ethical definitions (forget the means of their application) remains illusive. In talking about "justice," for example, do we favor John Rawls's justice of political fairness,[42] Harsanyi's utilitarian justice,[43] or Robert Nozick's libertarian justice? In thinking about morality do we look to Carol Gilligan[44] whose feminist critique still resonates across disciplines today, or Lawrence Kohlberg's rational progression of progressively thin, dispassionately logical ethical frames?[45] Common wisdom requires at least a measure of definitional agreement and that has been in very short supply at every level across the time period *of Principles*' various editions. Think about the many ways the idea of "autonomy" is defined and redefined by a cadre of authors.[46] And without clear, generally accepted definitions there is no method of resolution. Think about the unending debates over the appropriateness of abortion, euthanasia, eugenics, and physician-assisted suicide.

What a moment for a Hegelian seeking an opportunity for synthesis! Everywhere ideas contest in a range of disciplines and practices, all seeking but failing to create a more or less common ground. If ever there was a time for the ecumenical exploration of moral intuitions in social situations (and of the social situations that give rise to moral dilemmas)—this was it. Alas, like dyslexic supermen, *Principles*' authors and their intellectual inheritors all wore the guise of the common man (and woman) over the uniform of the superior philosopher. But the tattered undergarment of superiority always shone through because without it they'd just be . . . ordinary men and women.

And that's what bioethical founders were, ordinary men and women caught in the realities of their culture and society. As proponents of what they understood to be a common *American* morality, bioethicists became apologists for it, reflexively accepting its framework. The role of the bioethicist was not to question the social status quo or "speak truth to power," as Brody had it in an earlier quote, but to accept power and work within its permitted structures. "Even though we must be cautious about the tyranny of the modern, secular state," wrote Dave Thomasma in the 1990s, "its benefits in terms of individual freedom of expression are obvious."[47] The American ethic *Principles* advanced almost always promoted the latter but never really worried overmuch about its participation in the evils of the former. And it was there, in the tyranny of the modern secular state's economic priorities, that individual freedoms would either be promoted or truncated.

"There are moments in history when the very nature of class power, and the forms taken by its manufacture of the future, make questions of ethics and rhetoric—questions of representation—primary, or at least unavoidable."[48] Taken together, *The Belmont Report* and *Principles of Biomedical Ethics* were one of those moments. Their real role—fulfilled admirably—was to legitimate in medicine the forms of power and purpose inherent in the American politics of the day. The result promoted a political perspective as if it were a philosophical ideal, a brand of

American *real politik* as if it were universally acceptable and as rigorous as, well, Kant's *Critiques*. The test is not, perhaps, Brody's question—whether bioethics "speaks truth to power"—but whether it speaks truth at all.

Today, many bioethicists dismiss the principalist arguments of Beauchamp. They retain, however, a strong allegiance to *Principles*' assumption that the analytic method learned in philosophy is the appropriate road to the resolution of dilemmas arising in medical practice and research. They retain, in their criticisms, the general assumption that ethics is a rational thing whose referent is a morality that exists apart from the interpersonal and social contexts in which those dilemmas occur. At the least, there are few critiques out there that take the fundamental form of *Principles* as their concern. Chapters 7 and 8 will consider the manner in which the trained philosopher applies the general precepts and method of bioethics to questions of ethical concern. None of them could be labeled, like Gillon, disciples of *Principles* although their arguments share much of its core approach, and its values. The question becomes not whether that approach creates a common wisdom—it clearly doesn't—but whether it permits a broad "moral space," in Andres's words, for the consideration of differences.

7

Bioethics and Conformal Humans

"He insists he doesn't want to kill me," Harriet McBryde Johnson wrote of Princeton University bioethicist Peter Singer in 2003. "He simply thinks it would have been better, all things considered, to have given my parents the option of killing the baby I once was, and to let other parents kill similar babies as they come along and thereby avoid the suffering that comes with lives like mine and satisfy the reasonable preferences of parents for a different kind of child. It has nothing to do with me," she continued. "I should not feel threatened."[1]

That precise, lawyerly summation opened McBryde Johnson's 2003 *New York Times Magazine* essay, "Unspeakable Conversations," describing her meetings and lectures with Singer (figure 7.1) at Princeton. McBryde Johnson was an activist, author, and lawyer whose congenital spinal malformation required the use of a wheelchair and lifelong help with pedestrian daily activities. This meant, for her, a life that while different from the norm was in no way necessarily inferior. Singer, for his part, saw her life, and by extension those of others with limiting cognitive, physical, or sensory attributes, as if not natural tragedies then mistakes of nature that need not be accepted.

Their association, and presentations, were "unspeakable" because neither she nor Singer had the language to make explicable to the other the philosophy each sought separately to present. They thus talked at but not with each other. The meeting of these two different minds was not merely "unspeakable" but also unthinkable—a subject they could not together consider—because the lawyer Johnson and the philosopher Singer applied not only two different languages but two different types of thinking and two different definitional sets. There was therefore no

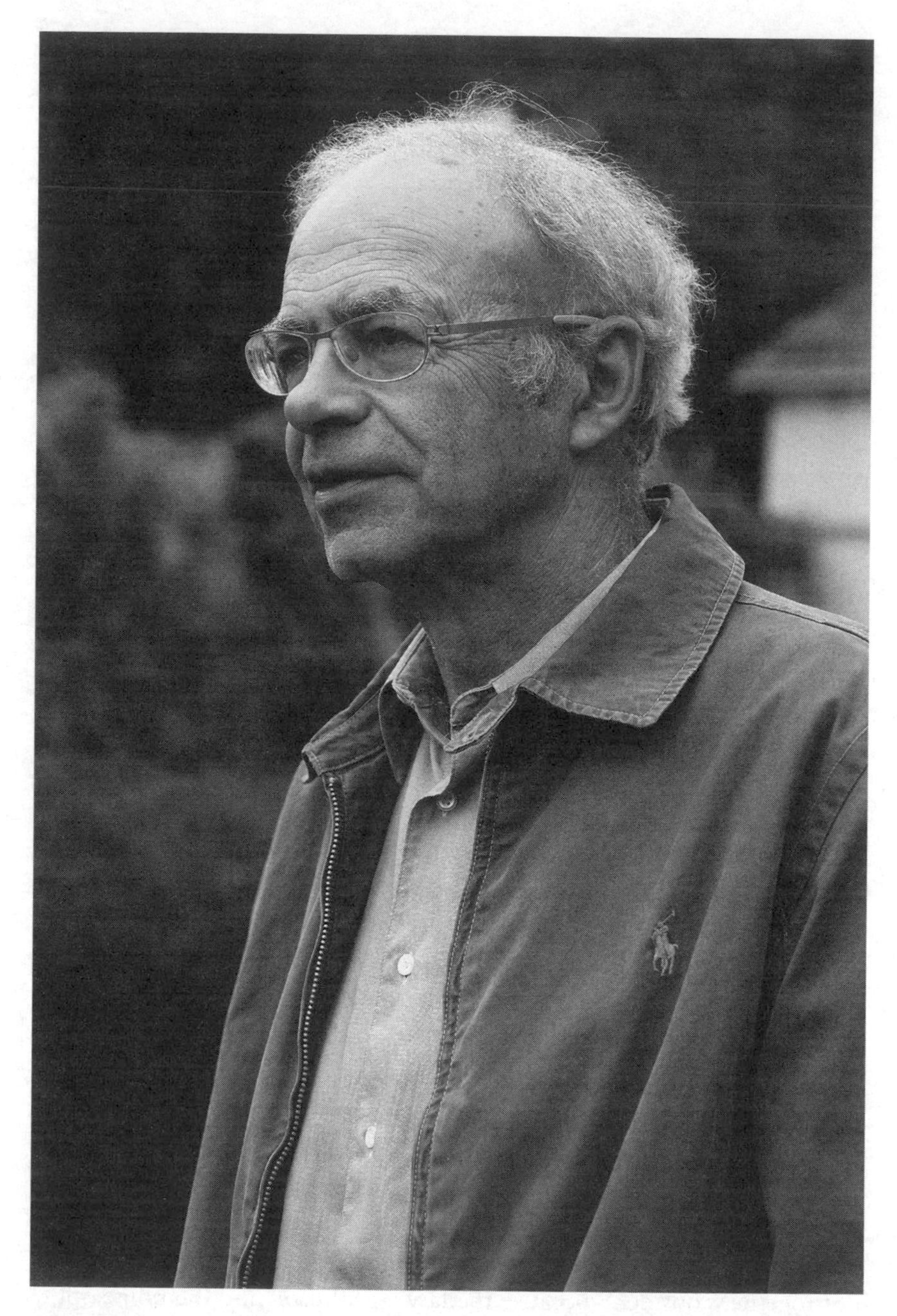

Figure 7.1
Peter Singer was the subject of Harriet McBryde Johnson's description of their meeting at Princeton University where Singer teaches. The opposing views of the two were sufficiently distinct to represent two fundamentally different perspectives on the human condition. *Source*: Ulrika Magnusson, photographer.

meeting of the minds, merely a passing glimpse of ideas that never really confronted each other.

Thinking about the shared failure of McBryde Johnson and Singer is a way to think about bioethics' blindness—prejudice may not be too strong a word—to issues of human diversity, of cognitive, sensory, and physical difference. What results is an implicit emphasis on productive, conformal normalcy rather than the range of human realities that exist in the community and in the clinician's world. And, too, it emphasizes the degree to which the assumption of a formal approach of disinterested rationality fails to confront the equally consistent, rational, but distinct perspective of those who argue from the experiential to the general. To see the problem one must first understand the exchange and its principal disputants—"debaters" would be too strong a word.

Disputants

What made the *New York Times* essay so delicious was that Singer is among the most influential of bioethicists, one whose writings are themselves the subject of independent scholarly study,[2] his *Practical Ethics* a standard text in university ethics courses.[3] As a self-described preference utilitarian, Singer is avowedly less interested in individual circumstance than in maximizing the sum quota of universal happiness while minimizing the sum quota of general suffering, as he understands them. Because he assumes limiting characteristics necessarily diminish an individual's happiness, and increase the suffering of both that person and his or her caregivers, why not, Singer asks, simply avoid (through abortion, euthanasia, and so on) the deficit these existences present? After all, he assumes, they must subtract from the totality of happiness by the suffering they impose individually.

Singer's general perspective, fairly summarized by McBryde Johnson, is representative of a class of bioethical argumentation. For example, another utilitarian, John Harris, similarly perceives the self-conscious decision to carry to term a fetus with a "harmed condition" (Down syndrome, deafness, spinal bifida, etc.) as harmful, and thus by implication ethically questionable.[4] In a similar vein, Jonathan Glover insists that "genetic disadvantage should come to be seen as injustice," and thus the avoidable birth of people like McBryde Johnson—those with inherent and limiting cognitive, physical, or sensory differences—becomes in his thinking if not a crime certainly an inequity.[5] In Glover's language "disadvantage" is any inheritable characteristic that results in a capacity that differs negatively from the norm. In building his argument Glover in turn references both Harris and an impressive host of other ethicist-philosophers.[6]

While some will reject Singer's (or Harris's) utilitarianism, and the conclusions from it, the argument he presents and represents shares much with the general bioethical perspective. None criticize Singer (or by extension others who agree with him) for his method of dispassionate, philosophically grounded analysis. His arguments are grounded in a belief in rationality as a criterion of the valued person and, too, in rationality as a kind of dispassionate discourse by which ethical issues are to be framed and then considered. Most bioethicists thus will accept Singer's methodology and many accept, to a greater or lesser degree, the criteria with which he weighs lives and their futures. With the exception of some "disability" theorists, in other words, the general landscape of the Singerian argument is broadly bioethical even if its particulars may be disputed occasionally by some.

McBryde Johnson writes about Singer not just because he is famous, or because the extremes of his views make him a convenient target, but also because Singer courteously invited her to Princeton to discuss their differences. Knowing his views are controversial, Singer goes out of his way to meet with those who do not agree with him. Time after time he has stood before hostile audiences, calmly arguing what seems obvious to him but is incomprehensible to many in the audience. And where it is comprehensible the arguments he advances seem to some brutish and distasteful. In post-lecture question periods few critics can articulate their objections in a way Singer the philosopher accepts as reasonable, or if reasonable then compelling. McBryde Johnson is only the best known of many who have unsuccessfully argued with Singer his Singerian point of view.

To simplify: Singer assumes a person with a physical, cognitive, or sensory difference must live less fully than the normal person. Because one rolls rather than walks, speaks with sign language rather than vocalizing, or reads by Braille rather than seeing words on the page (or screen) life must be less, and suffering must certainly be greater. By definition, if someone needs assistance in daily activities this must present a burden to the caregivers who assist the person in need. Burden and suffering are bad so why not avoid them? Why not go for normal, at the least?

As I understand him, Singer is the logical endpoint of bioethics as we have come to know it. He is not a particular fan of *Principles* and its methods but he is no critic of its principles transposed into a utilitarian calculus of total pleasure or suffering: Singer thus is for beneficence, justice, fairness, and nonmalfeasance, as he understands them. Their definition and interpretation, however, are filtered through a perspective in which we are all fungible, interchangeable elements of a greater totality. His focus is the big picture of sum gain, not the eccentricities and exigencies of the individual life. Singer is distinguished from others—for example, Glover—by the precision of his language and the clarity of his definitions. If you accept his definitions and you agree with his method then his conclusions seem necessarily to follow.

There is nothing unusual here. At least since Kant one or another kind of utilitarianism has been the reflexive response when vacuous ideals (in the sense that Kant's broad rational imperatives are empty) were applied to life's complex situations. Lifeboat ethics can be seen as a utilitarian context in which the needs of the many will always outweigh the desires of the fragile few. In the lifeboat or on shore a person's and society's choices should, as Kant said and Singer agrees, be based on some kind of universal value. Those are the ideas that philosophers seek to define and ethicists apply.[7] If you accept the assumption of scarcity that has been a motive force of bioethical advance, and if you accept bioethics' rationality—as a criterion of worth and a method of argument—then Singer's arguments become not only sensible but also an inevitable and logical conclusion. If and . . . if.

Singer sees the idea of human sanctity as at best outmoded baggage: "After ruling our thoughts and our decisions about life and death for nearly two thousand years, the traditional western ethic has collapsed."[8] Forget Kant's humanitarian ideals and the humanistic *Geist* of Hegel.[9] Singer, an early proponent of animal rights, takes the criterion of rationality in its broadest sense—most mammals think, at least to some degree—as a criterion of ethical protection. So too he assumes suffering irrespective of species membership is a crucial criterion in the ethics of our responsibilities. For Singer, humans are at best a special but not unique case within the general ethic he proposes.

While most bioethicists pay lip service to the idea of human worth and inclusiveness in practice, as we have seen, they draw tight a sphere of protected humanness to exclude the "pre-person" (the fetus before birth), the "post-person" (one who while alive is incapacitated and unable to participate socially), the fragile senior, and those others who fail this or that more or less utilitarian performance standard. Except for vitalists—who continue to believe in the sanctity of human life as an ordering ideal—and the disability activists who insist function is not the metric of individual importance—in the end most bioethicists are in-the-closet Singerians, at least in the lifeboat of scarce resources they assume we all necessarily inhabit.

McBryde Johnson

McBryde Johnson (figure 7.2) advanced a different ethical metric, embodying in her physicality the insistence that characteristics deviating negatively from the norm (she would not call them impairments) need not signal the personal or social failure of the life within. McBryde Johnson consistently denied the inherent suffering Singer assumed to be a necessary result of her condition, and by extension, of other persons with cognitive, physical, or sensory differences. She denied, too, the insistence that her life would have been happier or more satisfying or more socially productive were she—well, more like Singer, like you, or like me.

Here was the first barrier, the first insurmountable obstacle. Singer argued an ethic of at least normalcy in which the failure to meet its standard necessarily results in a life that is more burdensome (to others) and necessarily less fulfilling (for the person) than the average life. For him this is definitional and all else follows from those definitions. McBryde Johnson argued from the particular, her own experience and that of her friends, to insist Singer's assumptions did not meet the test of experience. Singer found the argument from experience not so much unconvincing as incredible. His very polite skepticism exemplified what Havi Carel has called the "striking feature of many healthy people—[the inability] to conceive of the lives of others" that are different from their own.[10] For McBryde Johnson, Singer's failure to accept her argument

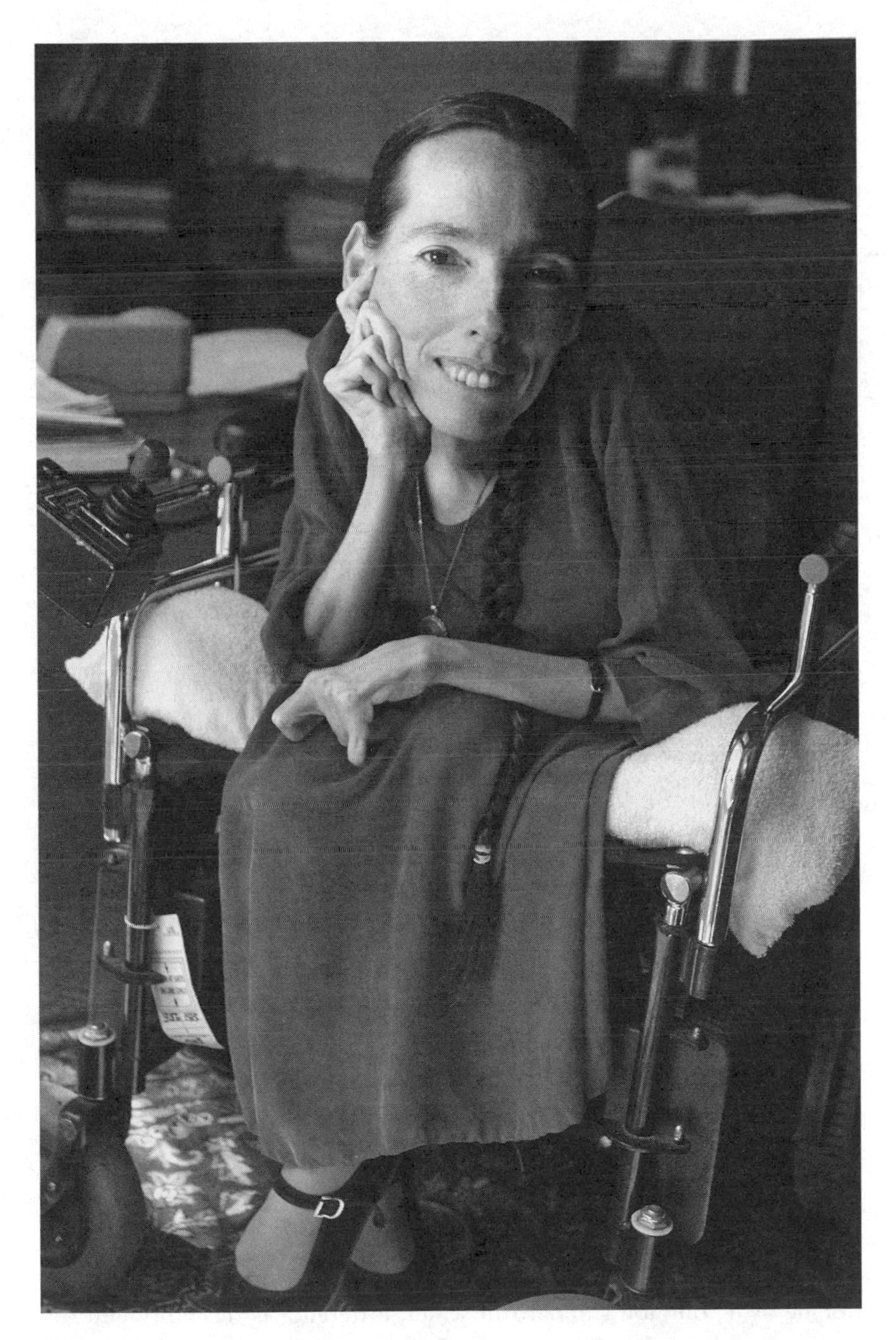

Figure 7.2
As author and lawyer, Harriet McBryde Johnson came to symbolize for many the argument that physical differences do not define necessarily either the quality of a life or its worth. *Source*: Wade Spees.

from experience was perhaps best perceived as a failure of moral imagination. In her article she was too polite to point out the very eugenic flavor of his conclusions or, as the next chapter argues, of the bioethics that may result from his assumptions.

After McBryde Johnson's death in 2008, Singer wrote a memorial in the *New York Times* titled "Happy Nonetheless" that infuriated her supporters.[11] Why ask the devil to praise the honorable fallen?[12] Indeed, others may have asked: Who better? Almost certainly, McBryde Johnson would have been either amused or irritated, depending on her mood. Her argument was always that familial and personal happiness are not defined by one's eccentricities or measurable characteristics but instead by a person's communal strengths. That she might need help in dressing was neither a necessary burden nor a failure in her life. Others might need her help in crafting a legal brief, perhaps, or in other activities where she excelled. That was, for McBryde Johnson, simply the diverse reality of a community of people, together. That one rolls rather than walks has no necessary bearing on the person's potential for happiness or social importance and thus should carry no weight in the accounts of benefits and burdens that utilitarians (and many bioethicists) typically advance. She was happy because she was McBryde Johnson, an author and lawyer and an embodied human being at ease with herself and in her community. That she used a wheelchair and needed help getting around in it was simply a fact of life, not a barrier to its quality. Nonetheless? Indeed.

Differences

In opposing Singer's normalcy McBryde Johnson was challenging a tradition that, as we have seen, stretches back to the nineteenth century and the birth of eugenics. She thus challenged as well, in the present, an established set of valuations whose adherents extend beyond the immediate world of Singer's influence. Contractarian justice theorists like John Rawls have been repeatedly criticized for a similar set of assumptions.[13] In his 1971 *A Theory of Justice*, Rawls assumed a normal range of functioning as a common standard in which difference is disability and the disabled are to be excluded from his definitions of political justice in modern society. Thus Rawls's "fair equality of opportunity" was only for those with similar characteristics and potentials.[14] Those whose cognitive, physical, or sensory characteristics deviate negatively from the norm were simply off the Rawlsian justice map. More recently, Norman Daniels invoked a similar idea of "species normal opportunity range," as a standard for his healthcare ethics.[15] Those with limiting characteristics are outside that range and thus largely beyond the bounds of justice and beneficence in the dispensing of scarce health resources. They can be discounted—like the Ashbury policy's seniors—in the lifeboat ethics of a world of limited resources.

And yet, the idea of a "normal opportunity range," like the Singerian equation of impairments with suffering, unhappiness, and disutility, is challenged by a generation of researchers. There is a wealth of social science that advances the type of argument McBryde Johnson presented in her Princeton lectures.[16] Brody summarizes the central conclusion of this literature by distinguishing "impairment" ("a dysfunction of the body") from the "handicap" that results from social constraints limiting the person with impairments. "Disability" becomes in this ordering the result of social policies that disadvantage persons with specific attributes rather than the inevitable consequence of individually limiting characteristics.[17] Differences exist, in other words, but it is the manner in which they are addressed or ignored by the community at large that makes them disabling and thus painfully burdensome.

"The importance of these distinctions is shown by research on quality of life as perceived by persons with disabilities," writes Brody. "Medical people [and most bioethicists] generally assume that the more severe one's impairment or disability, the worse the quality of life that will be experienced. This turns out generally to be untrue. Instead, one's quality of life is almost completely bound up with handicap. The extent to which society will or will not make accommodations."[18] It is this conclusion, defining disability as an unjust social outcome rather than a naturally disadvantageous reality that bioethicists from Callahan to Singer and Daniels do not so much contest as ignore. In doing so, they absolve society and themselves, as citizens and bioethicists, of any responsibility for the disability-creating failure of social support. It follows (although Brody does not make this point) that to the extent bioethics does not address the social elements that disable the person, it is complicit in their effect on persons of difference.

Traditional medical ethics advanced a general principle of care without qualification. Because bioethics does not, and because it has no overriding principle of human sanctity, bioethicists can and routinely do deny the ethical necessity of care for all as a human right. Because it takes scarcity as a fundamental position, and thus lifeboat ethics as its constructive starting point, those with cognitive, sensory, or physical limits (they can't row the boat!) will always be seen as less likely candidates for medical (and social) attention. This explains, at least in part, I think, why while hundreds of papers have been written in bioethics journals advocating a "right to die," and euthanasia as a right of rational individual choice, few have argued the right to "live with dignity despite difference."[19]

As a practical ethic, bioethics thus at once gives and takes away from the person of difference. "*Of course*" people like McBryde Johnson can choose the care they want but that choice need not be supported socially where assistance runs counter to economic realities or prevailing ideologies. *Of course* these impairments, deviations from the norm, must diminish life's quality, and of course, the requirements for care by definition will be burdensome both to the person himself or herself and to others. *Of course* our future would be better if their limiting conditions did not exist ("three generations of idiots is enough," as Oliver Wendell Holmes said). Anything else is . . . paradoxical and thus unbelievable.[20] People may say their life is fine, despite this or that limitation, but that is probably just rationalization. The old Hippocratic ethic and its "human centred western tradition" irrespective of capacities is out the window.[21] Modern neoliberal perspectives demand nothing less of its bioethics.

The Nondebate

McBryde Johnson's report of her meeting with Singer and his students made all this clear in a single moment of mutual incomprehensibility: "I told a story about a family I knew as a child," she wrote in her article, "which took loving care of a non-responsive teenage girl, acting out their unconditional commitment to each other, making all the other children, and me as their visitor, feel safe." Singer sought to clarify, for the purpose of the discussion, that one could know "absolutely" the teenager was not only persistently and totally unconscious but that "we can know, absolutely, that the individual will never regain consciousness." "Assuming all that," Singer asked, "don't you think continuing to take care of that individual would be a bit—weird?" "No. Done right, it could be profoundly beautiful."[22]

The best that could be mustered by the Princeton philosopher and the activist lawyer were the warring adjectives "weird" and "beautiful." The conversation between them began and ended with that unbridgeable difference. For McBryde Johnson, the nonresponsive teenager was simply . . . nonresponsive (and what teenager isn't?) but still a person who was a member of a family who cared for her. For Singer, she was a post-person maintained against all reason in a permanent vegetative state. That made of her a noncognitive, breathing artifact of the person who once was, and perhaps sentimentally, might have been. From this point of view the family members' continuing care was wasted effort (and a lot of effort was required). It was burden without return or benefit, at best weird if not also a tad insane.

The nonresponsive teenager lay at one end of a human continuum that stretches from the patient in a coma, to the person who is congenitally deaf or blind or mildly lame, to the super athlete or advanced thinker. In the middle of this broad spectrum sat McBryde Johnson in her wheelchair. She was undeniably smart and savvy and socially productive. She was also an exemplar of the kind of physical eccentricities signifying burden and harm to Singer, and by extension to others. Some, like McBryde Johnson, may seem to triumph over their limits but the individual hero's eccentric success only highlights the nature of limits themselves. Despite her protests Singer assumed McBryde Johnson's physicality must mean a lesser life quality, greater suffering, and thus a diminished happiness that any sane person would avoid. Rational parents would avoid imposing such a burden on their children-to-be, and on future generations, not to mention the onus of care with minimal return such parentage would require.

Phooey, said McBryde Johnson. Her parents did not regret her birth and she did not regret her life. She was Harriet McBryde Johnson and from the perspective of her wheelchair—and her parents' armchairs—that was more than good enough.

Lots of Weird

The persistently unconscious teenager of McBryde Johnson's story was more than a symbol. She was a reality, one of thousands of people continued in an unconscious state for shorter and sometimes long periods in the United States. Some are on ventilators and all receive nutrition and hydration support.[23] Over the years I have two or three times been introduced, as was McBryde Johnson, to unconscious family members maintained at home by their loved ones.[24] I have at other times consulted with and for families, as well as for hospital ethics committees, considering the continuation or termination of persons in similar unconscious states.

All this is important because how we think about the persistently unconscious teenager dictates how we think of others along the continuum of fragilities and difference: the fetus and the neonate, at one end of life's continuum, and the senior with advanced dementia or multiple diagnoses at the other.[25] More generally, how we think about them dictates how we think about "futility" as a rationale for noncare when medicine cannot return a person to some approximation of normal function.[26] Consciousness, futility, and the nature of personhood were central to the public and professional debates over the seven-year legal battle waged over the care or noncare of Floridian patient Terry Schiavo, for example.[27] Because she was as persistently unconscious as McBryde Johnson's teenager, Schiavo's husband sought to have her feeding tube removed so she might die of malnutrition and dehydration. Her parents, who insisted that death by dehydration and malnutrition was not in their daughter's best interests (thus assuming she had interests), were opposed.[28] In short, the focal point of the McBryde Johnson–Peter Singer debate had general consequence.

The Science

For all his philosophizing, Singer thinks of himself as a practical fellow.[29] "As a consequentialist, he writes, "my ethical arguments depend on a careful estimate of what the consequences of our actions are likely to be, and for that we must be guided by experience."[30] Here, too, most bioethicists join him in arguing consequential practicality in the application of the deep wisdom of their philosophy-grounded ethics. That philosophy insists a person is one in whom communicable, self-conscious awareness is demonstrable and thus evident. Those for whom such demonstrable capabilities are not in evidence are—less. But Singer is not a nurse, physician, or therapist daily engaged in the lives whose quality he judges. He does not live with persons of difference and his "estimates" are not so much practical as theoretical, intellectual constructs based upon little knowledge of applicable medical science and apparently, no experience in the thick complexity of the experiential real. There is thus no "ground truthing," as the physical scientist would say, no field check in which experiential investigation is used to confirm or deny a prejudice, supposition, or theory.

Singer was careful to preface his argument with the conditional assumption that "we can know, absolutely, that the individual will never regain consciousness." With this he assumed, first, that there is a single, precisely knowable consciousness against which can be opposed an equally certain reality of persistent unconsciousness that some call, to me inappropriately, a "vegetative state." Further, he assumed that a definitive state of appropriate consciousness could be accurately measured, assessed as to its presence or absence, and if present, accurately measured in terms of its relative strength. Thus he assumes, as a basis of argument, facts that are not only not in evidence but also that evidence disproves. Here he is in good bioethical company.

Ever since the Ad Hoc Committee of the Harvard Medical School created "brain death" as a criterion for the withdrawal of care,[31] the assumption has been that we indeed can make an accurate diagnosis differentiating the brain dead from the merely unconscious, damaged, but functioning, recoverable mind. Since 1968 reports of people assumed to be "vegetative" who unexpectedly awakened were sufficiently frequent, however, to give the public, if not most ethicists, pause. In different studies published in the 1990s the vegetative diagnosis was found to be wrong between 15 and 34 percent of the time. Cognitive activity was present in those assumed to be without, to be "vegetative." In some cases they were victims of incorrect diagnoses, of a science that promised a certainty it could not deliver.[32] In simple language, the 1968 Harvard Committee created a category for noncare whose easy determination has been proven to be false.

Recent advances in neuroimaging have made the debate more urgent but little clearer.[33] With magnetic resonance imaging (MRI) and more recently functional magnetic resonance imaging machines (fMRIs) "stylized graphics produced by tracking magnetic fields and electrons, not light, and encoded in colours that do not reproduce the grey matter, or the neurons, or sponginess and blood" are produced.[34] These are computerized transformations of aspects of the brain whose meaning are far from certain. "Prematurely applying [these as] an emerging assessment tool to these clinical, syndromic categories can potentially lead to diagnostic and prognostic confusion and category errors."[35]

In short, even the most advanced diagnostic tools of our day are incapable of accurately determining whether or what precise kinds of consciousness or feeling exist in the person. They cannot predict definitively what a future state of consciousness or feeling will be in either persistently or temporarily unconscious persons. Given our current state of neuroignorance the very idea of consciousness as a measured quality is up for grabs.[36] Despite the assumptions of most bioethicists, we cannot with any authority parse levels of sentience as if these were clear, distinct, definitive states that can be identified and measured with the same accuracy as, say, respiratory function.[37]

In the public debate over Terry Schiavo, bioethicists frequently displayed MRIs of her brain, insisting on that basis they could confidently argue the nonpersonhood of Schiavo and thus the appropriateness of withdrawing her nutrition and hydration.[38] But in fact the precise meaning of the fuzzy image returned by the computer algorithms that created the image was unclear.[39] Were there fleeting thoughts, sensations, might she suffer and not think? Who knew to any degree of certainty? The deeper question McBryde Johnson might have asked was: did it really matter?

All this is to say Singer argues from the start as if we can know that the nonresponsive teenager is unthinking and unsalvageable, but the only assumption he can make is that she (or he) was nonresponsive at the time of McBryde Johnson's introduction. If as many as 40 percent of all those diagnosed as being persistently vegetative are misdiagnosed,[40] and some thought forever dead to the world do wake up, there is nothing "weird" in hoping one's son or daughter, husband or wife, sister or brother, may be among those diagnosed as unsalvageable who are returned eventually to their community. It may be quixotic and unlikely but parenthood is, after all, an inherently and hopelessly quixotic state of being. Singer's "for the sake of argument" doesn't serve because there is no hard ground on which that argument can be made. Worse, it suggests a clinical certainty that is wholly uncertain, a good trick in debate if not, necessarily, in life-and-death ethics.

Rationality and Cognition

If rational cognition is the value Singer makes preeminent, Harvard neuroanatomist Jill Bolt Taylor (figure 7.3) presents a sense of the world from the perspective of an apparently unconscious or minimally conscious person. Taylor had a massive hemorrhagic stroke, eventually recovering to write about the experience after years of rehabilitation.[41] In the stroke, she lost for a time the Kantian, left-brain rationality that the authors of *Principles*, Singer, and most bioethicists, see as defining. Her report of the resulting consciousness that remained, and of its importance, is hard to dismiss. Her experiences are framed within the context of the neuroscience that is her life's work.

An fMRI (functional magnetic resonance image) produced immediately after the stroke would have shown massive areas of nonactivity,

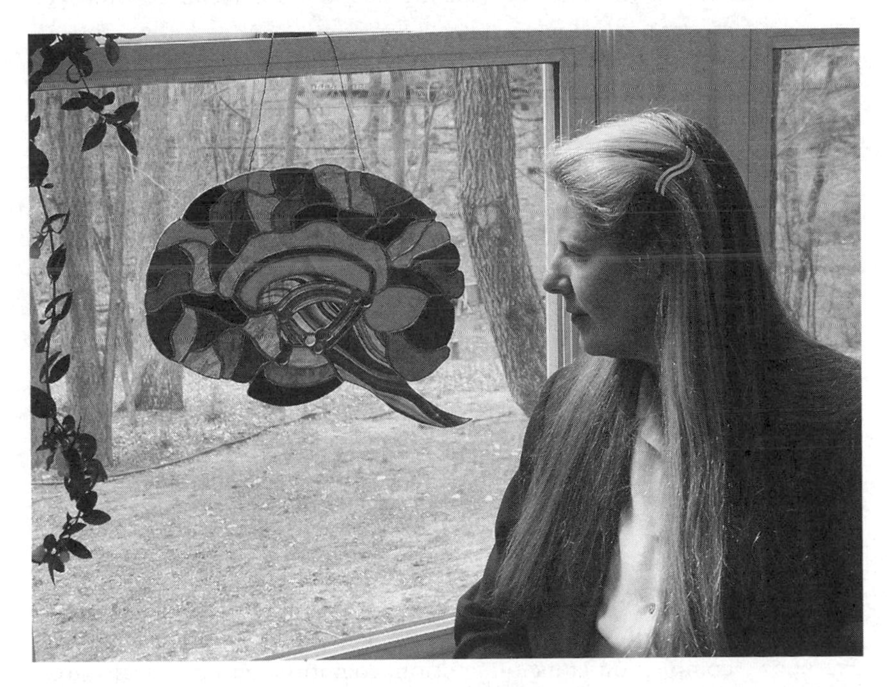

Figure 7.3
Following a severe stroke, Harvard neuroanatomist Jill Bolt Taylor went through years of rehabilitation and then wrote about her experience. In this photograph she considers a stained-glass construction in the shape of the human brain that she made. *Source*: Katherine Domingo, My Stroke of Insight, Inc.

or more precisely of diminished circulation, in those areas of the brain where the ethically all-important rational, self-conscious cognitive activity should be. There would have been, in the fMRI, patches of what we think of as neural activity (on the basis of blood flow) that appeared disconnected and intermittent. Jill Bolt Taylor was no longer a rational, thinking person. But in these extremes she was not "unthinking," she writes, but instead possessed of a very different kind of cognition (call it emotional awareness) that bioethicists do not credit, or if they do, not in the same way they value logical, rational thought processes.

And yet, Taylor describes in her stroke experience not a diminished sense of self but instead an expanded sense of the universal. It was nirvana-like, she writes nostalgically, and across the long period of rehabilitation she often wondered if a return to normalcy was itself a diminishment. It may or may not be that the unconscious teenager McBryde Johnson met was in a similar state. Because we cannot know, Singer's assumption for the sake of discussion becomes not a careful "what if," but, in its implication of knowledge that is unavailable, something of a cheat.

To anticipate: in the next chapter I argue that if we are unable to rigorously identify consciousness as a specific kind of neurological reality, we are at an even greater loss when it comes to rational intelligence as a definitional quality. It was during the eugenics of the early twentieth century that the American psychologist Charles Spearman conceived of intelligence as a single, unitary, biologic thing locatable in precise areas of the brain. As such, he believed, it could be tested as if it were, say, lung function.[42] This was Gall's phrenology updated to a new, noninvasive standard. And, today, bioethicists like Singer continue to assume that those who test below the norm on IQ tests (for example, persons with Down syndrome) are somehow less rational, less able, and thus probably less worthy of our care.

But just as consciousness remains a mystery so, too, does intelligence, except as a complex outcome of emotion, cognition, and physical status, all influenced by environmental and social circumstance. And so the easy assumption—one most bioethicists share with Singer—that we can make decisions based upon either intelligence or demonstrable cognitive activity is as false today as it was in Spearman's day. The post-person may be a person nonetheless,[43] the "dummy" a brilliant savant if given half a chance.

The Human

Singer would say, I think, as would many bioethicists, that McBryde Johnson's unconscious teenager is a human being but not a person and thus unworthy of care if there is no realistic hope of likely recovery and a return to rational personhood. That we know so little about persons in this state, and what we know seems to have been if not wrong then incomplete, argues for caution on the side of care. To do less is to deny the ethics that guided medical practice, and more broadly the social ethic that supported it, for millennia. As Michael Walzer put it: "The primary good that we distribute to one another is membership in some human community."[44] It was this ideal of an unequivocal membership deserving of care that in the early twentieth century was challenged first by Chicago's Haiselden, and later by Binding and Hoche in Germany. The belief in that community of humans and the importance of membership in it as both a good and an irrevocable right was similarly denied by the bioethicists for whom the nonresponsive teenager was best described, perhaps, as post-person, and thus dead for all practical purposes.

For Singer, however, and by extension for many contemporary bioethicists, Walzer's primary good is simply irrelevant. "Because membership of the species *Homo sapiens* is not ethically relevant, any characteristic or combination of characteristics that we regard as giving human beings a right to life, or as making it generally wrong to end a human life, may be possessed by some nonhuman animals."[45] Only speciesism, the advance of the human species as better and special, makes us value *Homo sapiens* above the animals we live with: a physician therefore should have no more moral or social standing than a veterinarian. If one does not put an unconscious dog or cat or cow on life support in hopes of its recovery, or maintain it in terminal distress, why do so for the unconscious teenager?[46] Here again, we have what Singer sees as illogical, incomprehensible and thus . . . weird.

Singer dismisses the ideal of human protectedness, and therefore rejects a duty to care on its basis. He substitutes in its stead the idea of suffering, the ability to feel and sense discomfort or pain (and in the inverse, joy and fulfillment) as the ethical criteria that should matter. He assumes the unconscious teenager and other post-persons do not have those capacities and thus their care can be dismissed as ethically unnecessary. And yet it was the capacity for thinking, albeit a different kind of thinking, and a capacity for emotion (albeit unexpressed) that Jill Taylor knew in abundance when her rational brain was in retreat following her stroke. The Singerian assessment of McBryde Johnson's presumed suffering (considerable) and enjoyment (necessarily diminished) similarly served his dismissal of the diversity of difference as anything but a negative to be avoided.

There is a problem here. We have no suffering meter either for mammals in general or for humans specifically—no precisely measurable, demonstrable criterion that could turn Singer's estimates of suffering (or happiness) into a firm measure of concern. We have his and other's assumptions based on a very incomplete science and a sense of the normal person's repugnance for the abnormal ("Look at her! What do you think? I hope she doesn't think or feel!").[47] All we have, in the end, is Singer's dismissal of the nonresponsive teenager's care as weird and his insistence that the rational living person, McBryde Johnson, must suffer (whatever she says) from her limitations in a way that should be avoided wherever possible.

McBryde Johnson knew she was a symbol, the very sign of the disabled, limited person. She thus stood as signifier of all those who, like her, would seem to the normal philosopher as limited and suffering. That assumption of the nature of her state, despite her repeated denials, was to her not simply ignorant but also prejudicial. Similarly, Singer and many other bioethicists extend their assumptions of the burdensome nature of difference to the burden of those who live with and care for those, like McBryde Johnson, who need help in daily life. But many carers see themselves as tasked, perhaps, but not onerously charged. Again, there is here a literature written by those who accept caregiving for fragile loved ones freely and gladly.[48] That is not to say there is no frustration, sadness, or stress. But in these writings the burden results not principally from the limitations of the fragile person but instead from the failures of social support and recognition.

It was this sense of the burdened caregiver and diminished care receiver that McBryde Johnson challenged by her very presence. Yes, she was in a wheelchair. Yes, she needed help in the performance of mundane daily activities. No, her parents did not feel her care had been an imposition. Nor did the personal assistant who traveled with her. Certainly her legal clients were not disadvantaged. And after all she, McBryde Johnson, was there, at Princeton, debating Singer and the philosopher ethicists-in-training he instructed. Talk about futility! What could be a more valuable if thankless task than that?

The Beautiful

McBryde Johnson thus reversed Singer's assumptions, insisting on the value of the person irrespective of capacity. She did this not with a rights-based argument or through the intellectual weighing, in the way of most bioethics, of "natural" and "diminished" capacities. Ethically and philosophically, she rejected the spirit of Singer's dispassionate methodologies. It was not that McBryde Johnson could not argue dispassionately and precisely. She was a lawyer, after all, and her briefs were, like her public articles, models of clear, logical thinking. Instead she chose a different approach, one whose language and substance advanced the argument that we are not fungible and we are not isolates. She chose the personal and emotional as her method of disputation—one perhaps un-Kantian, and some would say, unphilosophical: "I've decided to pound them with heart, hammer them with narrative and say 'y'all' and 'folks.' I play with the emotional tone, giving them little peaks and valleys, modulating three times in one 45-second patch. I talk about justice. Even beauty and love. I figure they haven't been getting much of that from Singer," she wrote in her famous essay.

Amazing, from the pages of *New York Magazine* the gimp in her wheelchair argues the value of the person as an emotional as well as self-consciously rational entity to the bioethicist. She insists that her physical state does not limit either her humanness or her personhood. She makes the argument in her person and through her history, a statement evidenced by her physical presence. In doing so, she implicitly criticizes and some would say refutes the bioethicist who insists upon the sanctity of the rational, self-conscious, individual self but finds himself incapable of accepting the argument of the rational, self-conscious individual who sits in her wheelchair on the podium with him. And to make it even better, McBryde Johnson resists the notion she is unique, or special, or heroic. She has in her writings tale upon tale of others who, like her, are happy and interested and socially integrated despite characteristics that limit their movement in our shared world. Wow.

Do not think of McBryde Johnson merely as an emotional if lawyerly disputant arguing her life, and that of her friends. Think of her instead as a philosopher, a phenomenologist and thus an intellectual descendent of Husserl's concrete account of the structures of the directly experienced. As such she spoke (and sometimes wrote) in the tradition of Maurice Merleau-Ponty for whom existence is not solely rational and cerebral, detached from the realities of daily living, but instead embodied in the lived world of the person. It was this experiential, lived world McBryde Johnson argued and which Singer ignored—or perhaps, poor Peter!—simply could not perceive and which most bioethicists dismiss in their deliberations. By rationality Singer meant a singular process of individual cognition divorced from emotion and experience while for McBryde Johnson, as for Isaiah Berlin, "Rationality is knowing things and people for what they are."[49] *That* was what McBryde Johnson sought to argue, the "are" of her lived reality (and the unconscious teenager's, and the teenager's parents and siblings, and their guests, and so on) as opposed to the "must be" of the ethicist's prejudicial musings.

From the perspective of her wheelchair McBryde Johnson was at once the message and the medium. Yes, her mobility was restricted but the truly burdensome disability came from her being discounted as at least equal on the basis of specific characteristics. That, as she presented it, was the ethical disaster. At Princeton she said this not baldly but indirectly; insisting on what Bruce Jennings called an ethics formed "in and through life lived in culturally meaning practices, not by abstract or escape from those practices."[50] She thus dismissed as if not inconsequential then at least insufficient the thinly abstract rationality of the bioethicist. Disagree? Why, just look at her sitting on the sheepskin pad of her wheelchair, her assistant waiting in the wings of the auditorium in case she was needed. They were there, together: What could be more human and honorable than that?

In building an argument from experience McBryde Johnson was not simplistic. She did not deny the realities of the nonresponsive teenager, or of her own physicality. She did not argue for the wheelchair as a superior way of living but instead as a legitimate way of being. She did not suggest persistent unconsciousness was a boon for the teenager. Instead she argued more generally and simply that limiting individual characteristics (she would not call them attributes) are not in themselves defining. For her, the discrete, existentially isolated, individual, rational being of bioethical imagining is a fiction, given what system biologists and relational psychologists like Allan Fiske describe as "the inherent sociability of homo sapiens."[51] We exist not as discrete beings but as social entities in families, neighborhoods, and communities in which all are dependent, one upon the other. In our relations we are emotional and personal rather than dispassionately rational isolates. The ethics McBryde Johnson proposed begins with this relational fact, and with caring as the natural metric of a human being irrespective of a person's limits.

Thus for McBryde Johnson the nonresponsive teenager's humanity, personhood, and thus the ethical importance of that life all are affirmed through the act of family care in an essential relationship irrespective of the unconscious adolescent's capacity. For Singer, as I understand him (and certainly for many other ethicists I know), relationships are thoroughly contingent, tenuous ties based on this or that individual's attributes at any moment. From that perspective care for the unconscious teenager (and, by extension, for a young McBryde Johnson) *was* weird. For McBryde Johnson both the teenager and the greater family's humanity, and thus their worth, were affirmed in their life together. They were validated (their humanity affirmed) as a unit when visitors like McBryde Johnson interacted with the teenager as a family member. From this perspective, personhood is a conclusion resulting from the caring an individual gives *or* receives. The bioethicists' appropriation (I would say misappropriation) of a kind of individualistic Kantian rationality as a metric of care outside of human worth was impeached as a result.

And while the highpoint of the nondebate was the nonresponsive teenager, the subtext was the manner in which all those with limiting characteristics are either accepted as they are or dismissed as inherently less worthy. Across a spectrum of human diversity that ranges from the unconscious teenager to the musical wunderkind or Olympic athlete, there sat McBryde Johnson on the sheepskin pad of her wheelchair as just another person. Normalcy doesn't matter, she said. Extremes are irrelevant. We are all simply people, together, and thus all equally worthy of care. From that perspective caring is redefined not as burdensome, as it must be for Singer, but instead as exemplary, an affirmation of humans as social beings, together.

Stephen J. Post

Had McBryde Johnson chosen to argue as an academic she might have called upon a range of others in support of her position. There are, for example, the relational psychologists like Alan Fiske who argues human behavior is interpersonally grounded rather than individually constructed.[52] Modern psychology's focus on individual development and later, isolated behavior divorced from familial and social relations are, from this perspective, inadequate. It comes out of the nineteenth-century ideals of radical individualism, a politic rather than a science. This idea, argued earlier by, among others, R. D. Laing in his *Self and Others*, is related to but distinct from the feminism whose landmark text was Carl Gilligan's 1982 *In a Different Voice*. There she argued what has become the essential message of feminist theory: moral choice is not a matter of disengaged logic divorced from human associations but always activated in a context that is interpersonal.

For a view from ethics there is Stephen J. Post who argued a more or less similar position[53] in his commentary on the famous legal battle fought in the early 1990s by the husband of eighty-six-year-old Helga Wanglie against her physician's insistence that continuing care was if not unseemly certainly unreasonable.[54] For most bioethicists the point was futility—the continued care of the unconscious octogenarian made no clinical sense. She would not recover and she was frail and cognitively unresponsive . . . why bother with the expense? Forget bioethics' insistence on patient (or surrogate) choice. Because Helga Wanglie would not improve there was no need for bioethicists or physicians to honor the informed preferences of her husband for his wife's continued care and treatment.

Underneath all this ran the arguments from scarcity rehearsed here in earlier chapters. Medicine is too costly and resources too slight to indulge individual whims if they will not enhance a productive person. Post's alternate perspective admired Mr. Wanglie's refusal to allow even persistent unconsciousness to impede the essential relationship that gave his life meaning. Love is not contingent and should be celebrated, Post implies, irrespective of the likelihood of clinical improvement. Post found a similar message in a 1993 newspaper story about a man whose wife was persistently unconscious and living at a skilled nursing facility. "He wheels her out into the nursing home TV room on Sundays to watch the Cleveland Browns games. She is on artificial feeding and sometimes requires ventilator support. They both wear the jersey of their favourite quarterback."[55] As David B. McCurdy wrote of Post, his arguments "lead him [Post] to see in affected persons a humanity transcending cultural views of personhood driven by rationality and productivity—'exclusory' views that deprive so-called non-persons of the moral protection of the 'do-no-harm' principle."[56]

Oliver Sacks

There is no better or more knowledgeable proponent of this ethic of the interpersonal, and of humanity as a protected class irrespective of capacity, than neurologist Oliver Sacks. "Reality is given to us by the reality of people, he wrote in *Awakenings*, his famous 1982 study of post-encephalitic patients. "Reality is taken from us by the unreality of unpeople."[57] His patients might have been in what he called a "Kantian delirium," living outside the normal sentient rhythms and identities of our world, but their loss of independent expression and self-actuated consciousness did not deny their personhood or their humanity.

Prior to their treatment with L-dopa (levodopa), Sacks was unsure of the status of the patients' awareness, their cognition. He did not know if they felt angst or joy in their near catatonic, fugue state. However, it did not matter to the medicine he and his coworkers practiced. The patients were maintained for decades in faint hope of a cure, or treatment, and in the belief that even in their neurologically limited state they were real, important, and deserving of care. That they endured with the help of hospital staff gave the patients a heroic rather than a tragic cast, Sacks argued. They were "made great by their endurance through affliction," and by extension so, too, were those who maintained them. Sacks's admiration for the general staff that cared for these patients was based on their having chosen this work when they could have done something else. The act of care affirmed not only the humanity of the lives in their charge but also, by extension, of the caregivers as well.[58]

Sacks thus critiqued both a type of medicine and an ethics based upon it in which the person is no more than the sum of his or her attributes at a moment. "What we do see, first and last, is the utter inadequacy of mechanical medicine, the utter inadequacy of a mechanical world view. These patients are living disproofs of mechanical thinking, as they are living exemplars of biological thinking."[59] That mechanistic thinking *is* bioethics today; one that assumes a simplistic formula of burden and benefit can be easily applied to the complex realities of care and treatment. It was Sacks's complex biological thinking and its insistence on a communal reality, and caring, that McBryde Johnson argued as the beautiful in terms of the unconscious teenager generally and her own life specifically. Yes, she needed physical assistance. No, she could not walk or run or kick her legs when swimming. Yes, she rolled rather than walked but, again, so what? "I enjoy my life," she wrote, "it's a great sensual pleasure to zoom by power chair on these delicious muggy streets." Poor you, she seemed to say, who only know the pedestrian experience of walking. It is this she argued to Peter Singer and the skeptics in his classroom, acolytes of the prince of normalcy confronted by the priestess of difference.

Kant and "The Beautiful"

We might with equal rectitude think of McBryde Johnson and Oliver Sacks (and, of course, Stephen J. Post) as philosophers of a Kantian cast. Kant writes about the beautiful as a conclusion disconnected from utility or purpose.[60] This beauty is not an objective property but a judgment whose universality rests on the recognition that *as* a judgment at least in theory it can and perhaps should be generally acknowledged. Thus this beauty is at once innate in a thing and at the same time is understood as greater than the individual case in which it is perceived to occur. This beauty has no a priori; it is instead an aesthetic judgment whose rationale is lodged in its referent. It need not be sentimental although it may be emotional.

It was this Kantian beauty that McBryde Johnson perceived in the care of the teenager without expectation of return, a lovely quality free of partisan interests (an insurance agent's, a philosopher's) and independent of functionality, which is to say, free of neoliberal accountancy. Its attraction lies not merely in its emphasis on the primary good of the essential relation between parent and child, brother and sister, nurse and patient, society and the person, but also in its insistence that the strength of those essential relationships can be shared across the greater community of family visitors like McBryde Johnson.

In transposing her story into that of a Kantian aesthetic the referent is not the unique isolate—the teenager in the bed—but the broader complex of parents and loved children living together. The beauty lies in the story's presentation of elemental relationships as the essential thing that gives meaning to all lives lived together irrespective of individual capacity at any moment. This perspective is advanced in opposition to those who assume all lives are contingent based on their capacities of the moment. It denies as a metric of care and ethical concern false calculations of benefit and burden, false because there is no calculus of commitment and love.

Most communitarians and utilitarians and all lifeboat ethicists ignore the essential relationship and focus instead on the contingent individual whose attributes at the moment and potential contribution to (or draining of) an imagined future resource state define that individual's worthiness. They see every one of us as a bundle of characteristics that define our utility so that when those are diminished our importance to society and in our lived worlds necessarily is diminished reflexively as well. We saw this, earlier, in the writings of Daniel Callahan who cared not a fig for what seniors had done and how they had contributed across their lives, only for what they might do for a future state to be peopled by the young. And why not? If you can't row the boat you don't get a seat in the lifeboat even if you've been rowing boats for years. In this vision we are all no more than the sum of our abilities at any one moment, creatures out of time and with a social history that is irrelevant to issues of care.

From McBryde Johnson's perspective, however, this argument is, to borrow Sacks's phrase, the real "Kantian delirium," a standard of worth based on contingent characteristics as if they existed outside the greater fabric of community and social interaction. For Sacks the unresponsive person is exquisitely human, and thus precious, in his or her fragility. "It is given to these patients," Sacks wrote, "through no wish or fault of their own, to explore the depths, the ultimate possibilities, of human being and suffering." Despite their apparent unresponsiveness they may teach us humanity, he continued; they may "lead us to a deeper understanding of the nature of affliction and care and cure."[61] For Sacks and McBryde Johnson (and Post, and so on) the important thing is not a simple EEG (electroencephalograph) reading but a complex relation, people together and not disparate isolates apart. It is that essentialness that is judged beautiful, and defining. It is . . . us.

All this was implicit in McBryde Johnson's report of her meeting with Peter Singer and his Princeton students. It was suggested, as well, in Sacks's classic study and in Post's critique. One may question the argument from communality and sociability rather than individuality but the whole cannot be dismissed as inconsequential, and certainly not as merely emotional. The argument of McBryde Johnson and by extension those others (Post, Sacks, and so on) *is* a distinct philosophy offering an alternative orientation from which a different ethic results. Its advantage is its "ground truthing," its grounding in the experiential. The resulting ethic, and its attendant morality, is clearly more in agreement with the traditional ethics of medicine than the bioethics that has sought to replace it. And at least in this reading it is, I think, more amenable to the wisdom of the Enlightenment, at least Kant's wisdom, than the modernist, neoliberal ethic in broad bioethical favor today.

Down Syndrome

A more prosaic, less famous example may serve to seal the argument, and this chapter. Again, Peter Singer provides the material. He is, he writes, willing to accept if not embrace a parent's decision to not abort but instead carry to term a fetus that in prenatal testing is shown to have Trisomy 21, that is, Down syndrome. "Many parents claim that their Down syndrome child enjoys life as much as their children without Down syndrome. If the couple believes that they would be just as happy with a child with Down syndrome as with a child without it, it could be rational for them to choose to continue a pregnancy after being told the foetus had Down syndrome."[62]

Singer's only interest is the prospective parents' belief they will be equally happy with a Down syndrome child as with another child without

Down syndrome. It is clear that while he would find such a choice "rational," and thus defensible, it would be for him at best curious. He is, after all, the prince of normalcy and thus assumes a person with Down, like a person in a wheelchair, must live a less full and thus diminished life that is necessarily more burdensome to those who live with them. He does *not* say "the person with Down syndrome will be a person worthy of respect and protection, by my definition, a thinking intelligent being who can know suffering." He acknowledges one might accept such a person as one would a rescue dog, perhaps, but not as an equal. Consequentially he sees it as neither wrong nor unreasonable to terminate a fetus with Trisomy 21.

Despite Singer's claim to thinking long and hard about his judgments and their consequences, his arguments in this arena are based not on experience in the phenomenological world but on the world he wishes to believe is real. He does not go to meetings of persons with Down syndrome or spend weeks in homes where a Down syndrome person resides. Singer argues about what he thinks the life of a person with Down syndrome, and those who love the person, must be like. His arguments on normalcy and difference are in the main largely ungrounded assumptions (I want to say prejudices) rather than thoughtful, consequential conclusions.

Thus he would presumably agree with those in the 1990s who assumed reflexively that persons with Down syndrome should not qualify for organ transplantation. They would, it was assumed, live less long and their contributions to society would be by definition less than those made by normal people. Consequentially, the utilitarians would say that given the scarcity of graft organs, they should go to paragons of normalcy who will better use them and better serve society at large.[63] Justice and its equities of opportunity are for the normal and the strong.

As a reality check, consider Dale Froese (figure 7.4), an adult member of the Canadian Down Syndrome Society (to which I belong). Dale does not see his chromosomal pattern with its tripled twenty-first chromosome as an impediment to his life or the characteristics of Down syndrome as a liability. "It is indeed good to be me," Froese writes. "I don't want anyone's pity. I don't want people to celebrate my successes. I just want to be me. My participation in the world as a friend, husband,

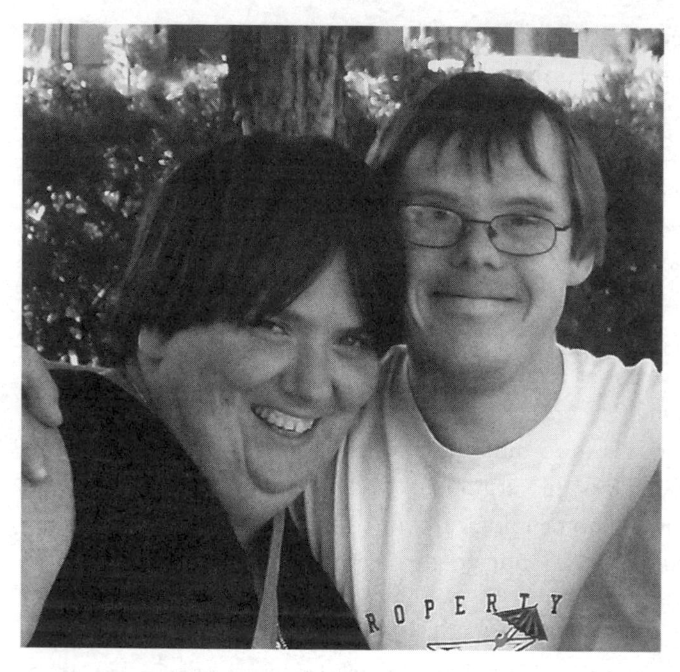

Figure 7.4
Dale and Leanne Froese are working members of the Canadian Down Syndrome Society. Dale argues that the assumption that their lives must be less because of Down syndrome, and their burden on family and society greater, is wrong. *Source*: Canadian Down Syndrome Society (CDSS).

employee and consumer enhance my feelings of belonging," he continues. "Although the world often sees me as being different, I refuse to see the world differently because I have a disability."[64]

That is precisely the perspective McBryde Johnson argued and Sacks articulated across their respective works. Froese sees himself as no more or less a member of the community than, for example, John Harris or Pete Singer. Froese engages the world to the best of his ability and that is the only thing that should be important. "I know people I am serving [at work] treat me a little differently. I am tolerant of this," he writes, "and try to change their perspectives by confidently completing my duties." Here one sees what to Singer was weird but was beautiful to McBryde Johnson. Froese is, as was McBryde Johnson, tolerant of those who see a personal characteristic as necessarily limiting. His response, like hers, is to be in the world and to interact with it, insisting in his (or her) embodied presence not his (or her) individual importance but the importance of relationships among those with whom he (or she) interacts in their respective communities.

Here one moves close to the heart of the matter. McBryde Johnson did not minimize the limits of her physicality. She simply insisted they were irrelevant to her personhood within the community of persons with whom she lived. For his part, Froese says the same about himself in his world. Froese serves food. McBryde Johnson worked as a lawyer. Neither the trebling of Froese's chromosome nor the eccentricities of McBryde Johnson's spine made them lesser persons in their communities. Their cognitive and physical characteristics had no fundamental bearing on the essential worthiness of the lives either led within a community of family and friends.

McBryde Johnson was clear about this in an undated piece asking, "When is life worth living?" She wrote: "I can undertake work that doesn't feed anyone's bottom line but satisfies my curiosity, my vision of justice, my sense of fun. Yet still, I have enough money to get everything I need and most of what I want." How many people with mundane physical traits can say as much? There is no shame (that most social of sentimentalities) in needing help or being limited in a way that requires assistance and, as McBryde Johnson wrote, "Without shame, there's no humiliation." Whether one has the physicality of McBryde Johnson or the cognitive abilities of Dale Froese the same is true. Shame, humiliation, and the emotional suffering that result are the consequence of being seen as a lesser being by dint of dependence, or difference. It is the disability that Brody described, one not inherent in the person but visited upon him or her by the prejudice of others who see them as, in Sacks's language, "unpeople."

Here, too, one may see a Kantian perspective, albeit different from the one that pretends to inform most bioethics. In his *Critique of Judgment*, Kant railed against the separation of mind and body: "The body is part of the self; in its togetherness with the self it constitutes the person."[65] That is the sentiment McBryde Johnson offered in opposition to the ethicist's person as a list of contingent abilities that define personhood or its lack at any moment. To separate function and person is to divide that which is indivisible. One cannot appreciate McBryde Johnson or Dale Froese as members of our world and simultaneously disparage their physical and genetic characteristics as making them unfit to be in the world. To do so denies their status as embodied persons. It denies their humanity, and the beauty that attends to the communities they support and that support them. Membership in these communities of experience at every level (family, neighborhood, society, species), irrespective of specific capacities, is the principle ethical good that McBryde Johnson and others argue.

Ethics, Redux

There was a time not too long ago when McBryde Johnson's argument would have been accepted as more or less commonplace, or at least as not unusual. It was the ethic that pervaded, for example, the rehabilitation wards I knew as a child in the polio years of the early 1950s. And, as chapter 8's review makes clear, it was the ethos of the early years of genetic exploration and testing of the 1960s and 1970s. But bioethics and the neoliberal arguments its ethicists typically advance put paid to all that. As bioethics took on authority, and its general argument gained legitimacy, court judgments shifted from a default assumption of the necessity to care and the sanctity of the person to one in which noncare was to become the norm. An early marker of this "dramatic sea change," as Post calls it,[66] was the case of Karen Ann Quinlan (whose persistent unconsciousness did not meet the Harvard Committee's criteria set), in which the courts at first denied her father's right to withdraw her life support.[67] Fifteen years later, the Helga Wanglie case marked the beginning of the time when noncare came to be argued as the default. By 1992–1993 the number of patients dying in the hospital's intensive care unit as a result of withheld therapies had risen to 90 percent.[68] By 1997 over 50 percent of all patients dying in the ICU at one San Francisco Hospital died as a result of the withholding or withdrawal of life support. The reasons for the deaths were typically "poor prognosis" and a resulting determination of "futility."

If humanness has no inherent value, if normalcy is the standard against which care and treatment are to be judged, then the failure to return persons to normalcy, or simply to keep them alive at the request of families, becomes weird and foolish. Why not jettison from the lifeboat all those who fail to meet a set of instrumental criteria, and as a result save the resources they might have consumed? The probabilistic becomes definitive ("poor prognosis") and care is deemed "futile" not simply because it is unlikely to significantly extend life but also because the person in his or her fragility is defined as imminently expendable. The resulting ethics makes of us all thoroughly contingent catalogues of our abilities at the moment. Our interpersonal and social histories become irrelevant and so, too, our place in the communities that we have sustained and that in need might sustain us.

Heroes row the boat; they don't just sit, taking up space. From this perspective there is no real groundwork for ethics except a utilitarian calculation of general good irrespective of individual need. Bioethics needed to disparage the traditional vocational ethics of medicine because it rested on a core value of interpersonal care and social service inimical to the ethics it sought to introduce. What Roy Porter called the history of medicine as a story for *The Greatest Benefit to Mankind* becomes something else entirely.[69] It becomes instead the story of the greatest benefit to the able, and especially the most able.

Humankind as a protected quality is, if we believe Singer, an irrelevant criterion of care. Human sanctity is more generally a good most bioethicists pay lip service to but ignore in their practical deliberations. For them, as for Singer, the value of each person is weighed at any moment, from pre- to post-person, on a simplistic scale of characteristics cast against the institutional backcloth of cost–benefit calculations. The ethics that results pretends to a protection of the individual but instead promotes selective care (whatever the person or surrogate might want) based on a criteria set that is, at best, incomplete. It promotes research as a future good even though that research may endanger human subjects who will not benefit from the research itself. It insists upon the rational isolate and the domain of his or her choice except when those choices—for example, Mr. Wanglie's—while clearly rational, are seen as inconvenient. We can't blame this on the Dead Germans the student in his Bob Marley tee-shirt dismissed. They would not, at least as I read them, have had much patience with the bioethics that insists upon them as a legitimizing source. The responsibility for this ethic is one we must take upon ourselves.

8

Research and Genetics: "For the Benefit of Humankind"

At least in theory, most bioethicists are, with Singer, "consequentialists" arguing an application of their understanding of what is good, right, and philosophically proper in relation to the science contributing to real situations they seek to order and regulate. Since its naming, bioethicists have claimed the necessity for a new medical ethic capable of managing issues arising from advances in the modern genetic science that began with James Watson's and Francis Crick's first description of the structure of DNA in the 1950s.[1] From them came the now famous double-helix structure in which two strands of sugar and phosphate molecules twist around each other like twin snakes around the staff of Asclepius.

The claim of bioethics—remember the opening paragraphs of *Principles of Biomedical Ethics*—has been that traditional medical ethics was necessarily incapable of adjudicating issues arising from this evolving new science. What was needed in bioethics was a "genethics" as James Nagel first called it in the 1980s, something "to incorporate the various ethical implications and dilemmas," as John Coggon recently put it, "with the technologies and applications that directly or indirectly affect the human species."[2] This raised the prospect of a cheerful eugenics in which bioethicists order not the care of people but the species at large. They become the arborists who prune and thus shape the human tree, deciding its future in the process. To do that would require a deep understanding of not simply the species, as we think it is and as we hope it might someday be, but also of the science that defines what we are and what we might become.

What, however, is the science on which bioethicists built their assumptions and how good is their understanding of it? To assess the bioethical claim that a new ethics was needed to answer questions raised by an advancing science we need a detour, not à la Beauchamp and Childress, into philosophical imaginings, but into the science itself, what it says and how it is to be understood.

New Sciences: Prehistory

The old medical ethic served very well for the first decades in which this new science came into being and into use. Its prehistory, one might say, begins in 1939 with the first published report of an unnamed hemolytic disease in newborns. It appeared that in rare cases the blood of the mother and the fetus was somehow incompatible. The reason became clear in the early 1950s when it was shown that the antigen that induced this incompatibility was the Rh factor, named in the 1940s by researchers who recreated the responsible agglutination effect by injecting into rabbits a serum based on Resus Macque blood.[3] Once the problem was understood, protocols to test for incompatible RH factors in the mother's amniotic fluid were developed. Where the test was positive, prophylactic measures to secure the health of the affected fetus were instituted.[4]

In 1956 tests of maternal amniotic fluid were sufficiently sophisticated to identify the presence or absence of the Barr body and thus to identify in utero the sex of the fetus. In 1959 the French pediatrician and geneticist Jérôme Jean Louis Marie Lejeune reported an apparently causal relationship between low levels of folic acid in pregnant woman and a higher incidence of neural tube defects in subsequent births. Also in that year Lejeune, building upon the insights of other researchers, was able to define the precise chromosomal profile of Trisomy 21. Testing of the amniotic fluid to identify Down syndrome, named after John Langdon Down who first described its characteristic appearance,[5] followed upon this discovery.

In the 1960s blood tests were developed that with a high degree of reliability could identify a series of markers for an expanding array of conditions, including Hemophilia A and Duchenne muscular dystrophy. In 1961, for example, American microbiologist Robert Guthrie developed a simple blood test for an error in metabolic function, phenylketonuria (PKU), causing significant neurological damage in newborns if they were not immediately given a special low-phenylalanine diet.[6] The test was first used as a diagnostic to identify young patients in whom PKU was manifest so they could be treated with dietary programs that would limit its effect.

Following quickly upon this diagnostic other tests were developed that could identify a range of congenital conditions including, in a partial list, glactosemia (GALT), maple syrup urine disease (MSUD), homocytstinuria (HCY), and later, congenital hypothyrodism and eventually sickle cell anemia. Again the goal was treatment: thyroid substitutes for those with hypothyrodism, for example, and a pneumococcal prophylaxis for infants with sickle cell anemia.[7] In 1963, Lejeune identified the genetic locus of another, rarer genetic condition, *cri du chat*. Named for the kitten-like cry of infants resulting form the eccentric development of a patient's larynx, the condition disappears naturally in about a third of affected children by the age of three.

The first seminal paper on the rapidly expanding range of diagnostic fetal testing was published in 1970.[8] All this work was of a kind that had powered medicine for centuries, the identification and then classification of symptoms in a manner permitting earlier diagnoses resulting in better care and treatment. Across the early years of the new science this remained the goal. The ethical end, as the World Health Organization made clear in 1968, was treatment: "The object of screening for disease is to discover those among the apparently well who are in fact suffering from disease. They can then be placed under treatment."[9]

Genetics and the Knowledge Industry

All this was fiercely Hippocratic, and Oslerian. Its focus was the patient and his or her care. There was no need for a new ethics unless the goal of patient care as the ethical focus of medicine was to be replaced with something else. That was exactly what happened when bioethics' "broader concept of benefit," as Pellegrino has called it,[10] substituted the perceived needs of the economy, and the lucrative knowledge industry, for the care of the patient as a primary good. Researchers saw the early identification of persons with eccentric phenotypes as a research opportunity rather than as the creation of a class of patients needing special care. Those arguing an Oslerian perspective insisting on patient care and protection as the *summum bonum* of medical practice increasingly were dismissed as obstructionist.[11]

One sees this in the debate over programs for the genetic screening of newborn infants in the United States. In 2006, for example, the American College of Medical Genetics recommended testing for twenty-nine core conditions as well as twenty-five secondary conditions. In theory, the goal was "the best interest of the affected newborn." There are, however, few treatment protocols for the majority of the fifty-four conditions identified in the screening panel. No benefit accrues to the infant's care; no special programs of support—for patients or their families—are necessarily enacted upon diagnosis. The testing of newborns thus does very little, in the majority of these fifty-four tested conditions, for the newborns whose biomarkers are collected.

The rationale behind testing for conditions for which no treatment exists (mandatory in some U.S. jurisdictions and in some conducted at the parents' expense) is thus not care but "biobanking," the identification of persons with conditions that make them desirable research subjects.[12] The very idea that screening should be restricted to conditions for which treatment is available, or where a patient and his or her family might be otherwise assisted by information on this or that condition, is merely the "old dogma" of the old medicinal ethics that, in the words of Alexander and Van Dyck, "dooms us to continual ignorance."[13] The sovereignty of patient care that underlay the old medical ethic becomes, from this perspective, merely an inconvenient obstacle to the needs of the knowledge industry and its future goods, whatever they might be.

Docile Bodies

The older ethic did not "doom" us all to continual ignorance, however. It balanced the goals of research and the necessities of treatment brilliantly across centuries of medical advances from the anatomy of Vesalius to the pathology of Morgagni to the clinical teachings of Osler and then the discoveries of Lejeune. Bioethics, at least since *The Belmont Report*, reversed the ethical order of the older ethic. The future goods to be gained by research became a principal and for some primary focus. The knowledge industry required an ethic in which "reasonable" (to the researcher at least) risks and harms to its subjects were permissible in studies that offered little or no hope of improved care to the patient.[14] The potential return—future saleable products—overrode the niceties of concern that, in the past, governed both medicine and its research.

In this imagining bioethics never argued the potential benefits of the research it promoted should be generally available.[15] Just as Ronald Reagan promised that tax cuts for corporations and the wealthy would trickle down, someday, to the eventual advantage of average citizens, medicine's new ethicists assumed that the fruits of *Belmont's* research-oriented ethic would sooner or later benefit the population at large. This would, of course, come through the marketplace where research companies with a successful product could name their price.

To date, the search for repairable genes underlying common causes of mortality has yielded few results in large part because it is rare that a single genetic variant can be used to alter a specific human ill: cancer, diabetes, Huntington schizophrenia, and so on.[16] In the end it does not matter overmuch, however, if the promise of a cure was false because research became an end to itself, an economically productive good largely divorced from issues of patient care. In this emphasis what was lost is the role of the physician as a guardian of patient well-being. The treating physician became either a research recruiter, or supervisor, or an obstruction whose concerns could be dismissed reflexively. The next step was to make patients if not eager then willing participants in research. The patient-cum-research subject had to be trained to accept his or her role as a research object. That was perhaps bioethics' most significant contribution to the whole: "The discipline of bioethics seeks to produce persons who are docile vis-à-vis the research establishment," writes Therese Lysaught.[17]

That is a serious charge for an ethic that in theory promotes autonomous patient choice. It brings forth Foucault's description of "docile bodies" as persons educated, coerced, or trained to do what officialdom wants in ways that serve the state and its interests, not the person.[18] Invoking Foucault argues that bioethics has created a narrow deliberative space whose assumptions permit only those questions whose answers lead in an officially acceptable direction. Research matters more than the people who are its medium of study. The population needs to be trained to accept this. And if they cannot be trained, perhaps they should be forced.

In 2005 bioethicist Rosamond Rhodes argued against existing research protocols that gave special weight to the protection of the vulnerable research subject. The bioethics program director and a professor of medical education at Mt. Sinai School of Medicine in New York City, Rhodes argued an ignorant public and an excitable public media were impeding a research agenda whose requirements should have priority."[19] In response to this "ethical catastrophe," Rhodes therefore proposed a program of compulsory research participation in which every U.S. resident would be obliged to serve as a research subject once every ten years. "Of course, autonomy would not be jettisoned," Lysaught commented dryly. "All research participants would have the freedom to choose which protocol they would participate in."[20]

Here we have Daniel Callahan's argument about seniors transposed to the research arena. Again scarcity—in this case of research subjects—compels the suspension of concern for the person. Again, there is an economic necessity—the growth of the research industry—as an implicit argument for this shift. And, again, we see the liberal ideal of personal choice suspended for those who may be so recalcitrant as to wish to put their care and treatment over the potential, future good of future generations who are to be, in theory, advantaged by their noncare.

Rhodes was not unique in her argument. Art Caplan promoted the idea in the 1980s[21] and more recently David Orentlicher advanced a similar position in The *Hastings Center Report* in 2005.[22] So, too, did John Harris, who argued "one might be able to articulate a civic obligation to participate in research and that indeed Rawlsian fairness itself might require it."[23] Since research requires numbers to make its studies possible, the rights of individual to not participate may fail in the face of the future collective who may someday benefit from today's research programs: "The rights and interests of research subjects are just the rights and interests of persons and must be balanced against comparable rights and interests of other persons," Harris argued.[24] Say goodbye to the ideal of the individual free to make his or her own choices, or the old ethical focus on the primacy of the patient in need. In this schema, the rights and interests of the research industry and its potential for saleable benefits to future persons not only balance but outweigh the rights of the person today.

Among the community of bioethicists none were so impolite as to note that advancing research need over patient choice and protection was exactly what had been criticized fiercely in experiments on humans at places like Tuskegee and Willowbrook. Nor did any object that the argument if enacted would violate, at least potentially, a range of international covenants set up after Nuremberg to inhibit objectifying research. To take one example, article 3.2 of the UNESCO 2005 Declaration on Bioethics and Human Rights stipulates "the interests and welfare of the individual should have priority over the sole interest of science or society."[25]

An Excitable Public

What excited the public and the media, much to the despair of Rhodes, were cautionary tales of relatively healthy human subjects who died as a result of participation in research projects approved by institutional review boards (IRBs) staffed in part by bioethicists. Among the best known of these in recent years in North America were the well-reported deaths of Jessie Gelsinger[26] and Ellen Roche.[27] Gelsinger, a relatively healthy nineteen-year-old with a genetically based liver condition, died in 1999 of a massive immune response to a virus used to deliver an experimental treatment. Roche was a healthy volunteer who died of a fatal reaction to a compound used in a study of a potential new treatment for asthma.[28]

These cases were not aberrations but instead exemplified a pattern of research excess. As early as 1980, *Science* reported the "NIH [National Institutes of Health] shaken by death of a volunteer" in a supposedly safe research program.[29] In 1985 there were reports of the deaths of other research subjects.[30] Just as nineteenth-century shipwrecks in the North Atlantic were seen as sad, even tragic, but disconnected events so, too, these were seen as unfortunate one-offs until the number of deaths was sufficient to make a pattern of malfeasance obvious. At U.S. Senate hearings convened after Gelsinger's death a witness from the NIH testified that over a seven-year period only 39 of at least 691 "adverse events" (patient illness or death) were "reported in a timely way."[31]

Bioethicists were ethically engaged here (I want to say complicit) in a number of ways. First, many had promoted research as a primary good whose future benefits outweighed the immediate needs of the person. Consulting bioethicists had stocked the research review boards that in theory had ethical oversight of the research programs. That participation promoted a "business model that," as Carl Elliott put it, "undercuts arguments for [bioethical] professionalism."[32] The result, Elliott later argued, was a credibility crisis for bioethics as anything other than tame publicists promoting as respectable the research industry and its agenda.[33] "Bioethicists have written for years about conflicts of interest in scientific research or patient care yet have paid little attention to the ones that might compromise bioethics itself."[34] In this and other writings Elliott generously assumed bioethics' focus was still medicine's old ethical goal: the care and protection of the fragile patient.

"The Therapeutic Misconception"

The principal goal of research is not the care or treatment of its test subjects although it is sometimes presented as such. This is what became known as the "therapeutic misconception" in which research participants—and often their physicians—"misunderstand the nature of the activity they have consented to."[35] Patients believe, or are led to believe, their participation in research programs may result in a therapeutic gain, or at least a better diagnosis. They assume at the least that participation in this or that research protocol will be safe. But the goal of the research is neither treatment nor diagnosis; patient safety, while desirable, is never guaranteed. If the patient doesn't get that it's his or her "misconception."

That "misconception" is, however, actively promoted. Consider, for example, a poster advertising a 2011 bioethical conference on a "moral obligation to participate in research" (figure 8.1). The importance of the idea is emphasized by the perhaps forty-point-sized sans serif font in which it is presented. The choice of font implies the issue is contemporary and modern. Had it been in Times Roman or Baskerville fonts the effect would have been different. Under the title, in bold, is the date and location of the conference at the University of Minnesota, Twin Cities Campus. The academic site adds legitimacy to the proposition and its discussion. Hold the meeting at a bingo hall and nobody will take it seriously. The names of the principal presenters are listed, down the right-hand column. Not surprisingly they include David Orentlicher and Rosamond Rhodes.

The message of the poster is delivered in the photograph that sits under the sans serif conference title. In it an African American physician or researcher bends forward in concentration, his attention riveted on the inner arm of a Caucasian woman, the patient. He leans forward and she looks down; together they are a portrait of mutuality and partnership in the scientific measurement of her health.

Wait! His second and third fingers are spaced apart, one at the distal end of her humerus, perhaps at the medial condyle, the other at the proximal end of her humerus at the inside of her elbow. But he can't take her pulse that way because there is no artery beneath the fingers. And he can't take blood pressure because he has no stethoscope with which to hear the ebb and flow of the blood. And even if he could do that there is no monitor with which to see the measurement he in theory is attempting to make.

So the whole is a sham and the African American in the white coat no doctor, just a poseur. But then, so is the faux patient who wears hospital identification around her neck and hospital garb, perhaps to reinforce the theme of the caring clinical encounter. She is probably a hospital worker, perhaps a nurse pulled from the corridor because someone thought she looked just right for the picture. And she does, her hair pulled back but a bit askew. Her body is relaxed—reflecting confidence in the doctor, and her attention on his faux testing as complete as his own. What gives the charade away is the large soda container with its carefully bent straw sitting negligently in her left hand. Even a first-year medical student would ask her to put it down before he began his examination.

The sham is carefully designed to project the idea of care and concern for the person, the mutuality of physician and patient. But what the program participants were being asked to consider had little to do with the mundane practice of medicine or the care of the person. Rather, it was an ostensible civic obligation that would mandate (and perhaps force) persons to serve as research objects to assist in the development of future medical resources to be sold commercially to those who in the future may be able to afford them. The brilliance of the image—like that of the proposition itself—is that it speaks of care, concern, and mutuality to promote an obligation in which care is largely irrelevant, concern for the patient and his or her choices minimal, and mutuality

University of Minnesota
Driven to Discover

Do people have a moral obligation to participate in research?

Conference
Wednesday, Oct. 12, 2011
8:30 am – 3:00 pm

Coffman Memorial Union, 4th Floor
University of Minnesota Twin Cities campus

Registration is free and open to the public

Do people have a moral obligation to participate in research? Thus far in the history of modern research ethics, the answer has been no. In the United States, since the aftermath of WW II the stance of research ethics with human beings has been primarily concerned with protection of human subjects, an ethic grounded in principles articulated in the *Belmont Report*: respect for persons, beneficence, and justice. Recently, however, there has been a small but growing and increasingly vocal literature challenging these long-held understandings.

This conference will explore the arguments for and against the claim that people have a moral duty to participate in research by some of the most prominent advocates on both sides of the question.

Objectives:

At the conclusion of this conference, participants will be able to:

1. articulate the major arguments for and against the claim that people have a moral duty to participate in research;
2. reflect on their own views regarding the claim that people have a moral duty to participate in research;
3. identify the implications for the way in which biomedical research will be taught and practiced should there be a paradigm shift in research ethics.

Who should attend?

Clinical researchers, research administrators, students, patients, members of society at large, IRB representatives and other regulatory bodies.

CONFERENCE SPEAKERS AND PANELISTS

JOAN LIASCHENKO, RN, PHD, FAAN
Professor
Center for Bioethics and School of Nursing
University of Minnesota

M. THERESE LYSAUGHT, PHD
Associate Professor
Department of Theology
Marquette University

DAVID ORENTLICHER, MD, JD
Professor and Co-Director
Center for Law and Health
Indiana University Schools of Law and Medicine

ROSAMOND RHODES, PHD
Associate Program Director and
Professor of Bioethics
The Bioethics Program; and
Professor of Medical Education
Mount Sinai School of Medicine

RICHARD SHARP, PHD
Director of Bioethics Research
Center for Ethics, Humanities, and Spiritual Care
The Cleveland Clinic

MARK YARBOROUGH, PHD
Dean's Professor of Bioethics
Bioethics Program
University of California Davis Medical School

This event has been designated by the Office of the Vice President for Research to satisfy the Awareness/Discussion component of the Responsible Conduct of Research (RCR) continuing education requirement.

REGISTRATION IS FREE AND OPEN TO THE PUBLIC

REGISTER NOW AT:
www.bioethics.umn.edu
email: bioethx@umn.edu
612-624-9440/F. 612-624-9108

For further information, contact
Candace Holmbo at holmb006@umn.edu.

Sponsored by:

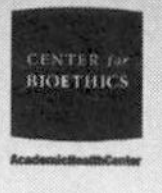

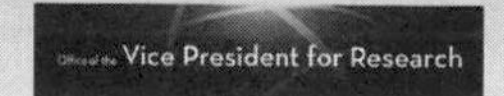

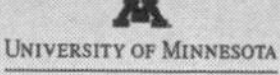

Clinical and Translational Science Institute
Driven to Discover℠

Figure 8.1
The obligation to participate in research is signified here by the caring physician with a concerned patient in close contact and association. But the research in which the patient is enrolled is likely to be an anonymous trial, not an intimate association. Care is not a priority. *Source*: University of Minnesota Department of Bioethics.

denied in the advance of an "obligation" to the future irrespective of the needs of the person today. Add to this the instruments of medical science—the blood pressure monitor in the background, the white coat of the doctor—and the whole becomes an indictment rather than a promotion.

Medicine as Research

The answer, to some bioethicists, is simple: divide ethics into different agendas, each with distinct priorities. "On the one hand, clinical research is seen as ethically distinct from medical care," Joffee and Miller wrote in 2008. "On the other hand, the obligations of investigators, especially in clinical trials, are thought to be grounded in the ethics of the doctor-patient relationship. To remove this incoherence, we need an entirely new conception of clinical research ethics—one that looks to science instead of the doctor-patient relationship and situates human subjects research in a continuum of biomedical research."[36] There is no continuum here, however. There is instead a clear rupture with the mandate to care on one side, and on the other, the research ethic in which patients are objects, ciphers in the database of a research program's results.

The division between patients whose care is primary and research subjects for whom care is a secondary concern began, as we saw, with *Belmont*. The problem was, and remains, the utility of patients as research objects typically rests upon the reality of their diagnosed conditions. Jessie Gelsinger was a valuable research subject *because* he had ornithine transcarbamylase deficiency. That made him a valuable resource for the phase I trial of a possible gene therapy treatment then under study. Ellen Roche was a healthy twenty-four-year-old before inhaling hexamethonium in a study on how the lungs of healthy people protect against asthma. She was important because she wasn't sick and thus served as a control until she became ill as a result of the drug trial. Sick to begin with or sick afterward, test subjects are patients and their care is under the supervision of physicians whose ethics, under bioethics, has its focus on future goods rather than present needs.

The problem is exacerbated in the United States where the doctor's office has become a recruitment field for many researchers. Patients are offered treatment, albeit experimental, that they could not otherwise afford if they agree to serve as research objects.[37] Depending on the trial protocol the research subject will receive a drug under study, a placebo, or a drug already accepted as standard treatment. When the test is completed, if the patient survives, the caring relationship terminates as well. Treatment is defined by, and bounded by, the research protocols the physician must follow. The "therapeutic relationship" that was at the heart of the old medical ethic extends only through the period of research and is bounded in its therapeutic nature by the research materials being tested.

"The distributive logic of the practice of [traditional] medicine seems to be this," wrote Michael Walzer, "that care should be proportionate to illness and not to wealth."[38] In its place bioethics instantiated Elliott's business model and for those physicians willing to participate made it a lucrative substitution. "The attraction for most physicians is that they can see that for each line item, the pharmaceutical companies are paying at least twice as much (and even up to five times as much) as an insurance company, or government agent would for the same services. Each office visit . . . generates two to three times the revenue as does seeing patients as part of standard [insured] medical visits."[39] From this perspective, the lack of universal health care in the United States is a research boon, funneling financially dependent patients into research programs as medical subjects. And—why not? *Principles* rejected out of hand medicine's traditional vocation of care and substituted a kind of professionalism that made of the nurse or physician a technician with no greater ethical responsibility than an insurance salesman.

None of this is to argue that research is not important. It is to say the demotion of the patient, and injunctions for the primacy of their care, in favor of a research agenda is ethically questionable and certainly unnecessary. Advances in medicine in the twentieth century were extraordinary well before bioethics' ascendancy, and during its early years. Lejune and the rest did not require the substitution of research priorities for patient protections. Indeed, they would have abhorred the suggestion. Nor did they require physicians to set aside their traditional goal of patient care and protection. The "ethical catastrophe" Rhodes feared lies not in the refusal of some to be objectified for the purpose of clinical trials but rather in the objectification of medicine as a commercial enterprise in which the patient in need is reduced to a research opportunity or a sales point.

Eugenics Redux

It is a small step from this research-oriented bioethic to the refashioning of the old eugenic argument in which pruning the human tree of undesirables is a reasonable service to future economies if not, as McBryde Johnson would have pointed out, to the pruned themselves. If all individuals can be objectified on the basis of their utility, and if future economies are more important than the lives of contemporary individuals, then why not simply engineer away those who are seen as deficient? This was the argument of *Buck v. Bell*, one that denied the security and sanctity of the person in favor of a rosier future economic state. It is also implicit in Van Rensselaer Potter's definition of bioethics as the "rational but cautious participation" in human evolution.[40]

Contemporary bioethicists like John Harris and Jonathan Glover advance this argument in books like the former's 2007 *Enhancing Evolution* and the latter's 2006 *Choosing Children: The Ethical Dilemmas of Genetic Intervention*. Their stated interest is the good of future humankind, the advance of the species. In the most polite way Glover and Harris argue for eugenic selection on the basis of, baldly summarized, the future person's own good (would you want to be a dummy?), the future parent's dreams (would you want to be the parent of a dummy?), and the future of the species in general (we won't want dummies here).

These and other, like-minded bioethicists share with transhumanists (for example, Nick Bostrom[41] and James Hughes[42]) the core eugenic belief that "human nature is improvable through the use of applied science and other rational methods."[43] Just as nineteenth-century phrenologists were sure they could identify criminal types by the bumps on their skulls, the new eugenicist is convinced he or she can identify the characteristics of persons by mapping out their genetic profiles. Prospective parents, the enhancement bioethicists say, should embrace embryonic selection technologies, and perhaps fetal abortion, because everyone wants babies that will be beautiful, healthy, intelligent, and thus someday successful. To accept less is to be a bad (or at least misguided) parent. And, too, we want a beautiful, healthy, smart citizenry. Because society *needs* the strong and successful rather than the damaged and weak, to seek anything else is bad citizenship. The insistence is that it is our right as species members—and perhaps our destiny—to take charge of the species' shared genetic inheritance to produce future generations of persons who will be like us, or perhaps even better endowed.

Here, again, is the promotion of future benefit as a primary, essential good. Here, too, is the dour view of normalcy and difference that pervaded the ethics of Peter Singer. Like the eugenics of yore, the whole rests on a tangle of assumptions that insist, first, that we know which characteristics should be promoted or restricted, and second, how to assure their broad promotion.[44] Alas, the science underlying this assumption is little clearer today than it was in the 1920s. Matti Häyry, a fan of Glover and Harris, summarizes the "science" of the new eugenics this way: "Children's inborn characteristics can be detected by prenatal and preimplantation tests; the molecular processes of the human body can be studied and modified; and changes can be introduced to our inherited and heritable features either individually or collectively."[45] By selecting for admirable "molecular processes," individuals can be engineered to become the type of person that enhancement enthusiasts wish our future selves to be. Rejecting potential persons whose characteristics we perceive as potentially unfavorable—a Dale Froese, for example—will remove those like them from the potential stock of future generations. They will not be missed because in their difference they necessarily will present an undesirable future burden. They will not be injured because they will never have been.

Evolution: Simple and Complex

Certain traits can be detected in the developing fetus, and for those who can afford it, during in vitro fertilization. What we can identify we cannot, however, modify. We cannot change the XX to an XY chromosome (or visa versa), altering the sex of the fetus; we cannot modify the tripled twenty-first chromosome to transform the fetus with Down syndrome into one with a regular chromosomal pattern. If there is to be male pattern baldness in the mature person the best we can do is put aside money for a good toupee or wig to be purchased in thirty or fifty years. If the gene for Huntington's disease is present the only choice is to abort the fetus (or terminate the embryo) or let it live with the knowledge of inevitable onset in adulthood if the person to be survives the vagaries of childhood, adolescence, and young adulthood.

That's it: we take it as it is or we kill it. If termination is chosen the result will not greatly affect our collective inheritance, however. Baldness will not disappear from the world. Nor will shortness, as much a result of parental diet and infant nutrition as it is of genetic predisposition. Disposing of potential persons with a genetic predisposition to Alzheimer disease or breast cancer will not rid future generations of these conditions. There are "wild" cases that appear spontaneously for reasons we do not understand. Down syndrome, for example, is a persistent genetic variation observed in all cultures and races. Thus to effect a change in the species' future the eugenicist would have to be like the farmer raising sterile, genetically modified plants. Each generation would have to be culled in an attempt to protect against the imposition of naturally recurring change.

More fundamentally, perhaps, contemporary eugenic ethics rests on the demonstrably invalid assumption that a simple positive correlation exists necessarily between specific traits and presumably desirable social outcomes.[46] It further assumes those traits are the sole result of a simple genetic signature rather than a complex of interrelated factors: economic, genetic, familial, social, and so on. Finally, this ethics assumes the effects of these conditions on the individual, and of the individual on society at large, are both immutable and easily described. Here, for example, are Savulescu and Sandberg on the governing theory: "Evolutionary theory predicts that genes promoting psychological and physiological traits that lead to a greater number of successful offspring will become more common over time."[47]

That Darwinian thesis "stands in its remarkable simplicity as an example of a single set of rules applicable to all biological systems."[48] The systems it attempts to order, however, are not simple but interrelated and complex. Each element of each system is subject to a complex range of deviations and exceptions that make hash of the presumably inevitable outcomes eugenic ethicists assume they can evaluate and then value. If evolutionary advance were as simple as enhancement enthusiasts assume, then all species members would have become as fleet as gazelles on the Savannah and as strong as our primate forbears in the forest. Simple Darwinian evolution would have bred these traits, generation by generation, until the undesirably slow and weak became extinct.

"Here again," writes Mark Witten, "scientists had it all wrong: they had assumed that a given disorder was the result of common mutations of a handful of genes."[49] In fact, the simple genetic profile is of limited value in predicting most future states. One reason is that our genetic profiles include genetic copy variations (CNVs), genes that seem normal but carry aberrations that may affect a range of characteristics. A single genetic copy variation can cause numerous differences. Conversely, one characteristic can be the result of a group of interacting CNVs.

Even were all this perfectly understood—and it certainly is not—it would not mean we could engineer the perfect future human because the characteristics that future human will need are unknown. What serves at any moment may not serve in the future; the environment tomorrow will require different abilities and responses from us than does our environment today.[50] Even where it possible to engineer a future human, the evolution and survival of the species therefore rests not on the limited breeding of a few exemplars whose attributes we today might admire but instead on a broad diversity of characteristics within the community of persons of tomorrow.[51] It is that diversity that has permitted the species to endure and progress.

This person has great vision and that one acute hearing, and perhaps perfect pitch. The first was most important to the hunter community in the day, the latter in the nighttime when vision was limited. It was not the exceptional individual's transmittable trait but rather the ability to capitalize on a diverse range of traits that assured the range of responses that permitted survival and promoted species evolution. The real key to human evolution and progress lies in the sociability of the species, its genius for cooperative interaction of persons with diverse capabilities. "Pleistocene evolution saw the emergence of human beings as intensely social species" whose sociability was the key to the cooperative behavior that permitted humankind to progress through the diverse abilities of its members.[52]

The problem for Darwin was altruism, the selfless behavior he saw in both animals and humankind by one species member for another. This kind of behavior seemed to him both pervasive and inimical to the game of survival in which each seeks to pass on his or her genes, building a better future. Evolution is more than a simple game of survival of the fittest, a zero-sum of "I win, you lose," and more one of cooperation in which altruism is the key to the mutual survival of the community.[53] Here one sees the failure of Darwinian theory as a simple program of the survival of the fittest. Its focus is the radical individual—the exemplary isolate—that was a common element in the social philosophy in Darwin's day. Darwin therefore saw altruism and cooperative behavior as a problem, a complexity whose reality he recognized but which he had trouble fitting into his argument. In retrospect he might better have seen them as the critical elements in species survival, with the "survival of the fittest" attribute a limited engine for species development within the context of species survival at large.

Certainly we see this to be true in humans. It was the ability to share emotions and ideas; to not only produce tools but also to transmit the secrets of their construction and use that distinguished humanity from its evolutionary ancestors. "Human evolution is not just a story of hunter-gatherers coping with a physical environment but one of *Homo sapiens* cooperating with each other to maximize species survival in the environments that effect them and they simultaneously effect through their patterns of behavior."[54] In that cooperation diversity was the key, a catalogue of characteristics each community could draw on in response to the challenges all community members faced.

Current research tells us that all species' communities have members with a diverse set of attributes that differentially serve the community. It is true of the ape and true, too, of the stickleback fish.[55] There are in all animal communities the adventurous and timid, those who act first and those who think first. Some are stronger; others are faster. All are needed if communal survival is to be assured. Were the "genetic challenge" more than a eugenic shill, if we could change everyone to reflect at least the mundane norm, it likely would be the death knell of the species. At issue is not, as Häyry has it, "rationality and the genetic challenge," but as Gregor Wolbring put it, "surviving [modern] eugenics in a technological world."[56]

Selection of a specific trait is a great way to create a hothouse flower. But making a rare orchid with pink tips on a purple petal doesn't transform the genus *Orchidaceae*. It simply creates a hothouse hybrid requiring continued protection to maintain its uniqueness. Were the eugenicists able to select replicable traits for future humans (and they can't, at least not yet) the result would be, at very best, hothouse humans. What we have in enhancement bioethics is not good science but to borrow Richard Lewontin's phrase, "biology as ideology," and an unscientific, unsavory ideology at that.[57] The error of the eugenic bioethicist is therefore fundamental, advancing a simplistic evolutionary model—one science has gone beyond—as if it were complete. The brightest, fastest, and strongest do not always survive, and if they do it is not solely on their own merit but rather through the support of the community at large.

Here we can see Singer and McBryde Johnson in a new light, albeit one that is more hers than his. They are equally valuable, equally critical elements in a society that seeks to understand itself and what it wants to be. McBryde Johnson saw this, I think. At the least it is implicit in her writings. Singer, like Glover and Harris, I suspect, never saw it at all.

Metaphor and Fact

Underlying the misuse of simplistic Darwinian arguments is the persistent mistaking of simple metaphors for complex referents. The metaphor is exclusory, its frame bending the tale of events to a single conclusion without reference to prior actions or causes. The metaphor of the lifeboat was but one example. We see again this mistaking of the metaphor for reality in the misappropriation of snippets of science as a guide to the ethics some seek to promote. Consider, for example, the promotional copy for a new book in 2010 stating that "as genes represent the 'blueprint' of an organism, their analysis and manipulation is a challenge to our understanding of human nature."[58]

It's a common idea that presents an egregious error. Blueprints are assumed to be complete descriptions of wholly understood systems whose potential (Heidegger would have said "ontology") is expressed in that description. In this reading, we assume to know exactly how a system will perform on the basis of its blueprint. The blueprint of a building's electrical system exhausts the nature of the system. If the wiring is as diagrammed we know exactly how the lights will work in the building . . . every time. One does not need to train the building to shine brightly at night; it does it when the right switches are tripped.

The human genome is not a blueprint, however. Reading it does not tell the tale of the human species or the individuals who are its members. A person's genetic profile (at least at the very coarse level at which we can interpret it today) at best describes potentials and potential limits. Whether those potentials are activated, let alone realized, will depend on a complex interplay of environmental, familial, and social factors that work together in a fashion that at present is at best very imperfectly understood. "A journalist once asked the behavioral psychologist Donald Hebb whether a person's genes or environment matter most to the development of personality. Hebb replied that the question was akin to asking which feature of a rectangle—length or width—made the most important contribution to the area."[59]

Inherited potentials must be activated in a conducive environment and then nurtured before they can be realized. Runners learn the tricks of running, gymnasts the secrets of balance, physicians the art of diagnostics not naturally but through years of tutelage and study. Some have the physiology to be great runners but to realize the potential for speed the person needs to run, run, and run. To perform well on the uneven parallel bars requires first an innate propioceptive sense, the perception of being in space, and then years of bruising, sometimes humiliating practice under the supervision of experienced instructors. Even if we could breed children with the potential speed at maturity of a gazelle, the innate balance of a chimpanzee, the strength of a gorilla, and the acumen of a William Osler, those potentials would become realized only after years of repetitive practice, study, training, and work.

To endure and then to excel requires not only natural attributes but as well a social environment that promote this or that excellence. Potential will mean nothing if the person does not have the desire to excel in a certain way. That, at least so far as we know, is not a genetic thing. The desire to excel is instead a complex outcome of individual interest, physical potential, and social encouragement. All this complexity of circumstance is ignored in the blueprint metaphor that assumes we are each a short set of simple traits whose provenance is completely understood and whose activation is inevitable.

Here, by the way of an aside, is the secret of the cloning debate. Even if we could make a viable perfect copy of this or that person's genetic profile his or her replicant would differ markedly in adulthood from the breeder's expectations. We develop in a family, community, and culture whose elements drive us forward or hold us back. Had Albert Einstein been cloned the resulting person might have become a schoolteacher who played the cello at night in the community orchestra, or guitar in a country music band. A Tiger Woods clone might grow up despising golf as a ridiculous waste of time ("But it gave you a good home, son"), choosing instead to spend his life in fashion design. Peter Singer's or John Harris's clones might choose to become scientists, disdaining parental philosophies as lacking the rigor of electron microscopy.

Intelligence

Intelligence exemplifies the kind of "trait" enhancement bioethicists seek to promote, a characteristic they wish to increase in future generations. It is also the kind of characteristic that some like Singer might choose to distinguish the worthy from the unworthy. What is meant by intelligence is unclear, however. At present, the best that might be achieved would be to breed high scorers on the Stanford-Binet intelligence test. The test's originator, nineteenth-century French educator Alfred Binet (figure 8.2), developed the first test as a diagnostic capable of identifying children in need of remedial education.[60] He was adamant this was not a measure of "intelligence," however it might be defined. Like Lejeune in the twentieth century, Binet sought not a sieve to separate the disposable from the worthy but an instrument that would promote additional care for those who needed it.

Early in the twentieth century, Stanford psychologist Charles Spearman conceived (incorrectly, we know today) of intelligence as a single, unitary, thing whose strength could be as precisely tested as if it were, say, visual acuity. Stanford University psychologists then transformed Binet's diagnostic into the now famous Stanford-Binet IQ test, thus constructing what they called "intelligence" as a testable thing. On this basis American psychologists created a number of categories of greater or lesser intelligence.

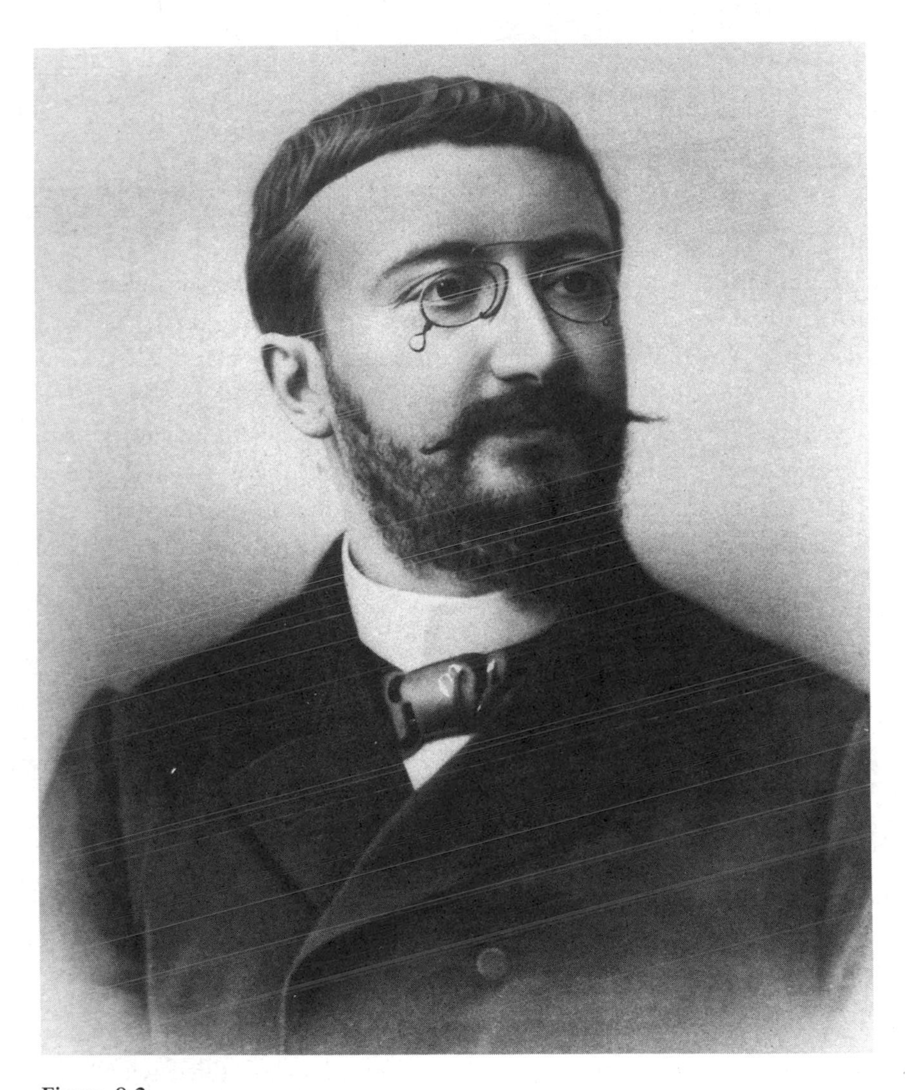

Figure 8.2
Psychologist Alfred Binet created the first "intelligence test" as a diagnostic to identify students who needed remedial help, not as a test of "IQ."

It was this type of intelligence test that Carrie Buck failed, resulting in her forced sterilization. Psychologists judged her IQ to be about 50, a "typical score for a low-grade moron."[61] Psychologists who retested her in the 1940s found, however, a woman of average intelligence who was simply poor and uneducated. Her sterilization, and that of others like her, did not save the United States from a moronic future. "It was not until the 1940s that the thesis that most retarded persons were born to retarded persons [the key tenet of sterilization programs] was flatly rejected.[62] When Stanford-Binet tests were applied to World War I army recruits something like 30 percent of the inductees were classified as moronic.[63] That did not prevent their service, of course. But to the surprise of army psychologists, many of the moronic recruits were found to be brave, clever, and resourceful. It turned out that test performance was as much a function of education, economic advantage, literacy, and social support as it was a measure of something innate.

Mensa

Those who today assume they can distinguish the intelligent from the intellectual failure are like the 1920s psychologists who assumed simple tests could measure the complex characteristics they sought to promote. Even where it possible to breed or otherwise select high IQ test scorers the result would not necessarily assure lives that were inherently more satisfying or persons more engaged, professionally or socially, in the community at large. Consider, for example, the Mensa society whose goal is "to identify and foster human intelligence for the benefit of humanity."[64] That beneficence is based on the belief that those who, like Mensa members, score high on intelligence tests are natural resources to be nurtured and esteemed. And yet, Mensa meetings are filled with high-scoring individuals whose social contributions have been at best minimal and whose personal achievements are at very best pedestrian. They may believe themselves especially worthy but that self-aggrandizing claim has no formal proof. Mensa members are good IQ test takers but any correlation between that skill and either personal happiness or social contribution appears at most incidental.

If we don't know what intelligence is, enhancement enthusiasts will respond, we know what it is not. Perhaps IQ tests are limited indicators of future performance, but science is on firmer ground with some genetic profiles—for example, Trisomy 21. We can identify in utero the fetus that will carry this genetic characteristic. We cannot say if the person who results will be "high functioning" college material or "low functioning" and in need of lifelong support. Not can we assume the person with Trisomy 21 will be less socially valuable, less an individual, or less delightful than another person with a normal chromosomal pattern.

If one is an enhancement bioethicist then Down syndrome people like Dale Froesce and his wife are obvious examples of the kind of persons we can ethically eject from the common gene pool. For a McBryde Johnson or for Froesce himself, however, Down syndrome is simply a common genetic variant normally occurring across the human experience and not to be reflexively dismissed. The Canadian Down Syndrome Society defines Down syndrome as a naturally occurring genetic pattern and not a disease. We make Trisomy 21 a burden by insisting upon a standard of normalcy that defines human intelligence in a manner that brooks no debate but also makes little hard sense.

For my part, I'd prefer to spend a week with the members of the Canadian Down Syndrome Society than any time at all with a congregation of Mensa members. The former are typically more engaged, more generous in their social imaginings, more interesting in their questions, and simply a lot more fun. Similarly, given a choice between the annual meeting of the Canadian Down Syndrome Society or that of the American Society for Bioethics and the Humanities I would prefer the former. Their intelligence while different in its application is no less acute, and certainly no less reasonable. And their sense of community membership and support, like Dale Froesce's, is for me preferable to the often-bitter, self-serving narrow divisions of bioethical academics.

Fungible Persons

One thus may reject the eugenics bioethicists and their dreams of species enhancement on the basis of their failure to grasp the complexity of the science they pretend to embrace. And, too, one may reject as unserviceable the standards they attempt to impose. There is, as well, a deeper failure shared by all those advance future economies over immediate, patient needs. Embedded in the cry for genetic direction is the assumption that none of us are uniquely valuable but instead that we are all interchangeable ciphers in the grand Foucauldian count of social constituency. Aborting this fetus or letting that person die doesn't matter because in the greater scheme of things none of us matter unduly. Thus we are free to choose the people who will matter if only we might know what characteristics they should have.

To argue otherwise is called, by some, the "Beethoven fallacy."[65] Its name comes from this question: if progressively deaf Beethoven had not been born would we have lost the benefit of his genius? Would the history of Western music have suffered as a result? Those who argue our fungibility do so in this way: without Beethoven another musical genius would have appeared, one no less majestic in his musical imagining. True, we would not have had Beethoven's Ninth Symphony but another composer would have written another equally transforming orchestral score. All this implies a kind of Platonic plane in which arts and science and philosophy are out there, waiting to be imagined. Who first imagines it, and how they do so, is an accident of circumstance on the way to the inevitability of knowledge and progress. Art, science, and philosophy are eternal and those who tap into them mere accidental agents of inevitable discovery.

The fallacy fails spectacularly, however. If we honor the work we must recognize the reality it presents: maybe someone else would have brought us a Beethoven-like musical transformation. And . . . maybe not. But it *was* Beethoven who did it as his hearing failed. Thus to assume that deafness is a necessary burden for the person and for society, a harm to be avoided, for example, is to ignore Beethoven's experience. Whether another musician would have been equally and similarly transformative is not only mere supposition but also, from this perspective, irrelevant. The point is that a guy who became deaf did the work and to assume deafness is a necessary impediment is thus false.

Equally important, what enhancement enthusiasts see as "impairments" are in cases like Beethoven's absolutely central to the work the "impaired" produce. The powerful chords and rhythms of Beethoven's Ninth Symphony are the work of a progressively deaf individual who felt more than heard the music he wrote and then conducted. He knew the audience's applause through the vibration in the floorboards beneath his feet at the symphony's premiere. The brilliant contemporary percussionist Evelyn Glennie's music is similarly grounded, her deafness resulting in a distinct, physically rhythmic, magnificent sound.

In a similar vein, the effects of Stephen Hawking's motor neuron disease have been a constructive impetus in the creation of the cosmology he has produced over the last forty years. "Some have attributed his great successes in cosmology to his enhanced cerebral freedom," write his biographers, "yet others have claimed that the turning-point in the application of his abilities was the onset of his condition, and that before then he was no more than an averagely bright student."[66] Hawking has said it was only after his diagnosis that he began his life's work in earnest.[67] The elegance of his equations and the lucidity of his prose arose in part, he has said, from the need to boil down and summarize in his mind equations that can be dictated to an assistant.

As a final example it is worth remembering the degree to which McBryde Johnson's writing and work was grounded in her embodied, experiential world. Not only did she write and lecture from the perspective of her wheelchair but, more important, she wrote and lectured about the experiential world she knew. It was that which propelled her into the specialty of disability law, championing those facing the challenges of social prejudice that she had known. Had she been physically normal it is unlikely she would have pursued her career path with such intensity. It is unlikely Peter Singer would have invited her to Princeton to debate were her legal area of expertise real estate, for example. Was she otherwise she thus would not have written her famous essay.

None of this is to argue for the proliferation of limiting characteristics. Hawking does not wish ALS on anyone. McBryde Johnson did not promote a degenerative spinal condition as an ideal way of being. Glennie does not ask those who hear her music to cover their ears, to be like her. These and other examples insist instead that cognitive, physical, and sensory differences, even where severe, are not an argument for the reflexive dismissal of this or that person or potential person on the basis of a single characteristic. The lives lived fully but with limits emphasize as well the complex social realities that advance or inhibit each person's potential within an enabling or disabling community. That is the arena beyond the simple that the eugenic ethicists in the main ignore.

For the Betterment of Humankind

To borrow a distinction from Heidegger, bioethicists in general appear to have misunderstood the human entity both ontologically (its *essentia*) and theologically (its *existential*).[68] We are not simple biochemical programs whose characteristics can be easily programmed. Genes do not operate in isolation. The human genome is where we start, not what we become in full. As genomicist J. Craig Venter put it: "We have, in truth, learned nothing from the genome other than probabilities. How does a 1 or 3 percent increased risk for something translate into the clinic? It is useless information."[69]

From the biochemistry of the individual cell itself to the height of the person in which the cell resides, the messages encoded in DNA are influenced and modified by a range of outside influences.[70] This is why monozygotic twins, identical at birth, come to be phenotypically distinguished over time on the basis of the effect of the physical and social environments in which they have lived.[71] More generally, active epigenetic mediation explains differences in body masses measured in the children of smokers compared to nonsmokers; body height in the children of mothers based on caloric intake during pregnancy.[72] "It's hard to tell in most natural populations whether inheritance is due to DNA sequence variation or epigenetic changes."[73]

"The empirical fruits of several decades of research in molecular, cell, and developmental biology have revealed that what distinguishes one biological form from another is seldom, if ever, the presence or absence of a certain genetic template but rather *when* and *where* genes are expressed, how they are modified, and into *what* structural and dynamic relationships their 'products' become embedded."[74] The gene is not a blueprint but a *set* of templates providing a range of differing instructions for potential characteristics whose specific activation results from a complex, epigenetic response to the environment.

In short, DNA isn't simple destiny. It is a critical element contributing to an individual's potential. The person becomes what he or she will be in relation to—and reaction to—the realities of the physical and social worlds in which he or she matures. Biology exists apart from neither culture nor environment but as an active agent in a process in which cultural and social influences are active and critical.[75] Bidirectional pathways of environment-human interaction proliferate, year by year as our science advances. The result is a messy complexity whose precise elements are at best only partially understood. "We have long assumed that talent is a genetic thing some of us have and others don't," writes David Shenk. "It turns out everything we are is a developmental process and this includes what we get from our genes."[76]

Our essential nature (Heidegger's *essentia*) is thus not firmly set at birth but an outgrowth of the communal processes of humans in association in the world we together create. "The betterment of mankind," the old eugenic promise, therefore lies not in the selective breeding of humans for this or that trait. It lies instead in the acceptance of diversity among peoples and the promotion of care for people irrespective of their differences. This was a perspective that was understood within the older ethic of medicine, one bioethics might have sought to embrace but instead, at least in the main, has ignored.

Enhancement enthusiasts are not wrong in their advancement of the human condition as an ethical ideal. But any serious attention to that goal demands participation in the "social evolution" that Van Rensselaer Potter's bioethics promised but his successors never really considered. Were the betterment of humankind a bioethical goal its ethicists would argue—as did eighteenth- and nineteenth-century physicians like Benjamin Rush and Rudolph Virchow—for social activism in the arenas of education, the environment (removing unhealthy pollutants), health care, and social infrastructure. These are the arenas in which hard, nurturing work would encourage the full potential of both present and future generations.

And here . . . there is science beneath the claim. For whatever it is worth, the average measured intelligence (IQ) increases as the presence of infectious diseases decreases.[77] The assumption is that infants who do not have to fight off diseases have greater metabolic resources available for cognitive development. Conversely, individual abilities—intelligence, for example—are lowered in the presence of preventable disease. Steen identifies thirty preventable illness or conditions that may lower the IQ scores of future generations of children. As well as diseases preventable by vaccination, these include the environmental effects of poverty on both the diet and the physical environment in which the child develops. It is for this reason, among others, that many biologists are so concerned about the effects of global warming on human environments.[78]

Similarly, height is directly responsive to the caloric intake of the mother during pregnancy. General measures of childhood development have been increasing in recent decades at a rate of one point every two years not as a result of better genetic breeding but in direct relation to the increasing levels of infant caloric intake.[79] In short, there is no better tomorrow if we ignore the needs of peoples—all peoples—today. There will be no better species if we ignore current people in hopes of some future, imagined über species. That this returns us to the environmentalism of Hippocrates and his insistence on the physical and social as determinants of health is neither incidental nor ironic. It just . . . is. And, of course, it is precisely this recognition of the complex relation of person to place—physical and social—that eugenic bioethicists, and the utilitarian in general, ignore.

Here, again, we return to McBryde Johnson's "beautiful" as a judgment transposed from the bedside of the unconscious teenager to a clarion call for a medical ethics of care. That beauty lies not in the phenomenology of the embodied person alone but in the *existentia* of the species community as diverse and communal. It insists upon an ethics that advocates for the flourishing of all irrespective of this or that person's idiosyncratic characteristics. Its grounding is in the potential of all rather than the independent qualities of the few. In seeing the interpersonal care of the unconscious teenager as beautiful, McBryde Johnson drew us toward what bioethicists have traditionally dismissed, or at least ignored: a human complexity that is at once biological, environmental, and social.

9

Choice, Freedom, and the Paternalism Thing

It may be that bioethics' foundation myth is merely that, a myth, its research emphasis debatable and its broadly principled assertions at best insufficient. Certainly its promise of careful argument, critical thinking and "wisdom" seems to be grounded in a suspicious tendency to the unproved assertion. There is, for example, its declaration that the traditional medical ethic was obsolete without any real consideration of what that ethic was or a detailed explication of its practical inadequacy. And, of course, there is the lifeboat ethic embraced from the start as if it was a natural state, assuring in the process that a type and class of avoidable lifeboat dilemma would be accepted as natural and thus inevitable.

All that may be true but, by golly, bioethics did put paid to the odious practice of medical paternalism in which arrogant physicians dictated treatment protocols irrespective of a patient's desires, and perhaps, best interests. If nowhere else, bioethics surely proved its worth in wresting control of medical decision making from physicians and giving it to patients or their surrogates. In so doing it affirmed the application of a social principle of individual freedom and choice in an arena, the practice of medicine, where it had been lacking. So what if bioethics doesn't, as its defenders promised, "bring moral order to the chaos of disputes regarding proper biological research and medical practice [note the order of importance]."[1] Its real service has been as a champion of autonomous patient choice and as a foe of medical paternalism, thus creating Margaret Walker's deliberative moral space—personal and general—Andres described in the quote reproduced, here, in chapter 1.

Paternalism, as bioethicists have construed it, is any interference in a person's freedom of action. It denies the person's idiosyncratically perceived best interests irrespective of whether others see the wisdom of those choices.[2] The argument was, and remains, that the patient as an independent consumer must be the sole arbiter of the treatment to be proffered. Physician cautions, conclusions, or recommendations are largely irrelevant, rather like those of a salesperson who might say, "I don't think that size eight shoes are best for your size ten feet but if that's what you want, grand. They're very handsome, indeed."

Bioethics built its business in part on the insistence that the old medical ethic created a class of imperious professionals whose arrogance demanded restraint. Paternalism was the hobbyhorse bioethics rode to the fore, the windmill its Don Quixotes sought to vanquish. In 2010, for example, the advertisement for a major academic conference made this self-congratulatory statement: "Twenty years ago, bioethics and law teamed up to defeat a common enemy—paternalistic medicine. Armed with new weapons . . . autonomy would reign, and doctors would do what they were directed to by patients, their advance directives, or their surrogates."[3] The conference celebrating this achievement was sponsored by as unanimous a chorus of voices as one can find in medical ethics: the American Society of Bioethics and the Humanities (ASBH), the American Society of Law, Medicine, and Ethics (ASLME), the American Bar Association (ABA), the *American Journal of Bioethics* (AJOB), Duke University, Emory University, and the University of Kansas.

The conference advertisement was jam-packed with assertions, notably that the old medicine ethics had been irremediably paternalistic, and deservedly vanquished by the newly armed bioethics and its legal partners in freedom. As a result, patient choice now reigned. Previous chapters of this book address elements of this mythology. But it is so pervasive, so embedded in bioethical lore, that it demands fuller attention here.

As we have seen, the charge of medical paternalism grew during a period in which primary responsibility for medical decision making was being taken from the physician and given to insurers, hospital committees, and other authorities. Bioethics inserted its constituents in this new model as expert valuators who would adjudicate questions of treatment. These new officials insisted with Callahan that while physicians might be valued for their technical expertise their judgments were suspect. Here, however, the problem was not that physician recommendations were expensive but that they were imperious in their application and thus antiliberal in their denial of patient freedoms.

Medicine was never particularly paternalistic, however. Since the days of the Greeks, physicians have argued to patients the acceptance of protocols with the best potential for treatment for this or that condition. Across the long history of the old tradition they rarely had the power to impose their will irrespective of patient wishes, however.[4] From the days of the itinerant Hippocratic physician until recently, medicine has been a fee-for-service, patient-supported practice. Imperious insistence would have been economically foolish, resulting in a patient's legitimate refusal to pay for a service he or she did not want. And, too, the insistence on payment for unwanted treatment would have diminished the trust of the patient and his or her family that was an essential element of medical practice. Without that trust, and the respect that resulted from it, physicians would not enjoy the praise of the community and the sense of social service that the Hippocratic oath promised as a reward for good medical practice.

Typically, egregious paternalism has occurred only when the needs of the state, or an employer, or a research program, were put before the needs of the patient. Where the physician is an employee of the state, and its focus is on cost and performance, the needs and wishes of the patient are necessarily devalued. We saw this in *Buck v. Bell* and in more recent years the Ashbury draft policy. And, too, where research needs trump patient care—for example, at Tuskegee and Willowbrook—the negotiated practice of medical decision making is similarly devalued. It is fairer to say that patient freedoms are diminished (paternalistically) when the old Hippocratic covenant is violated in favor of economic priorities and other non-care-related values.

Nancy Cruzan

Where "paternalism" has been argued the real subject has typically been something other than physician arrogance. Consider the case of Nancy Cruzan that the 2010 conference sought to celebrate as a triumph of bioethics in partnership with the law. On January 11, 1983, Nancy Cruzan was thrown from her car into a ditch after a horrific automobile accident. She barely survived and afterward remained until her death in a persistently unconscious state.[5] After four years without any visible improvement, Cruzan's husband and parents together sought the removal

thank you
NANCY BETH CRUZAN
MOST LOVED
DAUGHTER — SISTER — AUNT
BORN JULY 20, 1957
DEPARTED JAN 11, 1983
AT PEACE DEC 26, 1990

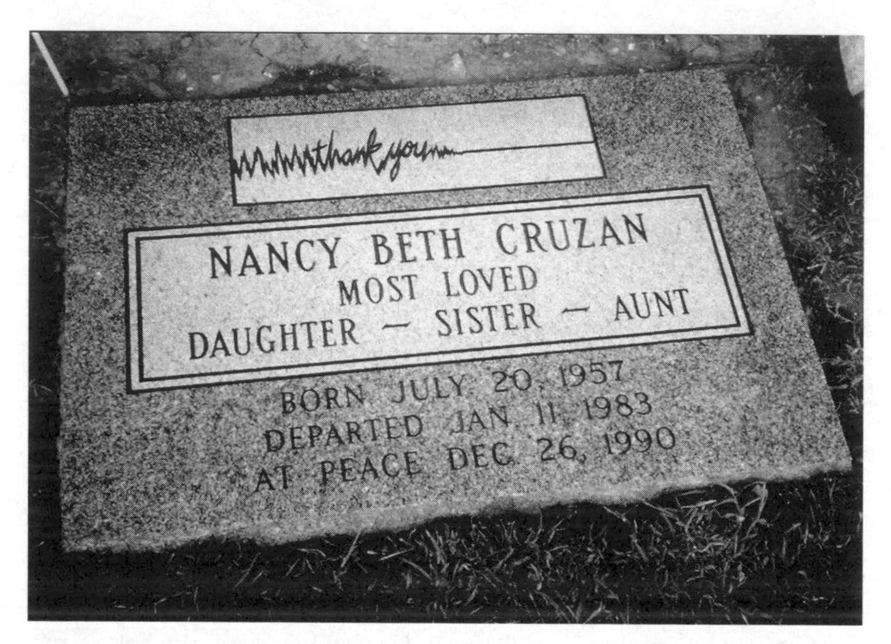

Figure 9.1
While the case of Nancy Cruzan is sometimes advanced as a victory against medical paternalism, the issue in law was the state's right to assert surrogates had to act as the incompetent patient would have required.

of her feeding tube in the belief that further maintenance was nonsensical; she was as good as dead. Hospital officials refused their request because they were uncertain of its legality. Legal statute required "clear and convincing proof" that a surrogate's order is not only in what a surrogate perceives as the patient's best interest but also, and equally important, in accord with the prior stated wishes of the person whose life they seek to end. The question in law, which made its way to the U.S. Supreme Court, was whether those requesting Nancy Cruzan's termination met the legal evidentiary standard (figure 9.1).

Hospital officials and attending physicians were willing to honor the family's request to remove Cruzan's feeding tube, thus ensuring her death, on presentation of evidence of the patient's prior wishes. They were bound, however, by laws whose rationale was clear: without such evidence any surrogate could insist on the discontinuation of support for a fragile relative whose maintenance was, for the surrogate, simply inconvenient. The issue in Cruzan was not physician paternalism but whether it was impertinent for society to "require that evidence of an incompetent's wishes as to the withdrawal of life-sustaining treatment be proved by clear and convincing evidence."[6] Writing for the majority, Chief Justice William Rehnquist argued the standard in law was not unreasonable and certainly not unconstitutional. The law asserts society's protective principle of the state's "life interest" in its citizens. In a land of checks and balances the general standard was a useful check against potentially inappropriate surrogate choices.

The Supreme Court thus upheld the standard benchmark of caution and rejected the family's request on the basis of insufficient evidence documenting Nancy Cruzan's prior wishes. The family eventually found what served as judicial proof and, once submitted to the courts, permission for the withdrawal of life supportive services was granted. Nancy Cruzan died eleven days after her feeding tube was removed on December 26, 1990. One year later, her father committed suicide on the anniversary of his daughter's death.

To clarify legal standards following the Cruzan imbroglio in 1990 Congress passed the Patient Self-Determination Act as part of the broad Omnibus Reconciliation Act of that year. It required institutions receiving Medicare or Medicaid funding to provide adult patients with information on their right to state their treatment or nontreatment preferences in advance directives that would be used to guide future care. The goal of the act was not to limit physician treatment but to provide patients with knowledge of the means by which they might give "clear and convincing evidence" of their future wishes to both physicians and relatives.

The case, and the act that was supposed to eliminate future problems, raised questions that remain exigent. "Since then," the conference organizers state in their literature, "many have come to believe that this policy structure was insufficient, fractured, or simply wrong headed. It has certainly been insufficient."[7] Do we want, for example, to think of the provision of food and fluids as no more than a clinical treatment that can be discontinued at the request of a surrogate? In 2004 the UN General Assembly adopted voluntary guidelines making nutrition a human right and since then its Right to Food Unit has sought universal acceptance of this idea. Shall it be a right for all except those incapable of standing up for themselves, perhaps a Jill Bolt Taylor in the immediate aftermath of her stroke?

Also unresolved were the bounds of surrogacy, of how far people can go on another's behalf and in their supposed best interests. This was an issue at law, and in ethical discussion of it, in the cases of Robert Wendland (2007) and Terry Schiavo (2005). And where surrogates disagree, who decides? Another problem is that living wills and advanced directives typically are written by persons in relative health about their expectations and wishes in cases of dire extremes they cannot imagine.[8] Can we really trust those choices? When a surrogate makes a decision that will result in the death of a fragile person over the physician's best judgment do we shrug and say, "Well, it's their choice?"

Buried in these uncertainties is the impertinent question: What was the new armament bioethics brought to this debate? The issue was legal and argued in law the role of the state in the protection of fragile persons and the limits of surrogacy on a fragile patient's behalf. The Cruzan case was never about high-handed, paternalistic physicians dictating conclusions irrespective of the patient's desire or needs. Rather, hospital officials referred a question of law to the law. The physician's role in this case was crucial but the choice of contested alternatives was set by social mores enshrined in statute. To the extent bioethicists engaged this as an issue of paternalism it was not the physician's, or medicine's, but rather the state's evocation of its "life interest" in the continuation of citizens and its goal to protect the fragile against unreasonable judgments.

This is not to deny excesses have occurred. Examples abound across these pages in the discussion of Carrie Buck, Jewish Hospital in New York City, Nuremberg, Tuskegee, Willowbrook, and so on. In all these situations, however, the problem was not the arrogance of the old medical ethic but its abandonment. In each case the physician's allegiance was not to the patient and his or her care, in the Hippocratic tradition, but to the state and its economic concerns, or to research and its future goods. In every case the problem lay in the objectification of the patient as either a research object or as a cipher in the utilitarian cost–benefit calculus of resource allocation.

Bioethics and Paternalism

Despite its insistence on the freedom of individual choice bioethics has been a signal promoter of paternalism at the cost of patient choice in the lifeboat ethic of scarce goods. Where scarcity reigns the presumptive right to care is diminished by the communal need to distribute limited resources where they might best serve future needs. In the lifeboat of scarce resources the determination of who lives and who dies is, as we have seen, the autocratic responsibility of the captain or first mate or whoever is in charge. Think, for a moment, of Callahan and his insistence that whatever they might wish, seniors should be denied all but comfort care so younger, more able folk might be better cared for by physicians. Callahan assumed seniors would be happy to give up their continuation in service of future generations. If they were not, however, his "communitarianism"—a kind of utilitarianism with a happy face[9]—could require it. Remember Dave Thomasma's embrace of the Ashbridge Draft Policy's reduction of service to seniors, irrespective of the levels of care Ashbridge patients requested, as "rational" in a world of resource limits. Remember Rosamond Rhodes whose idea of nonpaternalistic choice was to require people to choose between different research protocols requiring human subjects. Participation in tests as research objects, however, was to be mandatory.

Organ Transplantation

In their arguments bioethicists make the unrealistic assumption that science can speak precisely to the probable outcome of treatments and to the exact nature of a person's condition. They also assume, erroneously, that this perfect science exists outside any personal, social, or socioeconomic context that might influence the way a judgment of care or noncare is constructed. Their faith in a pure science that exists beyond the social constructions of its understanding is misplaced, however. Since the Ad Hoc Committee of the Harvard Medical School's 1968 definition of brain death, bioethicists have argued the withdrawal of life support is a natural course of action in the noncare of a physically alive but cognitively deceased post-person. The abandonment of that patient liberates hospital resources (another bed becomes available), and not incidentally, permits the potential provision of desperately needed donor organs.

Bioethical judgment based on the 1960 definition is, we now find, wrong. As Miller and Truog wrote in 2009, it makes no sense to argue the withdrawal of ventilation (or hydration and nutrition) does not directly cause the death of an unconscious patient.[10] The removal of a ventilator, typically accompanied by the injection of sedatives, is as directly the cause of respiratory and cardiac cessation as is the injection of potassium chloride in state executions. Nor, as we have seen, can one be certain those diagnosed as "brain dead" would not have survived and recovered. And yet, bioethicists do not call for changes in graft organ transplant policies. One would expect the enemies of paternalism and champions of patient freedoms at least would insist on informing the public of the ambiguities and uncertainties about "brain death," a now thoroughly contested where not absolutely devalued criterion. They do not do so, however, out of concern that, were patient families fully informed, they might choose further treatment rather than simply approve the withdrawal of care and then, hopefully, organ donation.[11] Patients living rather than being terminated would endanger organ supplies and generally tie up scarce hospital resources needed elsewhere for others. Thus it is better, bioethicists like Miller and Truog argue, not to tell people than let them make choices based on available knowledge. Paternalistic? Sure.

Similarly, Guggenheim Fellowship winner Dr. Lewis Cohen, a physician but not an ethicist, writes approvingly in support of ethical arguments to "reset default [clinical] standards" so that patient choices can be more easily ignored. "While this may seem like a step back in time to the era of paternalism, it is prompted by an appreciation of the flaw in overly relying on patient autonomy," he writes.[12] Cohen never explains what that flaw might be, however. His new standards would be carried out by a generation of physicians whose ethics are grounded not in the old Hippocratic injunction to patient care but a bioethics that assumes scarcity demands an ordered limit to patient choice (and thus survival) in the medical lifeboat of scarce resources. The result is a new bioethical paternalism whose principal focus is not patient care, or choice, but the utilitarian greater good.

A series of cases in which nontreatment is urged upon patients is now developing in various legal jurisdictions. One Canadian case before the courts at this writing serves as a convenient example of the many. In this case physicians rejected the wishes of a patient surrogate, a nurse, fighting for her elderly father's continued care. There was no doubt that the aggressive care she requested would prolong the patient's life. There was also little doubt he was nearing the end of his life. Were it simply a matter of paternalism by an arrogant doctor we would be shocked. But the real issue was the sense of scarcity and the resulting protocols of triage that made of it a kind of lifeboat case. As one law professor explained: "If the patient's life cannot be saved in a meaningful way and if intervention would deny resources that would benefit other patients. . . . Then the doctor is justified in clinical judgment to withhold treatment . . . clinical judgment is not negotiated with patients."[13]

There was no reason to assume the care of this patient would result in an inability to care for others *except* for the sense of scarcity bioethics has gifted to society at large and to medicine in particular. "Meaningful" becomes a simple judgment based on a set of contingent abilities rather than on patient or patient surrogate choices. The problem in this case was not simple physician arrogance or paternalism but the bioethical argument for the reflexive noncare of the fragile where resources are available but not infinite. Dave Thomasma would have called this "rational": *If* resources are limited, *then* the patient's desires (or the surrogate's) can be discounted if not simply ignored in the lifeboat of care. The physician's role becomes, in this context, not that of the Hippocratic patient protector but instead that of a resource administrator.

In the lifeboat ethic of bioethics the patient's wishes and choices *must* be secondary to some expert's valuation, to the first mate's vision of the greater good. And because the decision is typically made in extremes it is the physician who is called upon to enact the protocols of scarcity rather than to decide with a patient (or surrogate) on the best coarse of treatment. This is the last act of an ethical scenario that has reduced the sphere of physician responsibility, and of patient choice. Unpalatable choices are the result.

This is the tragedy of bioethics. It argues an ethic of individual choice but has created an ethos in which care decisions will be based not on patient needs or wishes but on the assumption of resource limits. It makes of health professionals crewmen, or at best first mates, forced to impossible choices in a lifeboat that is leaking and overloaded. Will they be like Alexander William Holmes and follow the dictates of superiors (ethicists, insurers, hospital officials, and pharmaceutical companies running drug tests, and so on)? Or, perhaps, will they, like John Messier, refuse the orders of superiors and then face the ruined careers that result when people challenge authority? Either way, the patient's desires, like those of the *William Brown*'s lifeboat passengers—not to mention those drowned with the sinking ship—are necessarily made inconsequential.

The Economics of Ethics

Deeply engrained in the bioethical *Zeitgeist* is the assumption that the market is the natural means by which choice is defined and the patient is merely a consumer of healthcare, a type of service like any other. He or she makes choices from a restricted set of available services and, as a consumer, expects those choices to be honored reflexively. Implicit in this consumerism is the assumption that the health-industry market will serve as not only an efficient distributor but also the appropriate regulatory mechanism by which excesses will be punished (by the "consumer") and efficiencies rewarded through increased profits (or state savings). Doctors are health workers expert in their field but no more qualified to make instrumental decisions than, say, the furniture salesperson urging a customer to purchase one brand of sofa over another.

This fits nicely with neoliberal dogma. The problem, Nobel Prize-winning economist Kenneth J. Arrow argued in 1963, is that market models applicable to the average competitive business—for example, the manufacture and sale of automobiles—do not apply to the medical-care industry.[14] Automobile sales are an open market in which a range of information sources provide the consumer with a wealth of data. Medicine is by definition a closed or partially closed market in which levels of data, information, and knowledge—three different but related things—are restricted or unavailable.

Markets: Open and Restricted

There is a competitive, open market in automobiles, one in which manufacturers are free to promote their products in as many ways as possible, offering a range of models at whatever price seems to them reasonable. If engineers and investors think they can build a better car, and especially a better car for less money, they are free to do so and then offer it for sale. Once dealerships are in place they can compete freely. That is what happened, for example, in the 1970s in North America when the sovereignty of continental automobile manufacturers (Chrysler, GM, and

Ford) was challenged first by Japanese manufacturers (Nissan, Toyota), and more recently by others (Kia, for example).

Consumers interested in purchasing a car may test drive a Kia, a Nissan, and a Ford. The potential buyer may read consumer reports comparing the different car models and talk to people who own this or that car about their experiences as owners. The purchaser makes choices based on generally available, easily comprehensible data on price, dealer support, owner experience, and so on. It is in this kind of market, Arrow writes, that competition best serves and consumerism reigns.

Medicine however, is a fiercely regulated, closed market in which competition is limited. First, a person who wants to practice medicine must undergo a recognized course of instruction that includes stringent testing. Then he or she must pass a series of standard examinations. The hopeful then must obtain the approval of a professional organization whose practice guidelines bound the limits of all practitioners. Similarly, hospitals and clinics where most practice is situated are regulated by law. Their performance is reviewed periodically for compliance to general standards. Depending on the services offered, the hospital or clinic must have a required complement of physicians and nurses as well as an approved laboratory, pharmacy, and surgical theater.

Ford can not deny Kia a showroom in Detroit but medical and hospital licensing authorities can deny the Koch Clinic a permit to operate in Michigan. And if they approve the Koch Clinic they can still deny Tom Koch the right to practice on the grounds that he has not taken the requisite courses or passed the required examinations.

Nor would any reasonable person wish medicine to be nonregulated, its clinics and hospitals open to any entrepreneur. To see what medicine would be like in a system of entrepreneurial freedom India provides a useful example. There patients are free to seek care from across a competitive environment of largely unregulated private clinics, hospitals, and laboratories. The result is "tens of thousands of misdiagnoses every year" and thousands of lives lost as a result.[15] There the Koch Clinic and its principal might prosper, especially if fee structures were set to attract the poor who can't afford a better option. In that environment the Koch Clinic would, of course, cut costs through the use of old, outdated equipment run by at best minimally trained and thus lower-paid personnel.

Trust and Faith

Another reason medicine doesn't answer to the protocols of the market is because "the customer cannot test the product before consuming it, and there is [therefore] an element of trust in the [patient-physician] relation" as a result.[16] I can't test out the orthopedic surgeon before my hip replacement; the cardiac surgeon before a stint is placed in my cardiac artery. I must trust in both the physicians engaged in these procedures and the hospitals where these procedures are to be performed. It was to engender trust that the Hippocratic physician swore always to put the patient's best interests first.

Today that trust must include not only the physician and the hospital but also the laboratory where tests are concluded and the pharmacies where prescriptions are filled. If I am on a blood thinner like Warfarin following a deep vein thrombosis I cannot spend several weeks testing the drug quality at different pharmacies, seeking at once the best product at the most affordable price. I have no standard for comparison (I can't test the drug's purity) and I need the drug *now*. And, of course, I have to trust that the drug prescribed is the best for me because I don't have the knowledge to debate the relative merits of Warfarin and, say, Fragmin (an injectible low molecular weight Heprin).

Discretion and Necessity

There is another difference, Arrow wrote: where automobiles are typically a matter of discretionary choice, medicine is a matter of exigent need. The liberty of deliberation available to the car buyer is absent in exigent medical situations. If I have a cardiac arrest I can't search around for a doctor I like but must take the doctor who receives me in the ER. I need to trust his or her clinical assessment (a myocardial infarction) and that the recommended treatment (angioplasty, bypass surgery, drug therapy, etc.) is the best alternative for me. Even were there time to deliberate, the average layperson lacks the background to intelligently weigh the potential benefits and risks of this drug or that procedure. "There is always an inequality of information as to production methods between the producer and the purchase of any commodity, but in most [non-medical] cases the customer may well have as good or nearly as good an understanding of the utility of the produce as the producer."[17] This is not the case in medicine.

The conditions of the marketplace and simple consumerism are not commensurate with the necessities of medicine or the realities of its practice. I must trust the practitioners—doctor, nurse, pharmacist, therapist, and so on—in a way I don't have to trust the automobile salesman. And in trusting the practitioner I also must trust the system of healthcare service and training within which he or she practices. It was this trust that the Hippocratic oath sought to justify through its creation of a class of practitioners dedicated to the care of society's members to whom they promised to first do no harm.

This idea of unequal knowledge and the necessity of trust has become a familiar trope in prime-time television medical dramas like *House, MD*. The patient is in distress and the physicians seek approval from the patient's surrogate for a risky procedure. "What does this mean?" the doctor is asked. "What are the options? Explain to me the alternative choices I might consider." The doctor, one eye on the patient's plummeting monitor levels, takes a deep breath and says, "Look. I could explain this but you wouldn't understand it without a background in neurology and pharmacology. And there isn't . . . time. Trust me, all you need to know is this is risky but it's the only choice that your sister [brother, child, spouse] has to not be quickly dead."

This is not to argue that all patients must surrender complete control of their treatment to any physician engaged in their care. Nor is it to argue physicians always know what is best. It is to say that the assumption of equalities of knowledge and of opportunities, and thus of informed decision making—the essence of consumerist choice—is inapplicable in the medical context. Doctors know things patients don't. And, of course, patients know things about their own lives and needs that doctors rarely perceive. It is in part the art of medicine to elicit from the patient the data a doctor or nurse needs to suggest treatment choices. Often what the patient says he or she wants' ("let me die") is not what is really wanted ("help me to live without pain or let me die"). Understanding the patient's wishes, explaining the nature of the clinical condition and negotiating the treatments to be employed are rarely simple. Buying a car is.

The U.S. Insurer

Finally, at least in the United States, patient choice is bounded from the start by a system that channels physician payment through insurers who restrict reimbursement to contractually engaged physicians. Where treatment is supported by federal monies (Medicare and Medicaid) the treating physician must be recognized as qualified by the appropriate agency. I may love Dr. Pasternak and believe in his care but if I am insured by Kaiser Permanente and Dr. Pasternak is on the Straub Clinic register then I cannot seek his services.

The health insurer, whose principal goal is a return on capital, not only restricts physician choice by the patient but also generally limits access to specific procedures and protocols. A doctor may wish to recommend "x" treatment but the insurer may refuse it on the basis of cost. The physician may be responsible for my care but the primary responsibility of the physician is to his employer's assessment of appropriately cost-efficient treatment alternatives. If I am a cancer patient with neurogenic or osteopathic pain the attending physician may know that the best possible treatment would be an intrathical pump delivering an opioid directly into the thical space (surrounding the spinal cord). The insurer may not support this therapy, however, because it requires a neurological procedure (under anesthesia) to insert a catheter and subcutaneous pump that, in turn, require several days of monitoring by computer telemetry. Indeed, the insurer may be reluctant to pay even for a neurolytic block, ordering instead a drug regime of Oxycodone even though it leaves me constipated, dizzy, mentally dull, and still aching.

Were bioethicists truly concerned with maximizing the care choices of the patient they would have fought long and bitterly against the health-care system that restricted patients in their choice of physicians, hospitals, and treatment plans based on insurer cost concerns. Bioethicists would have argued forcefully for a full range of treatment options based on the clinical needs of the patient rather than the economic goals of the insurer. They would have rejected arguments from scarcity promoted by Callahan as sufficient to reduce the care of persons (for example, seniors) irrespective of their wishes. They would have seen the relationship between patient and physician as complex rather than simple, a matter of distinct knowledge bases that may lead to misunderstandings and thus to dilemmas.

Certainly, were bioethicists to speak truth to power, as Brody insisted they should, they would have rejected the predicate assumption that the market is the ideal mechanism for the pricing and distribution of necessary care.[18] Instead they accept as natural, and naturally limiting, the system that makes medicine a market and the patient a consumer whose choices are bounded by his employment status and personal wealth. Certainly, if choice were the goal, or patient care, bioethicists would have been universally critical of a system in which the pharmaceutical industry is free to price life saving and life-prolonging products at a level beyond that which any but the richest patient (or insurer) can afford. Soliris, for example, is currently the most expensive drug in the world at almost $500,000 a patient a year.[19] It uniquely treats a rare blood disorder, paroxysmal nocturnal hemoglobinuria (PNH), which results in kidney failure. It is a live-or-die drug and health insurers and agencies often are understandably reluctant to spend the money for its distribution. In its first year of production, the producer, Alexion, reported $290 million in sales (more than a third of the cost of the drug's development) and a stock price increase of 130 percent principally resulting from Soliris's distribution.

Gleevic (Imatinib), the frontline drug for the treatment of chronic myelogenous leukemia as well as some gastrointestinal stromal tumors, costs (depending on dosage and supplier) up to $98,000 a year in the United States. In Canada, where drug costs are kept lower, the costs range up to $34,000 a year. Remicade (Infleximab) is a monoclonal antibody used in the treatment of autoimmune diseases like Crohn's disease and rheumatoid arthritis. Costs range in the United States from $1,500 to $2,500 per treatment. The drug is first administered twice in a month and after that every six to eight weeks. Some insurers refuse to pay the cost and patients must make do with older and less effective treatment alternatives even though they and their physician know the result will be less than optimal.

Were bioethicists concerned about patient care and patient choice they would, as a body, rail against the predatory pricing that makes choice the provenance of those wealthy enough to afford it. At the least they would insist that since at least half of the research and development costs of drug and other product development are federally supported, the prices of resulting products should be set at levels affordable to the public purse and the consumer.[20] Were they interested in care and treatment they would, at the least, insist on present need over possible future products and their attending profit. Instead they accept the market's rule—and where is the ethics in that?

Choice as Freedom

The simple ideal of individual choice that bioethicists advance under the rubric of respect for autonomy thus hides a nest of conflicts and limitations. The tensions that result are as old as the birth of modern capitalism in an expansive industrial age. They're found in the writings of Adam Smith and those of the father of utilitarianism, Jeremy Bentham. Certainly they are rife in the works of John Stuart Mill on whose works the authors of *Principles* relied in part.[21] As journalist, philosopher, and politician, Mill sought to advance a utilitarian theory of general good in which an individual's preference was both supreme and at the same time of minimal relevance. On the one hand, Mill was wholly committed to the sovereignty of the individual not as an absolute but as—how to say it?—an ideal as absolute as possible. He was, after all, not an anarchist. On the other hand, the Benthamite tradition that Mill embraced insisted upon the primacy of general utility over individual preference.

The enduring thrill of Mill (figure 9.2) is watching him scramble between these two poles. He wants individual will to triumph, but recognizes as preeminent Bentham's general measure of social right and wrong, the greatest good to the greatest number of people: 50 percent plus one. It would have been brilliant if the bioethicists of *Belmont* and *Principles* had chosen Mill as emblematic of this tension. Instead, they cherry-picked his ideal of individual choice as if it were unrelated to the utilitarian ideal in which individual need is at best secondary in the ordering of the general good.

Mill's writings present a fascinating pathology if not necessarily an appropriate groundwork for an ethics of anything, let alone of medical decision making. John Stewart's father was both an ardent follower of Jeremy Bentham and a fervent admirer of the French materialists. Utilitarianism was, in a real sense, the family business and the religion he sought to bequeath to his son. Believing in rationalism and materialism above all, he made of his son an experiment, a research object. How can one raise a child to be simply rational and therefore wholly unemotional in his or her thinking? In service of this trial-of-one Mill isolated his son from other children and raised him on a "carefully distilled intellectual diet, prepared by his father, compounded of natural science and the clas-

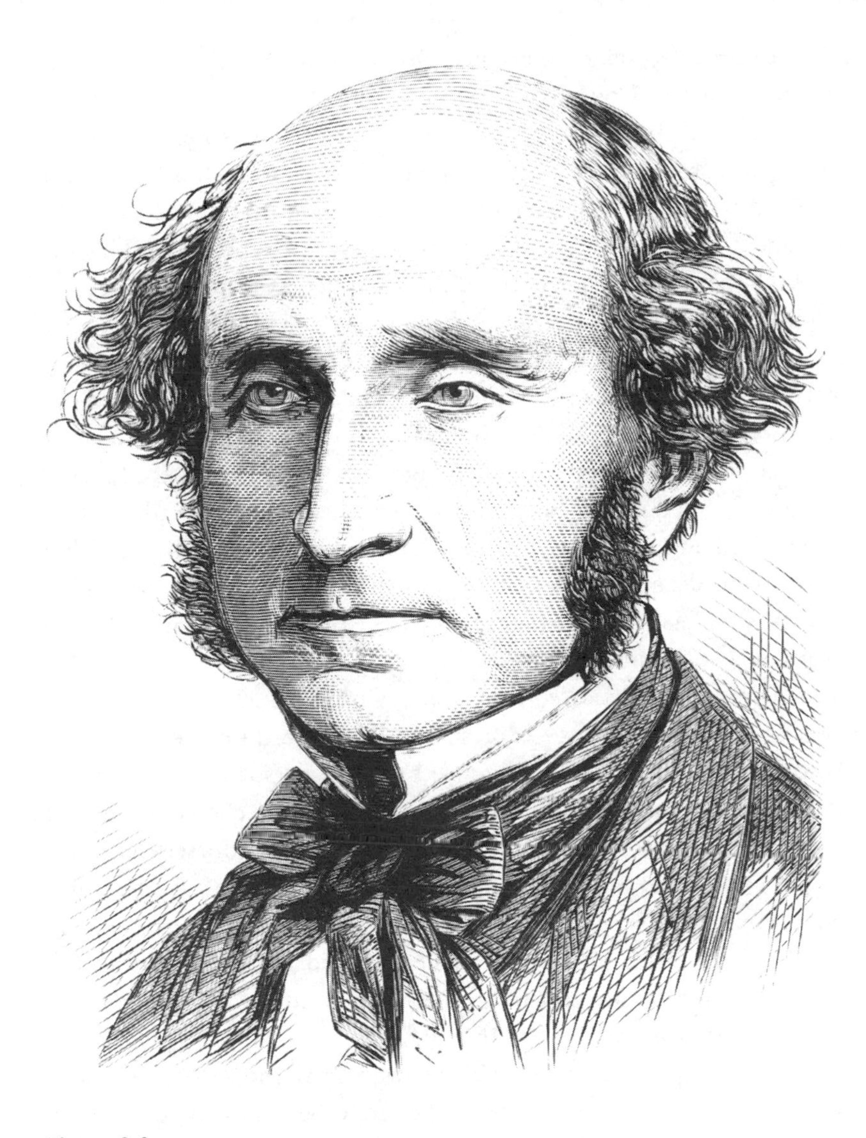

Figure 9.2
John Stuart Mill argued at once the unimpeded choice of the individual and the utilitarian virtue of the general good over that of the single person.

sical literatures. No religion, no metaphysics, little poetry . . . were permitted to corrupt his rationalist training."[22]

The young Mill was to be the embodiment of Kant's purely rational man (it was assumed then no woman could achieve this), no sentiment allowed. As such he was to be the practical Kantian preceptor, the embodiment of the Moral Folk Theory's practitioner. No wonder the adult Mill championed not only utilitarian schemes but also individual freedoms, especially the freedom of emotional, passionate speech over everything else. The boy whose associations were restricted, whose emotional and social growth were stunted, became the champion of nonrestriction. Where the lines might be drawn in Mill's writings are never really clear, however. They can't be because we never learn exactly what he meant by freedom except, perhaps, the old, vague generalities that Bentham had railed against but was always chary of defining. That freedom from disciplined definition must have been a relief for Mill, a liberation from his father's strictures and the isolation they imposed upon his early development.

Famously, Mill advocated an "arena within which the subject—a person or group of persons—is or should be left to do or be what he is able to do or be, without interference by other persons."[23] The greater that personal arena, the more the field of individual choice, the better we all would be. The idea was not unique to Mill, of course. Hegel, for example, considered and then dismissed it as promoting a limited, isolated sovereignty of self that was (like Kant's) abstract and formal, empty form without real substance: "If we hear it said that the definition of freedom is ability to do what we please, such an idea can only be taken to reveal an utter immaturity of thought."[24]

But Hegel emphasized what Mill ignored: real choice occurs not in isolation but rather within contexts that may be arbitrary, capricious, and well beyond one's control.[25] The arena in which liberty exists is bounded by economic, familial, political, and social circumstances. "The only part of the conduct of anyone for which he is amenable to society is that which concerns others," wrote Mill. "In the part which merely concerns himself, his independence is, of right, absolute. Over himself, over his own body and mind, the individual is sovereign."[26]

The problem is that little that we do, or choose, is independent of others. Medicine, for example, is a messy brew engaging on one hand, physicians, nurses, therapists, and the organizations that employ them within the greater socioeconomic system that licenses each and sets boundaries and standards for their performance. On the other hand are the patients, their employers (who in the United States buy their insurance packages), family members, friends, and neighbors who care about their lives and sometimes care for them in illness. What I choose affects others; what they choose affects me. Mill's freedom thus fails precisely in the way Isaiah Berlin described: "My individual self is not something which I can detach from my relationship with others, or from those attributes of myself which consisted in their attitudes toward me. For what I am is, in large part, determined by what I feel and think; and what I feel and think is determined by the feeling and thought prevailing in the society in which I belong of which, in Burke's sense, I form not an isolable atom, but an ingredient (to use a perilous but indispensable metaphor) in a social pattern."[27]

Mill's freedom therefore exists only within an extremely restricted arena of the socially possible. Its focus is not the context, however, but the choices made within that context. We are therefore *only* free to choose from what is available to us. We may want a treatment that in the context of scarcity and profit maximization is not available to us. Accepting that we lose the possibility of effective choice and Foucault's docility becomes the rule. The general result, Berlin says witheringly, is "a doctrine of sour grapes: what I cannot be sure of, I cannot truly want."[28]

It is this freedom that bioethics promotes, a Millian freedom from personal interference that is purchased at the price of indifference in a marketplace where choice is bounded by economic policy and its limits. "It is argued, very plausibly," writes Berlin, "that if a man is too poor to afford something on which there is no legal ban—a loaf of bread, a journey around the world, recourse to the courts—he is as little free to have it as he would be if it were forbidden by law."[29] Were the bioethicist to embrace this critique seriously he or she would argue for a context in which opportunities were defined broadly and not narrowly. But to do this bioethics would have had to abandon its neoliberal accountancy and insist instead on care as a humanist principle.

A serious treatment of medical ethics therefore resides not simply in the patient's simple preferences, or the physician's, but also across the interlocking levels of commercial and social realities that restrict or promote various treatment options. It was this, as we've seen, that powered the social physicians in North America—like Benjamin Rush—and the socially active researchers like Virchow. To ignore this and focus on personal freedom and choice alone is if not self-conscious then at least serious misdirection. It is the same as blaming a Swedish seaman obeying orders for the drowning of nineteenth-century Irish passengers sailing on an American ship in the North Atlantic. To do that is to be guilty of bad faith of the highest order.

IRBs

We see this at a different scale in the general failure of institutional review boards (IRBs) to provide any real protection for research subjects. In his review of a Minnesota case, Carl Elliott quotes from depositions by University of Minnesota IRB members on their role in a lucrative research trial in which a patient died. University officials unctuously assumed that the role of its IRB was, as *Belmont* promised, "to protect the rights and welfare of human research subjects"; however, the members of the IRB testified that they understood their role was only to assure that the pharmaceutical companies designing and paying for the trial had some plan or program offering at least some protection to the research subject. "If this were true," writes Elliott, "it would render IRBs worthless."[30]

Exactly so. To be fair, few IRB members have the background needed to intelligently question research protocols. Bioethicists tend to degrees in philosophy, not biostatistics and research design. In discussion in 2010 with an IRB member at the University of Toronto I was told she regularly is asked to approve research programs in which safeguards for patient safety are promised but rarely detailed in the researchers' proposals. It's a "black box," she said, "and we're to take it on faith." When I asked if this wasn't an abdication of her ethical responsibility to protect research subjects she shrugged unhappily as if to say sure, but what can you do? There is immense pressure to promote research that pays the university and its consulting IRB members as well. *Belmont* created the context in which one could accept the promise of subject safety without attention to the dangers that often result.

It didn't have to be this way, of course. Likewise, bioethicists arguing for the empowerment of the patient could have focused on the context of care and of health delivery. They could have taken as their role not compliant partnership in the research enterprise, but as research watchdogs whose single focus was patient protection and the social weal. That would have required courses in research statistics and in the arcania of science and social science, however, as well as the philosophy that was the primary subject of their studies. The result would have been an entirely different ethic from the one bioethicists claim today.

Another View

One can argue that IRBs are a paternalistic way to assert protection and control and where necessary to prevent, in the name of protection, dangerous or frivolous research programs from soliciting subjects. Their creation assumes that patients can't independently and intelligently choose programs with the best protocols; IRBs do so in their stead. That IRBs have been rife with failures does not mean, however, that paternalism is a bad thing. It is what society owes to its members, a concern for their safety in areas where peoples may not be able to choose intelligently for themselves.

Similarly, the paternalism that medicine is accused of is not always bad. As patients we want a physician who treats us with the care and concern given to a loved family member. And even where we disagree, on the basis of physician knowledge and training the decision to defer or deny a patient's wishes sometimes is the right thing to do.

Suicidal ideation, for example, is common among those who, normal yesterday, wake up today in a hospital room absent either limbs or limb sensation.[31] A resolute Millsian might say, give them what they want when they want it. It is their body and their choice. But in such cases we know what the patient does not: it takes time to process loss and to see the potential of a life unimagined in health. We know that more than two-thirds of all those with quadriplegia or paraplegia report, after two years, a quality of life that is acceptable and often fulfilling. Indeed, even patients with locked-in syndrome—total paralysis except perhaps the capacity to blink their eyes or move a finger—often report increasingly positive life quality over a long period of adjustment as long as communicative technologies are available.[32]

A refusal to support a decision for termination in the first months of a patient's radically altered state is good, even necessary, when based on medical experience and knowledge the patient—caught in the moment—will not and indeed cannot have.[33] To say "not yet" in these situations holds in abeyance a decision made in the midst of fear and the sometimes overwhelming sense of despair that attends drastic injury. Where the patient's choice is denied there is a hope that in the future the patient, with experience, will learn to accept and appreciate a life that while different still can be full and worthwhile. But for that to occur we need to recognize as a society an obligation to provide the physical therapy and social necessities that will make that possibility real.

For example, many proponents of euthanasia insist on a Millian "right" to die "with dignity" yet ignore the right to life with dignity despite restrictions. Without that as a prior guarantee the opportunity for a convenient, cost-efficient, speedy death is not a real choice but merely its pretense. And where is the ethics in that?[34] Were those bioethicists honest, they would insist on care and treatment first, on the potential of a life that can be full, if altered by circumstance, as a predicate "right" to a choice for early termination. That would be, however, a bioethic that admits to complexities of social circumstance and obligation that bioethics today does not perceive, or admit.

Here, again, we return to McBryde Johnson and her insistence on both the embodied self and on the nature of the communities that discourage, tolerate, or encourage persons of difference. To take this tact would be to focus on the social and cultural elements that restrict or promote choice rather than, as bioethicists have to date, on the ideal of choice without consideration of the contexts in which choices are made.

Public Health and Ethics

A step in the direction of a realistic, enlightened ethic is to emphasize that healthcare decisions are not only private and personal but also public because health choices are set within the public sphere. Bruce Jennings[35] argued something like this in an elegant essay on the idea of liberty beyond the Millian paradigm. Of *course* we reject individual preferences when they may harm the community. Few ethicists today would argue against quarantine strictures during an epidemic on the grounds they restrict individual liberty. We saw this briefly debated and then quickly laid to rest in the 2004 SARS (Severe Acute Respiratory Sundrome) outbreak in Toronto, Canada, for example. Public access to hospitals was restricted and strict protocols for those permitted entry were enforced.[36] Those exposed were confined to their homes. The question of individual rights and freedom of movement bowed to the necessary, community-protecting protocols of disease containment, as they have for centuries.

Similarly, at least in the United States, the fight against mandatory vaccination policies that protect communities against epidemic or pandemic intrusion was settled long ago in the 1895 U.S. Supreme Court decision *Jacobson v. Massachusetts*.[37] Compulsory vaccination in the midst of a smallpox epidemic might be coercive but it is necessary and thus permissible, the court ruled. "There is," the Supreme Court decision said, "a sphere within which the individual may assert the supremacy of his own will" but the boundaries of that sphere end, the court ruled, where the common good is overwhelming and self-evident. It then becomes the obligation of the community, the state, to assure the materials for public vaccination. In a similar way bioethics might have argued an expansion of health opportunities rather than accepting their truncation on the basis of malleable economic limits.

And so we come to this irony: the focus of the traditional medical ethic that bioethics sought successfully to supplant was grounded in the care and needs of the individual patient. It sought not overweening paternalism but informed care as its highest ideal. That care was rarely imposed but instead negotiated between patient and physician within the rules of the culture both ascribed to. In service of this ideal this ethic had to promote a relationship of trust between patient and physician to create a context in which care choices might be informed by the physician's best knowledge. The relational compact of physician and patient was grounded upon recognition by physicians of the importance of the individual to society at large, to a society of persons. To treat the person was to treat the society in which doctor and patient together lived. The ethics of this medicine was personal and individual in its focus but social and communal in its legitimating purpose. Its power lay in the knowledge of physicians and the duty of its application for the good of the human patient within society at large.

Bioethics sought to displace that ethic, branding it both practically inadequate and generally inimical to the radical freedom bioethics sought to promote. In doing so it advanced a context in which real choice was limited by economic constraints assumed to be immutable. In this construction, bioethics assumed as natural a neoliberal consumerism that does not necessarily serve the patient in distress. Its research ethic further displaced patient care as a medical priority and advanced generalizable, saleable commercial knowledge as a principal good. In doing so the physician's patient became the researcher's test object—an outcome that, in theory, *Belmont* was supposed to prevent.

In bioethics' advance of a philosophical perspective, bioethicists ignored, if they ever knew, a central premise of social psychology that "economic systems, political systems, religious systems, climate, and geography exert a distal yet important influence on human mind and behavior."[38] The geography of our lives and its landscape include both the choices we have and those we may want but that are restricted. It is not irrelevant to the ethical review of choices made or opportunities withheld. To ignore the complexity of context and history leaves us without alternatives. We are left only with the freedom of the leaky lifeboat where there is no choice at all for the passengers and no good choices available to the first mate and his crew.

And thus bioethicists become the thieves of virtue, "good careful people of the village" who seem to embrace loyalty and promote honesty, the people other villagers can trust. They seem . . . blameless and worthy. But these worthies, wrote Mencius, promote not virtue and care but the status quo in high-blown, pompous language: "They say, 'The Ancients! The Ancients!' as if that were an answer."[39] In this they are masters of misdirection. That, at least, is my free translation. In the end, Confucius put it best, perhaps: "Fine words and insinuating appearance are seldom associated with virtue." And in the end that is what bioethics has been, an insinuating appearance whose fine words promise a virtue this ethic cannot deliver. The grand themes of choice and freedom and care and knowledge bear little relation to the realities bioethics promotes. Because they are not considered they provide no palliative to the inequalities and inequities of the age that, for ethicists and philosophers, should be bioethics' focus and principal concern.

10

Complex Ethics: Toward an Ethics of Medicine

What went wrong with bioethics and why has it been such a failure? That it *is* a failure is an opinion shared by many of its practitioners. Bioethics is in crisis, wrote Richard Ashcroft in a special issue of *Bioethics* in 2010, its future in grave doubt because of weaknesses in its institutional form and a demonstrable lack of social relevance. "I don't think this is merely my own personal view," he wrote. "It is shared with many leading contributors to the field."[1] The editor of *Public Health Ethics*, Angus Dawson, declared in the same issue that "bioethics has no future, at least not in its present form."[2] Similarly, Miran Epstein argued bioethics has become irrelevant and as such too expensive to be continued.[3] Its allegiance to scarcity thus eventually becomes a reason for its dismissal in a world where financial resources are limited. For her part, Rita Macklin wrote that 2010 was the year future historians would mark as the beginning of bioethics' terminal phase if not the year of its demise.[4]

Others whose focus is specific rather than general offer similar critiques. In 2011, physician-ethicist Jeffrey Bishop critiqued the failure of current bioethical and medical perspectives on dying.[5] Invoking a Foucauldian critique he argued the mechanistic and materialistic perspectives of ethics as applied to medicine create a kind of nihilism evidenced in cases like that of Terri Schiavo. And, too, there are those searching for other evidence whose critique is not dissimilar but who find potential answers in the work of non-bioethicists like Charles Taylor.[6] None of this matters very much, however, when the programs of neoliberal accountancy—with its focus on economic and commercial concerns—dominate an atomized, individualistic world of negative freedoms. Philosophy becomes practically irrelevant in the face of state economics and corporate necessities.

It is thus no great surprise that by the end of the first decade of the twenty-first century bioethics had largely disappeared as a practical enterprise in all but name, and of course, institutional affiliation. And here, of course, in the institution and its neoliberal service, bioethics remains accepted, alive, and, to its practitioners, even useful. What began with the promise of a singular, unified biomedical ethic was fractured into a set of demi-demi-disciplines whose foci and priorities were sometimes contradictory and typically distinct in their priorities. Practitioners call it the "problem of equipoise,"[7] whose resolution has been to create one ethic for therapeutic care, another for clinical research, and a third, perhaps, for issues of public health.[8] That people might be at once patients needing care, research subjects as well as citizens whose state of health (or disease) is (or should be) the principal subject of public concern is ignored. If it were ever more than an imagining, bioethics as a singular ethic is simply gone.

The Failure

The extent of its failure is seen in the promises bioethics made and could not keep. It was to provide moral guidance based upon a "single canonical vision,"[9] as Engelhardt has it. Like Beauchamp and Childress's common wisdom that singular ethical imagining was to be a universal accepted by all who believed in ethical medicine practiced in a just social environment. To achieve this happy state all that was needed, bioethics insisted, was the appropriate application of an analytic methodology grounded in the writings of Enlightenment philosophers, especially Immanuel Kant. But Kant's brilliance, and that of his successors, was thinly theoretical, not practical or specific. Their arguments were never meant to serve as a map through the cultural mire of something as socially complex as medicine. The result, writes Daniel Hall, "rings hollow just to the extent that they [bioethicists] eschew normative notions of human flourishing in favour of procedures by which any 'rational" agent can resolve moral questions 'objectively' regardless of the virtues and practical wisdom that may (or may not) constitute their character."[10]

At the least, bioethics promised a methodology capable of constructing Walker's moral space, one in which a generally accessible language of analysis might be deployed to first define and then solve moral problems arising from medical practice and research. That philosophically grounded analytic approach promised, as former ASBH president Mark Kuczewski put it, to "lend a broader perspective to healthcare decision making than medicine affords."[11] The result was an academic version of Johnson's moral folk theory. In it the Kantian isolate—rational, unemotional, and uninvolved—would be the hero. But at the heart of that theory was a misreading of Kant, who was all about what we are and not what we are to do in this or that specific venue. Bioethicists from the start have argued "what we are to do" while assuming "what we are" is the unemotional, rational isolate of Kant's imagining, the individual agent of Johnson's moral folk theory.

But as the debate between Harriet McBryde Johnson and Peter Singer made clear there is more than one philosophy and more than one methodological approach. From the start, bioethics in the main eschewed the experiential reality and the phenomenological perspective that seek the broadest definition of humanness and human flourishing. Put another way, the philosopher-ethicist forgot to focus on the very things that are philosophically contentious, for example, the nature of human flourishing. Instead they argued as self-evident a thinly principled, wholly abstract ideal that was to be translated into an approach to complex, interpersonal sets of human associations. "What might otherwise have been thought to emerge gradually and naturally within our human consciousness—bottom up so to speak from concrete and specific nexuses," writes Stephen Erickson, "is now contrastingly construed as devolving, virtually by fiat, from more distant, abstract and generalized principles the residence and in most cases even the origins of which are largely bureaucratic and secular and institutional."[12]

Bioethics promised a medical ethic that was to be more complete and more adequate than the one it disdained and sought to replace. But from the get-go bioethics' primary interest was never the ethics of medicine and its practice. Its concern with the patient in his or her need always has been, at very best, secondary. From the debate over dialysis to the worry over the supply of research subjects, bioethics has been first and foremost about allocation in the context of a presumably natural scarcity of resources. It has always taken as given the morality of the lifeboat and the economics of its construction. Where the older medical ethic sought to argue a covenant of care within a social framework, bioethics argued a rationale for noncare and triage in a context of shortages whose causes bioethicists did not pause to explore.

At least since *Belmont* bioethics has promoted research as a future, productive good whose importance outweighs the immediate needs of the patient-cum-research subject. No wonder it sought to dismiss the older, Oslerian ethic in which the priority of research over patient care was rejected categorically. Bioethics attacked the older ethics of medicine not because it was inadequate but because its singular focus on patient care was at odds with the priorities of the knowledge industry and of governments whose neoliberal agenda has been economic and future-oriented, not patient-oriented and interpersonal.

The result is something philosophers from Kant to Foucault would condemn in its objectification of the person as a research object (Rhodes) or as an economic cipher (Callahan). The result was never the "common wisdom" of Beauchamp and Childress but instead the convenient wisdom of the neoliberal technocrat for whom the individual in need (and thus the necessities of care) is never more than a row on a spreadsheet of economic gain and loss.

Strangely, the demi-discipline of philosophically trained adepts who see themselves as bioethical experts has been largely without a conscience. Neither its signal organizations (like the American Society of Bioethics and the Humanities [ASBH]) nor its principal authors seem to take responsibility for their judgments. We're just a group of independent, free-thinking academics making arguments, said former ASBH president Hilde Lindemann. There is therefore no communal responsibility. As her successor Mark Kuczewski put it, bioethicists are merely guests in the house of medicine and not the real adjudicators of its application. No responsibility accrues. As Michael Corleone in the *Godfather* saga put it, it's nothing personal, just business.

"The field of bioethics must itself develop a conscience and dedicate itself to advocacy for those who have no money or power to offer this new profession," Kuczewski later wrote and here I of course agree. That was the point of Brody's clarion call urging bioethicists to speak truth to power, to advocate for the powerless. None have risen to the challenge because, as Kuczewski admitted, bioethicists from the start "aligned themselves with money and power."[13] Here bioethics lost the moral grounding that was to be its raison d'etre. Philosophy, as Socrates knew, is not about the easy embrace of money and power but rather its challenge and critique. Bioethics gave up a conscience—individual and collective—when it took on the convenient priorities of business and government. Bioethicists cannot speak truth to power when its practitioners are wholly in power's employ, advancing its agendas.

The result has been as damaging to the practicing bioethicist as it has been to both patients and physicians who have seen medicine reduced to a commercial transaction in which the ethical responsibilities of medical professionals are little different from those of an automobile salesman. It is no exaggeration to say bioethics has created a society of Francis Rhodes among the administrators, nurses, doctors, and social workers, who know the best they can do is not what is best for the patient but merely the best possible in unacceptably limited circumstances. Time and again practitioners—doctors, nurses, social workers, and others—have said to me they would if they could (for the care of this or that person) but all they can do is not enough and it makes them . . . sad. We make complicit the many who would provide care within a system that prevents prescription of the necessary drug (too expensive), or provision of the requisite rehabilitation (not covered). Burnout is the name we give for what happens when those who wanted to do the best they could for others find they can't even do the necessary.[14] Those who stay on the job become like old prison lags, the long-time prisoners who mop the floor and proclaim the institution fine because the floor is clean. There is no great honor in that, and less sanity.

Alternatives

It didn't have to be this way. "If the tradition of the virtues was able to survive the horrors of the last dark ages," writes Alasdair MacIntyre, "we are not entirely without grounds for hope."[15] Bioethics might have been that hope. When the scarcity of dialysis services arose in the 1960s it might have been the philosopher-cum-ethicist and not the politician who argued for a national program to ensure the salvation of all those with kidney disease who could benefit from this new treatment. The moral philosopher with his or her analytic tools might have pointed to the poliomyelitis years of the early 1950s when, irrespective of cost, many nations (Canada, Denmark, England, the United States, and so on) reflexively cared for young patients requiring extensive care, and later, rehabilitation. All they needed to have said was: "That care—both ventilation and rehabilitation—was good and the concern it demonstrated for human being and flourishing should be our model."

An ethic grounded in that history, and perspective, however, would have required the nascent bioethicist to focus not on shortages as a presumably natural limit but instead on the programs and policies that create shortages. In doing so they would have had to challenge the impersonal, future-oriented, trickle-down assumptions of the politics of their time. In their reflexive acceptance of the socioeconomic realities of the day, bioethicists embraced what in the end was one more politically convenient "practical ethic," in the original sense of an ethic of the efficient plantation whose owners never questioned the slavery that sustained them.[16] "Practical" becomes "efficient" and "acceptable" within a socioeconomic and political context whose assumptions and policies are never to be questioned. It accepts what is, leaving questions of the ethics and morality of the broader system aside.

Mark Kuczewski was wrong when he said bioethicists have been guests in the house of medicine. Rather, they have been strangers camped at the door of a practice whose realities few experienced or understood. As visitors they could have aligned themselves with their hosts' old medical ethic that argued for care as a social duty and an interpersonal virtue. They might have said that each generation must consider how to order relations between the healthy and the sick, the powerful and the weak. Their brief then would have been to mediate the necessities of care within the *realpolitik* of contemporary political wills. Instead what began within the best of liberal sentiments became just another neoliberal instrument that denied its best hopes in the name of an economics whose grounding principle is efficiency and whose focus is future good.

Alasdair MacIntyre warned of this in the 1980s when he wrote that "the barbarians are not waiting beyond the frontiers; they have already been governing us for quite some time. And it is our lack of consciousness of this that constitutes part of our predicament."[17] It is only a predicament if the realities are seen, however. Bioethics, to its shame, never looked although there were hints everywhere. "Values not only have a history," writes Catherine Belsey, "they also differ from themselves. They can therefore be changed in the future, if not in the light of a fixed idea (or Idea) of the good, at least in the hope that the trace of an alternative inscribed in them might one day be realized."[18] Here was where the philosopher turned ethicist might have begun, critiquing rather than accepting the values of officialdom. Here the analytic method and the history of ideas would have done some good. Instead bioethics took a set of thinly principled values as natural and complete without thinking overmuch about the manner in which their application might help create the problems bioethicists insisted they and they alone were best qualified to resolve.

Bioethics might have begun, as medicine did (and here the Greek conflation of person and society and their shared good could have been the intellectual baseline), with the idea of care as a right rather than a commodity whose provision is always contingent. *That* would have been the moment for the philosopher to invoke Kant's third categorical imperative from his *Groundwork on the Metaphysics of Morals*: "Now I say that man, and in general every rational being, exists as an end in himself, not merely as a means for arbitrary use by this or that will."[19] The analytic philosopher might have noted that whenever medicine went awry—whether in Germany or at Tuskegee or Willowbrook—it usually was because the focus had shifted from the needs of the fragile person to the priorities of the state (remember Carrie Buck) or the research industry. Then they might have joined Osler and his predecessors in advancing the needs of the patient in a way that philosophers from Socrates to Kant and Heidegger (and may I say, even Marx) would have approved.

The bioethics that might have been would not have sought to displace the older ethic of medicine but instead to expand upon its general moral vision. The old ethic was never complete, nor was it meant to be. Its broad strokes carried a general ethos, a few prohibitions, and a set of promises. The rest was to be filled in by those who in each society sought to find the best form of human service through the medicine of the day. Had bioethicists done this they might have created a moral space within which the balance between economic imperatives and human necessities could have been at least considered. In the face of neoliberal imperatives they would have spoken up as a social conscience in the old sense of Aquinas's "conscientia," applying knowledge (or at least moral vision) to activity. Then bioethics' appeal to "common wisdom" would have been neither an excuse nor a retreat but a thoughtful approach—a search at the least—that attempted to bring the best of the old medical ethic to the service of the best of modern society.

A Secular Ethics

Unforgivably, bioethics leaves largely unanswered the essential philosophical questions that lie at the heart of the issues it seeks to explore. Who are we, what do we believe to be important, and how do we convince others of that importance? If we deny the theology that made of humankind a good in itself, its individual members protected by the fact of their being, on what do we base our ethics of medicine or anything else? Without a strong and generally accepted core value as an a priori, perhaps all that is left is the brutal accountancies of the neoliberal. If that is true then liberalism becomes, as Isaiah Berlin put it, either anarchism or its fraternal twin, totalitarianism.

Bioethics teeters precariously between these two extremes. On the one hand some promote a libertarian, almost anarchist creed (autonomous choice, whatever he or she wants, whatever the situation). Others flirt with the totalitarian in the imposition of choices (lack of care for seniors) conceived as "duties" (to be a research subject) whose goal is not care of the person but future economic gain. Having rejected a theological core, bioethical philosophers have found no alternate center on which to base their thinking except, of course, the notion of the rational isolate in his or her imagining. But as we saw in the nondebate between Harriet McBryde Johnson and Peter Singer, rational peoples can imagine a variety of widely distinct, sometimes contradictory things.

At the least, bioethics might have started with Kant's great vision of humanity as an end in itself, and thus of humanity's members as subjects and never objects of accountancy who are means to some impersonally utilitarian end. That was McBryde Johnson's argument as it has been for many others. The historically minded might remember, for example, Montaigne: "Life should be an aim to itself," he wrote, "a purpose unto itself."[20] That simple statement stands as a counterweight to the neoliberal, consumerist reduction of us all (doctors and nurses and patients) to ciphers in a spreadsheet of production. Here, too, we might see as counterweight the "beauty" that McBryde Johnson promoted in a manner that resonates with the work of others like, in a partial list of those cited earlier, Stephen J. Post, Oliver Sacks, and Abraham Verghese. Let that beauty stand as a starting point for the bioethics that should have been and still might be should we choose it.

A robust ethics—of medicine or anything else—is a messy complexity in its various parts. There will be no simple answers, no easy referents to old truths easily dropped into the modern day. As the student in the Bob Marley tee shirt came to understand, philosophizing is like orienteering in a landscape one has never seen. The enthusiast has an abstraction and a general direction—a map and a compass—and then struggles through the brambles. If there is to be a bioethic rather than a neoliberal apologia cloaked in a philosophical veneer it will need a rethinking. The compass needs to be corrected and the map redrawn. Hopefully the result will be a place where virtue—however it is defined—is a common goal and not a commodity to be exploited by thieves of virtue as if it were their own.

Notes

Introduction

1. Tristram H. Engelhardt, “Confronting Moral Pluralism in Posttraditional Western Societies: Bioethics Critically Reassessed,” *Journal of Medicine and Philosophy* 36, no. 2 (April 2011): 244.

2. Albert R. Jonsen, “The Birth of Bioethics: The Origins and Evolution of a Demi-Discipline,” *Medical Humanities Review* 11, no. 1 (1997): 9–21.

3. Renée C. Fox and Judith P. Swazey, *Observing Bioethics* (New York: Oxford University Press, 2008), 7.

4. Many of these other histories are cited across this text. They include Albert R. Jonsen, The Birth of Bioethics,” Special Supplement, *Hastings Center Report* 23, no. 6 (1993) (November–December): S1–S4; Albert Jonsen, *The Birth of Bioethics* (New York: Oxford Unviersity Press, 1998); Fox and Swazey, *Observing Bioethics*; and most spectacularly, the foundation text of the field, Tom L. Beauchamp and James F. Childress, *Principles of Biomedical Ethics*, 5th ed. (New York: Oxford University Press, 2001). While not itself a history it is historical in its introduction and seminal in its bioethical perspectives, edition to edition. Elsewhere, there is a range of articles that have fleshed out the perspective.

5. Kyle B. Brothers, “Dependent Rational Providers,” *Journal of Medicine and Philosophy* 36, no. 2 (April 2011): 136.

6. John Law, *After Method: Mess in Social Science Research* (New York: Routledge, 2004).

7. Andrew Pickering, *The Mangle of Practice: Time, Agency, and Science* (Chicago: University of Chicago Press, 1995). The idea of a “mangle,” or “mess,” is used in the sociology of science and technology to describe the social, political, philosophical, and technical complexities that are entwined in the presentation of ideas, theories, and technologies.

8. Manfred B. Steger and Ravi K. Roy, *Neoliberalism: A Very Short Introduction* (New York: Oxford University Press, 2010), 9–12.

9. Oliver Rauprich and Jochen Vollmann, “30 Years *Principles of Biomedical Ethics*: Introduction to a Symposium on the 6th edition of Tom L. Beauchamp

and James F. Childress' Seminal Work," *Journal of Medical Ethics* 37, no. 8 (2011): 454.

10. The quotation from the first edition of *Principles of Biomedical Ethics* is cited in Rauprich and Vollmann, "30 Years," 455.

11. Harriet McBryde Johnson, "Unspeakable Conversations," *New York Times Sunday Magazine*, February 16, 2003, http://www.racematters.org/harrietmcbrydejohnson.htm (accessed January 18, 2008).

1 Dead Germans and Other Philosophers

1. The lecture on the ethics of data mapping and analysis is one I give frequently and to a range of graduate, undergraduate, and graduate classes in several disciplines. See Tom Koch, "'False Truths': Ethics and Mapping as a Profession," *Cartographic Perspectives* 54 (2006): 4–15.

2. James Wood, "The Fun Stuff: My Life as Keith Moon," *The New Yorker*, November 29, 2010, 65.

3. Michael Ignatieff, *A Life of Isaiah Berlin* (New York: Penguin Books, 2000), 88.

4. Ibid. Also see Bernard Williams, "Introduction," in *Isaiah Berlin, Concepts and Categories: Philosophical Essays*, ed. Henry Hardy (New York: Viking, 1978), xii.

5. Jill Lepore, "The Rise of Marriage Therapy, and Other Dreams of Human Betterment," *The New Yorker*, March 29, 2010, 97.

6. Wittgenstein, *Tractatus*, trans. C. K. Ogden, (London: Routledge & Kegan Paul Ltd., 1922), 4.11.2. Rather than the underlined, dog-eared print edition I have had for years, for this work I have used an online version of Wittgenstein's work and cite it in the references.

7. Larry R. Churchill, "Are We Professionals? A Critical Look at the Social Role of Bioethicists," *Daedalus* 128, no. 4 (1999): 255.

8. Ezekiel J. Emanuel, "Welcome and Plenary Lecture." Annual meeting of the American Association of Bioethics and the Humanities, Hyatt Regency Hotel, Washington, DC, October 15, 2009. In his plenary lecture Emmanuel emphasized the importance of bioethics—and bioethicists—in government and in policy.

9. For more on the relationship of bioethics and law, see, for example, Jonathan Montgomery, "Law and the Demoralization of Medicine," *Legal Studies* 26, no. 2 (2006): 185–210; also see Timothy James, "The Appeal to Law to Provide Public Answers to Bioethical Questions: It All Depends What Sort of Answers You Want," *Health Care Analysis* 26 (2008): 65–76. The greater literature here is quite vast.

10. Joseph Kaufert et al., "End-of-Life Ethics and Disability: Differing Perspectives on Case-based Teaching," *Medical Health Care and Philosophy* 23 (2010): 115.

11. Mark G. Kuczewski, "Disability: An Agenda for Bioethics," *American Journal of Bioethics* 1, no. 3 (2001): 37.

12. Mark G. Kuczewski, "Taking It Personally: Reflections on Living Bioethics and Medical Humanities," *ASBH Reader* (Summer–Autumn 2010): 4.

13. ASBH publications, http://www.asbh.org/publications/content/index.html (accessed June 14, 2011).

14. Kuczewski, "Taking It Personally," 13.

15. Audrey Kobayashi, "Paradoxes of Our Time," *AAG Newsletter* 46, no. 7 (2011): 3.

16. Tristram H. Engelhart, "Confronting Moral Pluralism in Posttraditional Western Societies: Bioethics Critically Reassessed," *Journal of Medicine and Philosophy* 36, no. 2 (April 2011): 244.

17. Daniel E. Hall, "The Guild of Surgeons as a Tradition of Moral Enquiry," *Journal of Medicine and Philosophy* 36, no. 2 (2011): 115.

18. Engelhardt, "Confronting Moral Pluralism," 244.

19. Ibid.

20. Kuczewski, "Disability," 37.

21. Harold Perkin, *The Rise of Professional Society: England since 1880* (London: Routledge, 1989); also see his *The Third Revolution: Professional Elites in the Modern World* (London: Routledge, 1996).

22. Talcott Parsons, *The Social System* (London: Routledge & Kegan Paul Ltd.), 1951.

23. See virtually anything Callahan has written in bioethics over the last three decades, especially his books of 1987 and 1990, discussed here in chapter 5.

24. Fox and Swazey, *Observing Bioethics.*

25. Jonsen, "Birth of Bioethics" (1993) and "Birth of Bioethics" (1997); Albert R. Jonsen, *The Birth of Bioethics* (New York: Oxford University Press, 1998).

26. Margaret Somerville, *The Ethical Imagination: Journeys of the Human Spirit* (Toronto: Anansi Press, 2006), 4. Similarly, there is her earlier work, *The Ethical Canary: Science, Society and the Human Spirit* (New York: Viking, 2000).

27. Howard Brody, *The Future of Bioethics* (New York: Oxford University Press, 2009), 193.

28. Kuczewski, "Taking It Personally," 36.

29. Charles Peters, "A Neoliberal's Manifesto," *Washington Monthly* (May 1983): 10, http://www.washingtonmonthly.com/features/1983/8305_Neoliberalism.pdf.

30. Daniel Callahan, "Why America Accepted Bioethics," *Hastings Center Report* 23, no. 6 (1992): S8.

31. T. J. Clark, *Farewell to an Idea: Episodes from a History of Modernism* (New Haven, CT: Yale University Press, 1999), 7.

32. For a good primer on neoliberalism, see Manfred B. Steger and Ravi K. Roy, *Neoliberalism: A Very Short Introduction* (New York: Oxford University Press, 2010).

33. Clark, *Farewell to an Idea*, 7. Because Clark writes from the perspective of art history, and the social histories that inform it, he is extremely clear in his treatment not only of modernism but also its fundamentally nineteenth-century antecedents.

34. Miran Epstein, "How Will the Economic Downturn Affect Academic Bioethics?" *Bioethics* 24, no. 5 (2010): 252.

35. Clark, *Farewell to an Idea*, 23.

36. This is a point made repeatedly by legal experts engaged in bioethical and health issues as well as by bioethicists with an interest in law. See, for example, James, "The Appeal to Law." For the "demoralizing" effect on the practice of medicine of this bioethical turn, see Montgomery, "Law and the Demoralization of Medicine."

37. Oliver Rauprich and Jochen Vollman, "30 Years *Principles of Biomedical Ethics*: Introduction to a Symposium on the 6th Edition of Tom L. Beauchamp and James F. Childress' Seminal Work," *Journal of Medical Ethics* 37, no. 8 (2011): 455. Here they quote from the sixth edition of Tom L. Beauchamp and James Childress, *Principles of Biomedical Ethics* (New York: Oxford University Press, 2011), 3.

38. Mark Johnson, *Moral Imagination: Implications of Cognitive Science for Ethics* (Chicago: University of Chicago Press, 1993), 7.

39. Alasdair MacIntyre, *After Virtue: A Study in Moral Theory*, 2nd ed. (Notre Dame, IN: University of Notre Dame Press, 1984). MacIntyre talks about the Enlightenment enterprise as a general failure in which, of course, Kant figures prominently.

40. Charles Taylor, *Hegel and Modern Society* (New York: Cambridge University Press, 1979). In considering Hegel it is necessary, in Taylor's first chapter, to pay close attention to Kant and his antecedents. For the nonphilosopher, it's a first-rate introduction.

41. Tom L. Beauchamp, "History and Theory in 'Applied Ethics,'" *Kennedy Institute of Ethics Journal* 17, no. 1 (2007): 60. Beauchamp here is reacting to the work of Robert Baker and Lawrence McCullough, "Medical Ethics' Appropriation of Moral Philosophy: The Case of the Sympathetic and Unsympathetic Physician," *Kennedy Institute of Ethics Journal* 17, no. 1 (2007): 3–22.

42. Baker and McCullough, "Medical Ethics' Appropriation."

43. Isaiah Berlin, *Four Essays on Liberty* (New York: Oxford University Press, 1969), 138.

44. Jon Tilburt, "Shared Decision Making, after MacIntyre," *The Journal of Medicine and Philosophy* 36, no. 2 (2011): 150. Tilburt nicely summarized McIntyre's critique of Kant and the entire Enlightenment enterprise: "Alasdair MacIntyre argues that the task of grounding morality in a reason that

stands outside of traditions, ultimately failed and led to a kind of moral fragmentation."

45. Berlin, *Four Essays*, 156.

46. Taylor, *Hegel and Modern Society*, 79.

47. John Law and Annemarie Mol, "Complexities: An Introduction," in *Complexities: Social Studies of Knowledge Practices*, ed. J. Law and A. Mol (Durham, NH: Duke University Press, 2002), 2.

48. Beauchamp and Childress, *Principles of Biomedical Ethics*, 1.

49. Clark, *Farewell to an Idea*, 242.

50. Beauchamp, "History and Theory," 61.

51. Peter Singer, "All Animals are Equal," In *Applied Ethics*, ed. P. Singer (New York: Oxford University Press, 1986), 215–228.

52. Margaret C. Nussbaum, *Frontiers of Justice: Disability, Nationality, Species Membership* (Cambridge, MA: Belknap Press 2006), 346–352.

53. Nicole Gerrand, "The Misuse of Kant in the Debate about a Market for Human Body Parts," *Journal of Applied Philosophy* 16, no. 1 (1999): 59–67.

54. Jean-Christophe Merle, "A Kantian Argument for a Duty to Donate One's Own Organs. A Reply to Nicole Gerand," *Journal of Applied Philosophy* 17, no. 1 (2000): 93–101.

55. Rosemond Rhodes, "Rethinking Research Ethics," *American Journal of Bioethics* 5, no. 7 (2005): 7–28.

56. Gerrand, "Misuse of Kant."

57. ASBH, "Lifetime Achievement Award."

58. Brody, *Future of Bioethics*, 4.

59. Hilde Lindemann, "Speaking Truth to Power," *Hastings Center Report* 40, no. 1 (2010): 44–45.

60. Margaret U. Walker, "Keeping Moral Space Open," *Hastings Center Report* 23, no. 2 (1993): 33–40.

61. Judith Andre, *Bioethics as Practice* (Chapel Hill, NC: University of North Carolina Press, 2002), 69. Cited in Brody, *Future of Bioethics*, 5.

62. John Evans, *Playing God: Human Genetics Engineering and the Rationalization of Public Bioethical Debate* (Chicago: University of Chicago Press), 72–76. For a discussion of Evans, see Therese M. Lysaught, "Docile Bodies: Transnational Research Ethics as Biopolitics," *Journal of Medicine and Philosophy* 34, no. 4 (2009): 393–394.

2 Something Old

1. *American Heritage Dictionary of the English Language* (New York: Houghton Mifflin, 1973).

2. Andrew A. Michel, "Psychiatry after Virtue: A Modern Practice in the Ruins," *Journal of Medicine and Philosophy* 36, no. 2 (2011): 186–211, 180. The idea of ethics as describing "rules" of behavior was only introduced much, much later.

3. Tom Koch and Sarah Jones, "The Ethical Professional as Endangered Person: Blog Notes on Doctor-Patient Relationships," *Journal of Medical Ethics* 36, no. 6 (2010): 371–374.

4. Talcott Parsons, *The Social System* (London: Routledge & Kegan Paul Ltd., 1951).

5. Harold Perkin, *The Rise of Professional Society: England since 1880* (London: Routledge, 1989).

6. Harold Perkin, *The Third Revolution: Professional Elites in the Modern World* (London: Routledge, 1996); Herbert M. Swick, "Toward a Normative Definition of Medical Professionalism," *Academic Medicine* 75, no. 6 (2000): 612–616.

7. Fabrice Jotterand, "The Hippocratic Oath and Contemporary Medicine: Dialectic between Past Ideals and Present Reality," *Journal of Medicine and Philosophy* 30, no.1 (2005): 107–128.

8. Tom L. Beauchamp and James F. Childress, *Principles of Biomedical Ethics*, 5th ed. (New York: Oxford University Press, 2001), 1.

9. Tristram H. Engelhardt, "Managed Care and the Deprofessionalization of Medicine," *The Ethics of Managed Care* (Dordrecht: Kluwer Academic Publishers, 2003), 100.

10. Peter Singer, *Hegel: A Very Short Introduction* (New York: Oxford University Press, 1983), 20.

11. Jonathan Montgomery, "Law and the Demoralization of Medicine," *Legal Studies* 26, no. 2 (2006): 201; Joseph M. Jacob, *Doctors and Rules: A Sociology of Professional Values* (London: Routledge, 1988).

12. Thomas Percival, *Medical Jurisprudence or a Code of Ethics and Institutes Adopted to the Professions of Physic and Surgery* (Manchester, UK: 1794), sec. 1L 8. Also quoted in Miran Epstein, "How Will the Economic Downturn Affect Academic Bioethics?" *Bioethics* 24, no. 5 (2010): 230.

13. Michael Walzer, *Spheres of Justice: A Defense of Pluralism and Equality* (New York: Basic Books, 1983), 86.

14. G. A. Cohen, *Why Not Socialism?* (Princeton, NJ: Princeton University Press, 2009), 11–12.

15. American Medical Association, *Principles of Medical Ethics* (Chicago: American Medical Association, 1957), sec. 6, http://www.ama-assn.org/resources/doc/ethics/1957_principles.pdf (accessed February 21, 2012); also cited in Epstein, "Economic Downturn," 230.

16. Daniel E. Hall, "The Guild of Surgeons as a Tradition of Moral Enquiry," *Journal of Medicine and Philosophy* 36, no. 2 (2011): 118.

17. Robert Bartz, "Remembering the Hippocratics: Practice, and Ethos of Ancient Greek Physician-Healers," In *Bioethics: Ancient Themes in Contemporary Issues* (Cambridge, MA: MIT Press, 2000), 15.

18. For a review, see Elliott A. Krause, *Death of the Guilds: Professions, States, and the Advance of Capitalism, 1930 to the Present* (New Haven, CT: Yale University Press, 1996).

19. Perkin, *Rise of Professional Society*; also see William M. Sullivan, "Medicine under Threat: Professionalism and Professional Identity," *Journal of the Canadian Medical Association* 162, no. 5 (2000): 673–675.

20. This rather intriguing suggestion comes from a web page created by medical historian Keith Blayney, "The Caduceus vs the Staff of Asclepius," 2005, http://drblayney.com/Asclepius.html#hygiene (accessed June 27, 2011).

21. L. Gluckman, "The Caduceus—A Further Interpretation," *New Zealand Medical Journal* 111, no. 1070 (1988): 281–282. It is worth noting there is a huge, erudite, and conflicting literature on the history of the caduceus and its meaning at various times in history.

22. The broad history of the interrelationship of activist medicine, medical data, and advancing science is reviewed in Tom Koch *Disease Maps: Epidemics on the Ground* (Chicago, IL: University of Chicago Press, 2011).

23. James H. Cassedy, *American Medicine and Statistical Thinking, 1800–1860* (Cambridge, MA: Harvard University Press, 1984), 27. Cassedy's history concerns the progressive use of public health data in the development of American medicine and public health. For a review, see John H. Warner, "Review: James H. Cassedy, *American Medicine and Statistical Thinking, 1800–1860*," *Medical History* 29, no. 4 (1985).

24. Koch, *Disease Maps*, 80.

25. Gregg Mitman and Ronald L. Numbers, "From Miasma to Asthma: The Changing Fortunes of Medical Geography in America," *History and Philosophy of the Life Sciences* 25, no. 3 (1993): 393.

26. Tom Koch, "Mapping the Miasma: Air, Health, and Place in Early Medical Mapping," *Cartographic Perspectives* 52, no. 4 (2005): 27.

27. James Jameson, *Report on the epidemick cholera morbus* . . . (Calcutta: Government Gazette Press, by A. G. Balfour, 1819), http://pds.lib.harvard.edu/pds/view/7095430 (accessed February 21, 2012). This was the first authoritative report on cholera as a new potentially epidemic disease.

28. Privy Council, "Instructions and Regulations Regarding Cholera, Issued under the Authority of the Privy Council," in *Annual Register or a View of the History, Politics, and Literature of the Year 1831* (London: Baldwin and Cradock, 1832), 357–360. For a discussion, see Geoffrey Marks and William K. Beatty, *Epidemics* (New York: Charles Scribner's Sons, 1976), 197.

29. George Rosen, *A History of Public Health* (Baltimore, MD: Johns Hopkins University Press, 1993), 44–45.

30. R. J. Morris, *Cholera 1832: Social Response to an Epidemic* (London: Croom Helm, 1976), 28–29.

31. Lancet, "History of the Rise, Progress, Ravages, Etc. of the Blue Cholera of India," *Lancet* 17 (1831): 241–284. The article was unsigned but presumably the work of the journal's editors.

32. Michael Ryan, *Manual of Medical Jurisprudence, Second Edition* (London: Sherwood, Gilbert, and Piper, 1836), viii, http://www.archive.org/details/amanualmedicalj00ryangoog (accessed January 18, 2012). The whole of Ryan's landmark text is available online in a variety of electronic formats.

33. Still, the best history here is Martin S. Pernick, *The Black Stork: Eugenics and the Death of "Defective" Babies in American Medicine and Motion Pictures since 1915* (New York: Oxford University Press, 1996).

34. Pernick, *Black Stork*, 29.

35. For the flavor of the debate see, among the proponents, Timothy E. Quill, "Death and Dignity: A Case of Individualized Decision Making," *New England Journal of Medicine* 324, no. 10 (1991): 691–694; or Timothy E. Quill and Margaret P. Battin, *Physician-assisted Dying: The Case for Palliative Care and Patient Choice* (Baltimore, MD: Johns Hopkins University Press, 2004). For differing views, see Tom Koch, "Living vs. Dying 'with Dignity': A New Perspective on the Euthanasia Debate," *Cambridge Quarterly of Healthcare Ethics* 5, no. 1 (1996): 50–60; and Tom Koch, "On the Subject(s) of Jack Kevorkian, MD: A Retrospective Analysis," *Cambridge Quarterly of Healthcare Ethics* 7, no. 4 (1998): 436–441.

36. Pernick, *Black Stork*, 7.

37. *Buck v. Bell* (1927) 274 U.S. 200.

38. Stephen J. Gould, *The Mismeasure of Man* (New York: W. W. Norton, 1981), 335–336.

39. Benno Müller-Hill, " Lessons from a Dark and Distant Past," *Bioethics: An Anthology*, second ed. (Malden, MA: Blackwell Publishing, 2006), 235.

40. Arthur L. Caplan, "Misusing the Nazi Analogy," *Science* 309, no. 5734 (July 22, 2005): 535.

41. Jonathan Glover, *Choosing Children: The Ethical Dilemmas of Genetic Intervention* (New York: Oxford University Press, 2006), 29.

42. Pernick, *Black Stork*, 163.

43. Ian Hacking, "Why Race Still Matters," *Daedulus* 134, no. 1 (2005): 104.

44. Karl Binding and Alfred Hoche, *Permitting the Destruction of Unworthy Life* (Leipzig: Verlag von Felix Meiner, 1920). I have relied on a translation by Walter Wright, Patrick G. Derr, and Robert Solomon, published in *Issues in Law and Medicine*. For an interesting perspective based on a partial translation of a section of the text, see Robert Baker and Lawrence B. McCullough, "Medical Ethics' Appropriation of Moral Philosophy: The Case of the Sympathetic and Unsympathetic Physician," *Kennedy Institute of Ethics Journal* 17, no. 1 (2007): 13–17.

45. Karl Binding and Alfred Hoche, "Permitting the Destruction of Unworthy Life: Its Extent and Form," trans. Walter Wright, Patrick G. Derr, and Robert Solomon, *Issues in Law and Medicine* 8, no. 2: 255.

46. Baker and McCullough, "Medical Ethics," 14.

47. Ibid., 17.

48. Ibid.

49. Sarah Wise, *The Italian Boy: A Tale of Murder and Body Snatching in 1830s London* (New York: Henry Holt and Co., 2004), 6–7.

50. Ruth Richardson, *The Making of Mr. Gray's Anatomy: Bodies, Books, Fortune, Fame* (New York: Oxford University Press, 2008), 116–122.

51. Michael Bliss, *William Osler: A Life in Medicine* (New York: Oxford University Press, 1999), 352–353.

52. Joseph J. Fins, "A Leg to Stand On: Sir William Osler and Wilder Penfield's 'Neuroethics,' *American Journal of Bioethics* 8, no. 1 (2008): 40.

53. Nuremberg Military Tribunals, *Trials of War Criminals before the Nuremberg Military Tribunals under Control Council Law* (Washington, DC: Government Printing Office, 1989), 181–182.

54. This is the source of Arndt's famous characterization of the "banality of evil": Hannah Arndt, *Eichman in Jerusalem: A Report on the Banality of Evil* (New York: Viking Press, 1963).

55. For a recent review of some of these covenants, see Fabrice Jotterand, "Human Dignity and Transhumanism: Do Anthro-Technological Devices Have Moral Status?" *American Journal of Bioethics* 10, no.7 (2010): 45–52.

56. Harald Schmidt, "Whose Dignity? Resolving Ambiguities in the Scope of 'Human Dignity' in the Universal Declaration on Bioethics and Human Rights," *Journal of Medical Ethics* 33, no. 10 (2007): 578–584.

57. Raymond A. Vonderlehr, "Untreated Syphilis in the Male Negro: A Comparative Study of Treated and Untreated Cases," *Journal of the American Medical Association* 107, no. 11 (September 12, 1936): 856–860.

58. Britt Russert, "'A Study in Nature': The Tuskegee Experiments and the New South Plantation," *Journal of Medical Humanities* 30, no. 3 (2009): 156.

59. Therese M. Lysaught, "Docile Bodies: Transnational Research Ethics as Biopolitics," *Journal of Medicine and Philosophy* 34, no. 4 (2009): 384–385.

60. Rebecca Skloot, *The Immortal Life of Henrietta Lacks* (New York: Broadway Paperbacks, 2011), 29–30.

61. Stephen Napier, "A Regulatory Argument against Human Embryonic Stem Cell Research," *Journal of Medicine and Philosophy* 34, no. 5 (2009): 497.

62. Robert Dingwall and Vienna Rozelle, "The Ethical Governance of German Physicians 1890–1939: Are There Lessons from History?" *Journal of Policy History* 23, no. 1 (2011): 29–52.

63. The details of the polio epidemic in the United States are well described by Barry Trevelyan, Mathew Smallman-Raynor, and Andrew D. Cliff, "The Spatial Dynamics of Poliomyelitis in the United States: From Epidemic Emergence to Vaccine-Induced Retreat, 1910–1971," *Annals of the Association of American Geographers* 95, no. 2 (2005): 269–293.

64. Edmund Sass, "The History of Polio: A Hypertext Timeline," 2005, http://www.cloudnet.com/%7Eedrbsass/poliotimeline.htm (accessed November 24, 2006).

65. Ger L. Wackers, *Constructivist Medicine* (Maastricht, NL: Universitare Pers Maastricht, 1994), 137–138.

66. Tom Koch, "Were Polio to Return Today . . . ," *Journal of the Canadian Medical Association* 178, no. 9 (2008): 1244, http://www.cmaj.ca/content/178/9/1244.full.pdf+html (accessed December 12, 2011).

67. Edmund Pellegrino, "The Metamorphosis of Medical Ethics: A 30-Year Perspective," *Journal of the American Medical Association* 269, no. 9 (1993): 1158.

68. Naomi Rogers, *Dirt and Disease: Polio before FDR* (New Brunswick, NJ: Rutgers University Press, 1996), 2.

3 Something Newer

1. Shana Alexander, "They Decide Who Lives, Who Dies," *Life Magazine* 53 (1962): 102–125.

2. David J. Rothman, *Strangers by the Bedside: A History of How Law and Bioethics Transformed Medical Decision Making* (New York: Basic Books, 1991), 150–151.

3. Edward R. Murrow, "Harvest of Shame," *CBS Reports*, November 26, 1960.

4. For an excellent discussion of scarcity and of the importance of Harry Pearson's arguments, see David Harvey, *Social Justice and the City* (Cambridge, MA: Basil Blackwell, 1973), 113, 139.

5. Albert R. Jonsen, "The Birth of Bioethics," Special Supplement, *Hastings Center Report* 23, no. 6 (1993): S1–S4.

6. Ibid., S2. In his works Jonsen reviews the questions and issues that arose in the early years of organ transplantation and summarized here in the text.

7. Immanuel Kant, *Foundations of the Metaphysics of Morals (Grundlegung zu Metaphysik der Sitten)*, trans. Lewis W. Beck (New York: Macmillan Publishing Co., 1785/1959), 47. I have relied on various translations of Kant's work, online and in print. For citation purposes, I include the one I own and use most frequently.

8. Jeffrey H. Bishop, *The Anticipatory Corpse: Medicine, Power, and the Care of the Dying* (Notre Dame, IN: University of Notre Dame Press, 2011), 154. Bishop provides a thorough and comprehensive review of the relationship between the Ad Hoc Committee and the issue of organ transplantation.

9. Ad Hoc Committee of the Harvard Medical School, "A Definition of Irreversible Coma: Report of the Ad Hoc Committee of the Harvard Medical School to Examine the Definition of Brain Death," *Journal of the American Medical Association* 205, no. 6 (1968): 37–40.

10. Alexander M. Capron, "Anencephalic Donors: Separate the Dead from the Dying," *The Hastings Center Report* 17, no. 1 (1987): 7–9.

11. Michael J. Broyde, "The Diagnosis of Brain Death: Correspondence," *New England Journal of Medicine* 345, no. 8 (2001): 617.

12. Henry. K. Beecher and Henry I. Dorr, "The New Definition of Death: Some Opposing Views," *International Journal of Clinical Pharmacology, Therapy and Toxicology* 5, no. 2 (1971): 120–124. This article, which began as a paper presented by Beecher in 1970 to the American Association for the Advancement of Science, developed a life of its own. It has been cited since in scores of books and journal articles.

13. See, for example, Calixto Machado et al., "The Concept of Brain Death Did Not Evolve to Benefit Organ Transplants," *Journal of Medical Ethics* 33, no. 4 (1997): 197–200.

14. Miran Epstein, "The Political Economy of Death and the History of Its Criteria," *Reviews in the Neurosciences* 20, nos. 3–4 (2009): 294.

15. Robert Veatch, "From Forgoing Life Support to Aid-in-dying," Special Supplement, *Hastings Center Report* 23, no. 6 (1993): S7–8, http://www.questia.com/googleScholar.qst?docId=5002196576 (accessed June 20, 2011).

16. Kant, *Foundations of the Metaphysics of Morals*, 46.

17. Charles Taylor, *Hegel and Modern Society* (New York: Cambridge University Press, 1979), 4–5, 78–79.

18. Richard M. Titmuss, *The Gift Relationship: From Human Blood to Social Policy* (New York: Vintage Books, 1982).

19. Karl Binding and Alfred Hoche, "Permitting the Destruction of Unworthy Life: Its Extent and Form," trans. Walter Wright, Patrick G. Derr, and Robert Solomon, *Issues in Law and Medicine* 8, no. 2: 249.

20. Nicole Gerrand, "The Misuse of Kant in the Debate about a Market for Human Body Parts," *Journal of Applied Philosophy* 16, no. 1 (1999): 59–67.

21. Jean-Christophe Merle, "A Kantian Argument for a Duty to Donate One's Own Organs. A Reply to Nicole Gerand," *Journal of Applied Philosophy* 17, no. 1 (2000): 93–101.

22. Robert E. Cranston et al., "The Diagnosis of Brain Death," *New England Journal of Medicine* 345, no. 8 (2001): 616–618, 616.

23. See, for example, Nancy L. Childs, Walter N. Mercer, and Helen W. Childs, "Accuracy of Diagnosis of Persistent Vegetative State," *Neurology* 43, no. 8 (1993): 1465–1467.

24. Nicholas D. Schiff, "Hope for 'Comatose' Patients," *Cerebrum* 5, no. 4 (2003): 7–24; Joseph J. Fins, "A Leg to Stand On: Sir William Osler and Wilder Penfield's 'Neuroethics,'" *American Journal of Bioethics* no. 8, no. 1 (2008): 37–46.

25. Here see Robert D. Truog, "Is It Time to Abandon Brain Death?" *Hastings Center Report* 27, no. 1 (1997): 29–37. Robert D. Truog and W. M. Robinson, "Correspondence," *New England Journal of Medicine* 345, no. 8 (2001): 617 http://www.nejm.org/doi/full/10.1056/NEJM200108233450813 (accessed February 22, 2012).

26. Allan Kellehear, "Dying as a Social Relationship: A Sociological Review of Debates on the Determination of Death," *Social Science & Medicine* 66, no. 7 (2008): 1535.

27. Robert D. Truog and Franklin G. Miller, "The Dead Donor Rule and Organ Transplantation," *The New England Journal of Medicine* 359, no. 7: 674, http://www.nejm.org/doi/full/10.1056/NEJMp0804474?query=TOC (accessed June 20, 2011).

28. Franklin G. Miller and Robert D. Truog, "Rethinking the Ethics of Vital Organ Donations," *Hastings Center Report* 38, no. 6 (2008): 38-46, 42, http://www.maceyleigh.net/articles/ethics_of_vital_organ_donations.pdf (accessed June 20, 2011).

29. See, for example, Richard D. Lamm, "New World of Medical Ethics: Our Duty Lies Both to the Individual and the Population," *Vital Speeches of the Day* 59 (July 1, 1993): 549–553.

30. Richard D. Lamm, "Columbus and Copernicus: New Wine in Old Wineskins," *Mount Sinai Journal of Medicine* 56, no. 1 (1989): 1–10; Richard D. Lamm, "Saving a Few—Sacrificing Many, at Great Cost," *New York Times*, August 2, 1989, 23.

31. Richard D. Lamm, "Copernican Health Ethics," Annual Meeting of the American Society of Bioethics and the Humanities, Marriott Denver City Center, Denver, CO, October 26, 2006.

32. Richard D. Lamm, "Doctors Have Patients, Governors Have Citizens." *Narrative Matters: The Power of the Personal Essay in Health Policy*, ed. Fitzhugh Mullan, Ellen Ficklen, and Kyna Rubin (Baltimore, MD: Johns Hopkins Press 2006), 34–41.

33. Ibid.

34. "Gov. Lamm Asserts Elderly, If Very Ill, Have 'Duty to Die,'" *New York Times*, March 29, 1984, A16, http://www.nytimes.com/1984/03/29/us/gov-lamm-asserts-elderly-if-very-ill-have-duty-to-die.html (accessed February 22, 2012). Following a 1993 report on Senate testimony by Hillary Rodham Clinton, *New York Times* editors added a note to this (and other) electronic file stories on Lamm in which he claimed his position was misquoted, misunderstood, or misstated.

35. T. J. Clark, *Farewell to an Idea: Episodes from a History of Modernism* (New Haven, CT: Yale University Press, 1999), 8.

36. Daniel Callahan, *Setting Limits: Medical Goals in an Aging Society* (New York: Simon and Schuster 1987), 15.

37. Ibid., 36.

38. Ibid., 111. In correspondence Callahan denies that his vision of the "good city" is based on productivity, or that his communitarianism is anything but benign. But he also insists his is not an ageist perspective, merely one in which the vision of the elderly focuses on the future needs of society rather than their own.

39. For more on Callahan and communitarianism, see Daniel Callahan, "Why America Accepted Bioethics," *Hastings Center Report* 23, no. 6 (1993): S8–9.

40. Tom Koch, *Scarce Goods: Justice, Fairness, and Organ Transplantation* (Westport, CT; : Praeger Books, 2001), 181.

41. Daniel Callahan, *What Kind of Life? The Limits of Medical Progress* (Washington, DC: Georgetown University Press, 1990), 253.

42. Ibid., 255.

43. Ibid., 115.

44. For a brief perspective on the literature of physician self-knowledge, see, for example, William Reichel, "Physician Know Thyself," *Journal of the American Board of Family Practice* 12, no. 3 (1999): 258–259.

45. Roger Crisp, Tony Hope, and David Ebbes, "The Asbury Draft Policy on Ethical Use of Resources," *British Medical Journal* 312, no. 7045 (1996): 1528–1533.

46. David C. Thomasma, "The Asbury Draft Policy on Ethical Use of Resources," *Cambridge Quarterly of Healthcare Ethics* 8, no. 2 (1997): 249.

47. For a later entry in the gerontological reaction to Callahan and Lamm's arguments, see, for example, Ellen M. Gee and Gloria M. Gutman, *The Overselling of Population Aging: Apocalyptic Demography, Intergenerational Challenges, and Social Policy* (New York: Oxford University Press, 2000).

48. Robert H. Binstock and Stephen G. Post, *Too Old for Health Care? Controversies in Medicine, Law, Economics, and Ethics* (Baltimore, MD: Johns Hopkins University Press, 1991).

49. The term "greedy geezers" was first given currency in Henry Fairlie, "Talking 'bout My Generation," *The New Republic* 28 (March 1988): 19–22.

50. John L. Hess, "Social Security Wars: Confessions of a Greedy Geezer," *The Nation* 250 (April 2, 1990): 437–439.

51. Stephen Katz, *Disciplining Old Age: The Formation of Gerontological Knowledge* (Charlottesville: The University Press of Virginia, 1996), 6.

52. For a popular rendition of this perspective, see Eloise Salholz, "Blaming the Voters; Hapless Budgeteers Single Out 'Greedy Geezers,'" *Newsweek* 116, no. 18 (October 29, 1990): 36. For a more academic discussion of the diffusion of "greeder geezers" as an excuse for other social problems, see Robert H. Binstock, "Another Form of 'Elderly Bashing,'" *Journal of Health Politics, Policy and Law* 17, no. 2 (1992): 269–272.

53. Elizabeth A. Binney and Carroll L. Estes, "The Retreat of the State and Its Transfer of Responsibility: The Intergenerational War," *International Journal of Health Services* 18, no. 1 (1988): 83–96.

54. Daniel Callahan, "The Economic Woes of Medicare," *New York Times* blog, November 13, 2008 (accessed December 28, 2009), http://newoldage.blogs.nytimes.com/2008/11/13/heart-surgery-how-old-is-too-old/?scp=2&sq=Daniel%20Callahan&st=cse.

55. Bill Bytheway, "Unequal Aging: The Untold Story of Exclusion in Old Age," *Sociology of Health and Illness* 32, no. 6 (September 10, 2009): 967. Bytheway was reviewing a then recently published book by Paul Cain and Malcolm Dean, *Unequal Aging: The Untold Story of Exclusion on Old Age* (Bristol, UK: 2009).

56. Thomas R. Malthus, *An Essay on the Principle of Population, as It Affects the Future Improvement of Society* (London: J. Johnson, in St. Paul's Church-Yard, 1798), 4, http://www.esp.org/books/malthus/population/malthus.pdf (accessed July 19, 2010).

57. Ibid., 44.

58. Sarah Green, "Innovations 'R' Us." *The Scientist* 24, no. 12 (2010): 13, http://classic.the-scientist.com/article/display/57823/ (accessed February 28, 2012).

59. John Markert, "The Malthusian Fallacy: Prophecies of Doom and the Crisis of Social Security," *The Social Science Journal* 42, no. 4 (2005): 555–568.

60. Ernst & Young, *The Economic Contributions of the Biotechnology Industry to the U.S. Economy*, Biotechnology Organization, 2000, 1, accessed December 18, 2011. http://www.bio.org/articles/economic-contributions-biotechnology-industry (accessed January 15, 2012). For a more focused, state-level review, see Allan G. Helvesi and Kenneth B. Bleiwis, "The Economic Impact of the Biotechnology and Pharmaceutical Industries in New York State," Office of the Comptroller Report 11-205 (Albany, NY: Office of the Comptroller, 2005), http://www.docstoc.com/docs/69310177/The-Economic-Impact-of-the-Biotechnology-and-Pharmaceutical (accessed August 22, 2011).

61. AdvaMed, "The Medical Technology Industry at a Glance," Advanced Medical Technology Association (2004), 2, http://www.omnex.com/training/iso13485/articles/ADVAMED-Medical-Device-Industry-Facts.pdf (accessed December 2, 2008).

62. Louis Lasagna, "Mortal Decisions: The Search for an Ethical Policy on Allocating Health Care," *Science* 43:6 (1991), 43–44.

63. Ibid., 43.

64. David C. Thomasma, Tommi Kushner, and Steven Hellig, "From the Editors," *Cambridge Quarterly of Healthcare Ethics* 8, no. 3 (1999): 263.

65. Paul T. Menzel, *Strong Medicine: The Ethical Rationing of Health Care* (New York: Oxford University Press, 1990).

66. Rothman, *Strangers by the Bedside*, 32.

67. John F. Kilner, *Who Lives? Who Dies? Ethical Criteria in Patient Selection* (New Haven: Yale University Press, 1990).

68. U.S. Senate Special Committee on Aging, *Who Lives, Who Dies, Who Decides: The Ethics of Health Care Rationing*, Hearing before the Special Committee on Aging, 102nd Congress, 1st Session (Washington, DC: U.S. Government Printing Office, 1991).

69. Koch, *Scarce Goods*, 195–198; Tom Koch, *The Wreck of the William Brown* (Camden, ME: McGraw-Hill Marine, 2004), 188–189.

4 Lifeboat Ethics

The story of the *William Brown*, and the subsequent trial, *United States v. Holmes*, is based on my 2003 book *The Wreck of the William Brown*. A complete list of references describing the wreck, the political machinations, and the trial is included there. Quotes of court testimony are taken from trial reports of the day. The testimony of survivors is taken from either court testimony or depositions given to U.S. and British consuls in Le Havre, France. Today those depositions are preserved in the The National Archives, Kew, Richmond, Surrey, UK.

1. Nathaniel Philbrick, *In the Heart of the Sea: The Tragedy of the Whaleship* Essex (New York: Viking, 2000).

2. *United States v. Holmes*, 1842.

3. George Lakoff and Mark Johnson, *Metaphors We Live By* (Chicago: University of Chicago Press, 1980), 10.

4. John R. Wallace, "Sortal Predicates and Quantification," *Journal of Philosophy* 62, no. 1 (1965): 8–13.

5. Howard Adler Jr. and John A. Francis, "Proximate Cause: A Growing Limitation on Civil RICO Actions," 13 *RICO Law Reporter* 1 (1991), 443. http://www.dgslaw.com/documents/articles/273380.pdf (accessed December 28, 2011).

6. United States Code 18 U.S.C., Chapter 96 § 1961–1968.

7. Govind Persad, Alan Wertheimer, and Ezekiel. J. Emanuel, "Principles for Allocation of Scarce Medical Interventions," *The Lancet* 373, no. 9661 (2009): 423–431.

8. Norman Daniels, *Just Health* (New York: Cambridge University Press, 2008). For a discussion, see Benjamin Sachs, "Lingering Problems of Currency and Scope in Daniel's Argument for a Society Obligation to Meet Health Needs," *Journal of Medicine and Philosophy* 35, no. 4 (2010): 403–406.

9. Robert N. Butler, *Why Survive? Being Old in America* (New York: Harper & Row, 1975), 4.

10. Miran Epstein, "How Will the Economic Downturn Affect Academic Bioethics?" *Bioethics* 24, no. 5 (2010): 230.

11. David Harvey, "Population, Resources, and the Ideology of Science," *Economic Geography* 40, no. 3 (1974): 272. Scarcity, in Harvey's analysis, is a central tenant of Western economic theory underlying assumptions of demand, production, and pricing.

12. Here a recent article on the history of scarcity in petroleum production and distribution is especially useful. See Mathew T. Huber, "Enforcing Scarcity: Oil, Violence, and the Making of the Market," *Annals of the Association of American Geographers* 101, no. 4 (2011): 816–826.

13. *Congressional Record*, 118th Congress, September 30, 1972: 33, 008.

14. Ger L. Wackers, *Constructivist Medicine* (Maastricht, NL: Universitare Pers Maastricht, 1994), 137–138.

15. Jill H. Fisher, *Medical Research for Hire: The Political Economy of Pharmaceutical Clinical Trials* (New Brunswick, NJ: Rutgers University Press, 2009), 15.

16. Tom Campbell, "U.S. Has Much to Learn from Our Health Care," *Toronto Star*, July 19, 2009, A15, http://www.thestar.com/article/668161 (accessed December 28, 2011).

17. Bob Evans and Marko Vujicic, "Political Wolves and Economic Sheep: The Sustainability of Public Health Insurance in Canada," in *Public-Private Mix for Health* (Oxford: Radcliff Publishing Ltd., 2005), 125.

18. Paul Farmer and Nicole Gastineau Campos, "Rethinking Medical Ethics: A View from Below," *Ethics and Infectious Disease* (Malden, MA: Blackwell Publishing, 2006), 261–284.

19. Immanuel Kant, *Foundations of the Metaphysics of Morals (Grundlegung zu Metaphysik der Sitten)*, trans. Lewis W. Beck (New York: Macmillan Publishing Co., 1785/1959), 4. The same distinction is made in Kant's *Groundwork of the Metaphysics of Morals*, trans. H. J. Paton (New York: HarperCollins Publisher, 1785/1948).

20. Charles Taylor, *Hegel and Modern Society* (New York: Cambridge University Press, 1979), 75–76.

21. Peter Singer, *Hegel: A Very Short Introduction* (New York: Oxford University Press 1983), 42.

22. Kant, *Groundwork of the Metaphysic of Morals*, §75.

23. This, Kant wrote, he learned from Rousseau who put "the honor of humanity" above the desire for knowledge. See Catherine Chalier, *What Ought I to Do? Morality in Kant and Levinas* (Ithaca, NY: Cornell University Press, 1998), 12–13.

5 Biopolitics, Biophilosophies, and Bioethics

1. For a discussion of the relationship between ethics and politics, see Raymond Geuss, *Philosophy and Real Politics* (Princeton, NJ: Princeton University Press, 2008), 1–2.

2. T. J. Clark, *Farewell to an Idea: Episodes from a History of Modernism* (New Haven, CT: Yale University Press 1999), 102.

3. Daniel Callahan, "Why America Accepted Bioethics," *Hastings Center Report* 23 no. 6 (1992): S8.

4. Shelley Tremain, "Foucault, Governmentality, and Critical Disability Theory," In *Foucault and the Government of Disability* (Ann Arbor: University of Michigan Press, 2005), 4. Written from the perspective of critical disability theory, Tremain's introduction in this volume is a good first reading on Foucault.

5. Michel Foucault, *The History of Sexuality,* vol. 1: *An Introduction*, trans. Robert Hurley (New York: Random House, 1978), 144.

6. Warren T. Reich, "How Bioethics Got Its Name," Special Supplement, *Hastings Center Report* 23, no. 6 (November–December 1993): S6–S7.

7. John Harris, *Enhancing Evolution: The Ethical Case for Making Better People* (Princeton, NJ: Princeton University Press), 2007.

8. The history of this nineteenth-century conflation of state economic objectives and scientific programs is well described by Anson Rabinbach in his *The Human Motor: Energy, Fatigue, and the Origins of Modernity* (New York: Basic Books, 1990).

9. R. F. Kimball, "The Great Biological Generalization," *Quarterly Review of Biology* 18, no. 4 (1943): 364–367.

10. This history is elegantly described in Lenny Moss, *What Genes Can't Do* (Cambridge, MA: MIT Press, 2003).

11. David Shenk, "Is There a Genius in All of Us?" *BBC News Magazine*, January 12, 2011, http://www.bbc.co.uk/news/magazine-12140064 (accessed June 26, 2011).

12. Kenneth S. Ramos, "A Vision That Challenges Dogma Gives Rise to a New Era in the Environmental Health Sciences," *Environmental Health Perspectives* 113 (2005): 162–167.

13. Moss, *What Genes Can't Do*; Paul A. Wade and Trevor K. Archer, "Epigenetics: Environmental Instructions for the Genome," *Environmental Health Perspectives* 114, no. 3: A140–A141.

14. Bruce Jennings, "From the Urban to the Civic: The Moral Possibilities of the City," *Journal of Urban Health: Bulletin of the New York Academy of Medicine* 78, no. 1 (2001): 93.

15. Robert Baker and Lawrence B. McCullough, "Medical Ethics' Appropriation of Moral Philosophy: The Case of the Sympathetic and Unsympathetic Physician," *Kennedy Institute of Ethics Journal* 17, no. 1 (2007): 3–22.

16. Tom L. Beauchamp, "History and Theory in 'Applied Ethics,'" *Kennedy Institute of Ethics Journal* 17, no. 1 (2007): 57.

17. Baker and McCullough, "Medical Ethics' Appropriation," 5.

18. Beauchamp, "History and Theory," 57.

19. Peter Singer, *Hegel: A Very Short Introduction* (New York: Oxford University Press, 1983), 42.

20. National Research Act 1974 (July 12) Pub. L. 93–348.

21. *The Belmont Report: Ethical Principles and Guidelines for the Protection of Human Subjects of Research* (Washington, DC: U.S. Government Printing Office, 1979), http://ohsr.od.nih.gov/guidelines/belmont.html (accessed January 8, 2009), summary.

22. For this and other, similar instances, see Rebecca Skloot, *The Immortal Life of Henrietta Lacks* (New York: Broadway Paperbacks, 2011), 129–130.

23. *William A. Hyman v. Jewish Chronic Disease Hospital* (1965) 268 N.Y.S. 2nd 397.

24. Skloot, *The Immortal Life*, 133.

25. *Salgo v. Leland Stanford Jr. University Board of Trustees* (1957) Civ. No. 17045, First Dist. Div. One.

26. *The Belmont Report*, 4.

27. James A. Anderson, "Clinical Research in Practice: Reexamining the Distinction between Research and Practice," *Journal of Medicine and Philosophy* 35, no. 1 (2010): 48.

28. Howard Brody, "Are There Three or Four Distinct Types of Medical Protection?" *American Journal of Bieothics* 6, no. 4 (2006): 51–53.

29. Winston Chiong, "The Real Problem with Equipoise," *American Journal of Bioethics* 6, no. 4 (2006): 47.

30. Trisha Phillips, "From the Ideal Market to the Ideal Clinic: Constructing a Normative Standard of Fairness for Human Subjects Research," *Journal of Medicine and Philosophy* 36, no. 1 (2011): 79–106.

31. Jill H. Fisher, *Medical Research for Hire: The Political Economy of Pharmaceutical Clinical Trials* (New Brunswick, NJ: Rutgers University Press, 2009), 7.

32. Miran Epstein and Mark Wilson, "Consent in Emergency Care Research," *The Lancet* 373, no. 9785 (July 2011): 26.

33. Nina Hallowell et al., "Healthcare Professionals' and Researchers' Understanding of Cancer Genetics Activities: A Qualitative Interview Study," *Journal of Medical Ethics* 35, no. 2 (2009), 113–119. The idea of a "misconception" or "misunderstanding" of research that needed participants who would not benefit was first described in Paul S. Applebaum, Loren H. Roth, and Charles W. Lidz, "The Therapeutic Misconception: Informed Consent in Psychiatric Research," *International Journal of Law and Psychiatry* 5, nos. 3–4 (1982), 319–329.

34. Fisher, *Medical Research for Hire*, 45.

35. Miriam Shuchman, *The Drug Trial: Dr. Nancy Olivieri and the Science Scandal That Rocked the Hospital for Sick Children* (Toronto: Random House Canada), 2005.

36. Ian Roberts et al., "Effect of Consent Rituals on Mortality in Emergency Care Research," *Lancet* 377, no. 9771 (2011): 1071–1072, http://www.thelancet.com/journals/lancet/article/PIIS0140-6736(11)60317-6/fulltext (accessed July 7, 2011).

37. Zachary M. Schrag, *Ethical Imperialism: Institutional Review Boards and the Social Sciences, 1965–2000* (Baltimore, MD: Johns Hopkins University Press, 2010).

38. Joseph J. Fins, "A Leg to Stand On: Sir William Osler and Wilder Penfield's 'Neuroethics,'" *American Journal of Bioethics* 8, no. 1 (2008): 40.

39. Beauchamp, "History and Theory," 61.

40. Immanuel Kant, *Foundations of the Metaphysics of Morals* (*Grundlegung zu Metaphysik der Sitten*, trans. Lewis W. Beck (New York: Macmillan Publishing Co., 1785/1959), ix.

41. Therese M. Lysaught, "Respect: Or, How Respect for Persons Became Respect for Autonomy," *Journal of Medicine and Philosophy* 29, no. 6 (2004): 668.

42. Beauchamp, "History and Theory," 61.

43. *The Belmont Report*, 1979.

44. Albert R. Jonsen, "The Birth of Bioethics," Special Supplement, *Hastings Center Report* 23, no. 6 (1993) (November–December): S3.

45. Fisher, *Medical Research for Hire*, 16.

46. Laurence B. McCullough, "Introduction," *Theoretical Medicine* 4, no. 2 (1983): 227–229.

47. Robert Bartz, "Remembering the Hippocratics: Practice and Ethos of Ancient Greek Physician-Healers," in *Bioethics: Ancient Themes in Contemporary Issues*, ed. Mark G. Kuczewski and Ronald Polansky (Cambridge, MA: MIT Press, 2000), 12.

6 Principles of Biomedical Ethics

1. Robert Dingwall and Vienna Rozelle, "The Ethical Governance of German Physicians 1890–1939: Are There Lessons from History?" *Journal of Policy History* 23, no. 1 (2011): 969.

2. Oliver Rauprich and Jochen Vollmann, "30 Years *Principles of Biomedical Ethics*: Introduction to a Symposium on the 6th Edition of Tom L. Beauchamp and James F. Childress' Seminal Work," *Journal of Medical Ethics* 37, no. 8 (2011): 582–583.

3. Mark Johnson, *Moral Imagination: Implications of Cognitive Science for Ethics* (Chicago: University of Chicago Press, 1993), 7.

4. Raanan Gillon, "Transplantation and Ethics," in *Birth to Death: Science and* Bioethics, ed. David C. Thomas and Tommi Kushner (New York: Cambridge University Press, 1996), 106.

5. Raanan Gillon, *Philosophical Medical Ethics* (Chichester, NH: Wiley, 1986).

6. John D. Arras, "The Hedgehog and the Borg: Common Morality in Bioethics," *Theoretical Medicine and Bioethics* 30, no. 1 (2009): 14. http://pages.shanti.virginia.edu/jda3a/files/2009/11/Common-Morality-PDF1.pdf (accessed June 27, 2011).

7. Tom L. Beauchamp and James F. Childress, *Principles of Biomedical Ethics*, 5th ed. (New York: Oxford University Press, 2001), 1.

8. Daniel E. Hall, "The Guild of Surgeons as a Tradition of Moral Enquiry," *Journal of Medicine and Philosophy* 36, no. 2 (2011): 118. The fellowship pledge can be found at the Guild's website: http://www.facs.org/fellows_info/statements/stonprin.html#fp (accessed January 10, 2012).

9. Obviously, the wording changes slightly depending on the translation.

10. Sherwin B. Nuland, *Doctors: The Biography of Medicine* (New York: Alfred A. Knopf), 307.

11. Bruce Jennings, "From the Urban to the Civic: The Moral Possibilities of the City," *Journal of Urban Health: Bulletin of the New York Academy of Medicine* 78, no. 1 (2001): 93.

12. *Roe v. Wade* (1973) 410 U.S. 113. Often overlooked in debates *over Roe v. Wade* in the abortion controversy is the degree to which it insisted upon the personal rights of persons to make decisions about their bodies. To the extent that *Roe v. Wade* is retrenched as an abortion document, the idea behind it—the

right of individuals to make decisions about their own bodies—will be limited as well.

13. Cristina Luiggi, "The Philadelphia Chromosome, circa 1960," *The Scientist* 24 (12): 84, http://classic.the-scientist.com/article/display/57846/ (accessed January 18, 2012).

14. Renée C. Fox, "Is Medical Education Asking Too Much of Bioethics?" *Daedalus* 128, no. 4 (1999): 3.

15. Hall, *Guild of Surgeons*, 118.

16. Paul Farmer and Nicole Gastineau Campos, "Rethinking Medical Ethics: A View from Below," *Ethics and Infectious Disease* (Malden, MA: Blackwell Publishing, 2006), 261–284.

17. Oliver Sacks, "Epilogue," *Awakenings*, rev. ed. (London: Picador, 1982), 242–255.

18. Abraham Verghese, "The Calling," *New England Journal of Medicine* 352, no. 18 (2005): 1844–1847.

19. Tom L. Beauchamp, "History and Theory in 'Applied Ethics,'" *Kennedy Institute of Ethics Journal* 17, no. 1 (2007): 60.

20. Johnson, *Moral Imagination*, 7.

21. Beauchamp, "History and Theory," 60.

22. Charles Taylor, *Hegel and Modern Society* (New York: Cambridge University Press, 1979), 75.

23. Isaiah Berlin, *Four Essays on Liberty* (New York: Oxford University Press, 1969), 138.

24. Taylor, *Hegel and Modern Society*, 4. In writing about Hegel and his legacy Taylor must, of course, first deal with Kant and his legacy. It was, after all, Kant's works that challenged Hegel and to which he reacted in his writings.

25. Taylor, *Hegel and Modern Society*, 78.

26. Catherine Chalier, *What Ought I to Do? Morality in Kant and Levinas*, trans. J. M. Todd (Ithaca, NY: Cornell University Press 2002), 17.

27. Chalier, *What Ought I to Do?* 14–15.

28. Immanuel Kant, *Groundwork for the Metaphysics of Morals*, ed. Lara Denis, trans. Thomas K. Abbott (Orchard Park, NY: Broadview Press Ltd., 1785/2005), 53.

29. Chalier, *What Ought I to Do?* 5.

30. Dana J. Lawrence, "The Four Principles of Biomedical Ethics: A Foundation for Current Bioethical Debate," *Journal of Chiropractic Humanities* 14 (2007): 34–40, 34.

31. Fabrice Jotterand, "Human Dignity and Transhumanism: Do Anthro-technological Devices have Moral Status?" *American Journal of Bioethics* 10, no. 7 (2010): 45–52. Here Jotterand's review of international human rights charters and covenants, and especially the Universal Declaration on Bioethics and Human Rights, is useful.

32. Therese M. Lysaught, "Respect: Or, How Respect for Persons Became Respect for Autonomy," *Journal of Medicine and Philosophy* 29, no. 6 (2004): 675.

33. David C. Thomasma, "Anencephalics as Organ Donors," in *Biomedical Ethics Reviews, 1989*, ed. James M. Humber and Robert F. Almeder (Clifton, NJ: Humana Press, 1990), 35.

34. David C. Thomasma and Eric H. Lowey, "A Dialogue on Species-specific Rights: Humans and Animals in Bioethics," *Cambridge Quarterly of Healthcare Ethics* 6, no. 4 (1997): 435.

35. This literature has grown over the years. For an early article in this writing stream, see, for example, Nancy L Childs, Walter N. Mercer, and Helen W. Childs, "Accuracy of Diagnosis of Persistent Vegetative State," *Neurology* 43, no. 8 (1993): 1465–1467. In the same vein, see Keith Andrews et al., "Misdiagnosis of the Vegetative State: Retrospective Study in a Rehabilitation Unit," *British Medical Journal* 313, no. 36 (1996): 13–16.

36. Paul W. Schoenle and W. Witzke, " How Vegetative Is the Vegetative State? Preserved Semantic Processing in PVS Patients—Evidence from 400 Event-related Potentials," *Neuro Rehabilitation* 19, no. 3 (2004): 29–34.

37. Bruno Latour, *We Have Never Been Modern*, trans. Catherine Porter (Cambridge, MA: Harvard University Press, 1993), 21.

38. Charles L. Bosk, "Professional Ethicist Available: Logical, Secular, Friendly," *Daedalus* 128, no. 4 (1999): 47–68.

39. Arras, "Hedgehog and the Borg," 13.

40. Rauprich and Vollmann, "30 Years," 582–583. Here they quote from the sixth edition of *Principles*, 3.

41. H. Tristram Engelhardt Jr., "Confronting Moral Pluralism in Posttraditional Western Societies: Bioethics Critically Reassessed," *Journal of Medicine and Philosophy* 36, no. 2 (April 2011): 264.

42. John Rawls, *Justice as Fairness: A Restatement* (Cambridge, MA: Belknap Press, 2003).

43. John C. Harsanyi, "Can the Maximin Principle Serve as a Basis for Morality? A Critique of John Rawls's Theory," *The American Political Science Review* 69, no. 2 (1975): 594–606.

44. Carol Gilligan, *In a Different Voice: Psychological Theory and Women's Development* (Cambridge, MA: Harvard University Press, 1982), 198. And in citing Gilligan I cite as well the feminists whose work followed from her writing.

45. See, for example, Lawrence Kohlberg, "The Claim to Moral Adequacy of a Highest Stage of Moral Judgment," *The Journal of Philosophy* 70, no. 18 (1973): 630–646.

46. For a taste of the inability to precisely define autonomy, and the many autonomies that result, see Rebecca L. Walker, "Respect for Rational Autonomy," *Kennedy Institute of Ethics Journal* 19, no. 4 (2009): 339–366.

47. David C. Thomasma, "Bioethics and International Human Rights," *Journal of Law, Medicine & Ethics* 25 (1997): 295–306.

48. T. J. Clark, *Farewell to an Idea: Episodes from a History of Modernism* (New Haven, CT: Yale University Press, 1999), 103.

7 Bioethics and Conformal Humans

Early drafts of this chapter were presented in a 2010 lecture series at the University of Toronto, Centre for Bioethics, and later that year as a Wellcome lecture, at the University of Manchester, Centre for Social Ethics and Policy.

1. Harriet McBryde Johnson, "Unspeakable Conversations," *New York Times Sunday Magazine*, February 16, 2003, http://www.racematters.org/harrietmcbrydejohnson.htm (accessed January 18, 2008). This article reporting on her visit to Princeton and Peter Singer developed a huge footprint on the Web where it was mirrored by a number of authors. For a separate discussion, see Tom Koch, "Enhancing Who? Enhancing What? Ethics, Bioethics, and Transhumanism," *Journal of Medicine & Philosophy* 35, no. 6 (2010): 685–699. A related argument is in my article "Eugenics and the 'Genetic Challenge,' Again: All Dressed Up and Just Everywhere to Go," Special Issue: Review of Matti Häyry's *Rationality and the Genetic Challenge*, *Cambridge Quarterly of Healthcare Ethics* 20, no. 2 (2011): 1–13.

2. For a general review of Singer's philosophy, see Hyun Höchsmann, *On Peter Singer* (Belmont, CA: Wadsworth/Thompson Learning, 2002). For a focused treatment of an element of the Singerian argument, see Charles C. Camosy, "Common Ground on Surgical Abortion?—Engaging Peter Singer on the Moral Status of Potential Persons," *Journal of Medicine & Philosophy* 33, no. 6 (2008): 577–593.

3. Peter Singer, *Practical Ethics*, 2nd ed. (New York: Cambridge University Press, 1993). One may, as I do, believe Singer to be wrong-headed and yet admire him. The work here is brilliantly clear, comprehensible, and forceful.

4. John Harris, *Enhancing Evolution: The Ethical Case for Making Better People* (Princeton, NJ: Princeton University Press, 2007), 88–94. Parents are responsible for the genetic makeup of their offspring and if ethically responsible should seek the best potential for those children.

5. Jonathan Glover, *Choosing Children: Genetics, Disability, and Design* (Oxford, UK: Clarendon Press, 2008), 61.

6. Among those Glover draws upon in his citations are, for example, Allen Buchanan et al., *From Chance to Choice: Genetics and Justice* (Cambridge, UK: Cambridge University Press, 2000).

7. Singer, *Practical Ethics*, 318.

8. Peter Singer, *Rethinking Life and Death: The Collapse of Our Traditional Ethics* (New York: St. Martin's Griffin, 1994), 1.

9. Charles Taylor, *Hegel and Modern Society* (New York: Cambridge University Press 1979), 79–81.

10. Havi Carel, *Illness: The Cry of the Flesh* (Stocksfield: Acumen, 2008), 46.

11. Peter Singer, "Happy Nonetheless," *New York Times*, December 28, 2009, MM34, http://www.nytimes.com/2008/12/28/magazine/28mcbryde-t.html?_r=1&ref=magazine (accessed March 24, 2010).

12. Stephen Drake, "Peter Singer's "Tribute" to Harriet McBryde Johnson—and Paul Longmore's Response," *Not Dead Yet* news commentary, January 13, 2009, http://notdeadyetnewscommentary.blogspot.com/2009/01/peter-singers-tribute-to-harriet.html (accessed January 13, 2012).

13. This is a frequent and well-rehearsed complaint of feminist and disability-based ethicists. See, for example, Eva F. Kittay, *Love's Labour: Essays on Women, Equality, and Dependency* (New York: Routledge, 1999), 80. Similarly, there is Margaret C. Nussbaum, *Frontiers of Justice: Disability, Nationality, Species Membership* (Cambridge, MA: Belknap Press, 2006), 103–104.

14. John Rawls, *A Theory of Justice* (Cambridge, MA: Belknap Press, 1971), 73.

15. Norman Daniels, *Just Health* (New York: Cambridge University Press, 2008).

16. For a somewhat dated but still useful review of these materials, see my "Life Quality versus the 'Quality of Life': Assumptions Underlying Prospective Quality of Life Instruments in Health Care Planning," *Social Science & Medicine* 51, no. 3 (2000): 419–428; and its companion paper "Future States: Testing the Axioms Underlying Prospective, Future-oriented, Health Planning Instruments," *Social Science & Medicine* 52, no. 3 (2001): 453–466.

17. Howard Brody, *The Future of Bioethics* (New York: Oxford University Press, 2009), 161–162.

18. Ibid.

19. Tom Koch, "Living vs. Dying 'with Dignity': A New Perspective on the Euthanasia Debate," *Cambridge Quarterly on Healthcare Ethics* 5, no. 1 (1996): 50–60.

20. Gary L. Albrecht and Patrick J. Devlieger, "The Disability Paradox: High Quality of Life Against All Odds," *Social Science and Medicine* 48, no. 8 (1998): 977–988. For a response, see Koch, "Life Quality versus the 'Quality of Life.'"

21. Singer, *Rethinking Life and Death*, 169.

22. This is a condensed telling of the full passage in McBryde Johnson's 2003 article. Material in quotation marks attributed to Singer are from the article. The text around summarizes other materials in an attempt to keep the quoted materials at a reasonable length.

23. Jeffrey Spike and Jane Greenlaw, "Ethics Consultation: Persistent Brain Death and Religion: Must a Person Believe in Death to Die?" *Journal of Law, Medicine & Ethics* 23, no. 3 (1995): 20–23.

24. For a description of one of my meetings with a presumably unconscious person, see Tom Koch, "Showtime," in *Watersheds: Stories of Crisis and Renewal in Our Everyday Lives* (Toronto: Lester Publishing, 1994), 13–49.

25. Agnieszka Jaworska, "Respecting the Margins of Agency: Alzheimer's Patients and the Capacity to Value," *Philosophy & Public Affairs* 28, no. 2 (1999): 105–138.

26. John K. Davis, "Futility, Conscientious Refusal, and Who Gets to Decide," *Journal of Medicine & Philosophy* 33, no. 4 (2008): 356–374; Tom Koch, "End of Life, Year, after Year, after Year," *Journal of the Canadian Medical Association* 181, no. 11 (2009): 868.

27. Timothy Quill, "Terri Schiavo—A Tragedy Compounded," *New England Journal of Medicine* 352, no. 16 (2005): 1630–1633.

28. Tom Koch, "The Challenge of Terri Schiavo: Lessons for Bioethics," *Journal of Medical Ethics* 31, no. 7 (2005): 376–378.

29. Singer, *Practical Ethics*, 3.

30. Peter Singer, "Ethics and Disability: A Response to Koch," *Journal of Disability Policy Studies* 16, no. 2 (2005): 132.

31. Ad Hoc Committee of the Harvard Medical School, "A Definition of Irreversible Coma: Report of the Ad Hoc Committee of the Harvard Medical School to Examine the Definition of Brain Death," *Journal of the American Medical Association* 205, no. 6 (1968): 85–88.

32. Nancy L. Childs, Walter N. Mercer, and Helen W. Childs, "Accuracy of Diagnosis of Persistent Vegetative State," *Neurology* 43, no. 8 (1993): 1465; also see Keith Andrews et al., "Misdiagnosis of the Vegetative State: Retrospective Study in a Rehabilitation Unit," *British Medical Journal* 313, no. 36 (1996): 13–16.

33. Tom Koch, "Images of Uncertainty: Two Cases of Neuroimaging and What They Cannot Say," in *Advances in Neurotechnology: Ethical, Legal and Social Issues*, vol. 1: *Philosophical Premises in Application*, ed. James Giordano (Boca Raton, FL: CRC Press, 2012).

34. Catherine Belling, "Graphic Brain-Imaging," *Atrium* 6 (Winter 2009): 2–7.

35. Joseph J. Fins et al., "Neuroimaging and Disorders of Consciousness: Envisioning an Ethical Research Agenda," *American Journal of Bioethics-Neuroscience* 8, no. 9 (2008): 3–12. See also Joseph J. Fins, "Neuroethics and Neuroimaging: Moving toward Transparency," *American Journal of Bioethics* 8, no. 9 (2008): 46–52.

36. Paul W. Schoenle and W. Witzke, "How Vegetative Is the Vegetative State? Preserved Semantic Processing in PVS Patients—Evidence from 400 Event-related Potentials," *Neuro Rehabilitation* 19, no. 3 (2004): 29–34.

37. Guy Kahane and Julien Savulescu, "Brain Damage and the Moral Significance of Consciousness," *Journal of Medicine & Philosophy* 34, no. 1 (2009): 6–26.

38. This was a commonplace practice for several years when issues of Terry Schiavo's care or noncare were debated in panels and discussion sessions at the annual meeting of the American Society for Bioethics and the Humanities.

39. Koch, "Images of Uncertainty."

40. For example, the case of locked-in patient Ron Houben. See Shanon Firth, "Locked-in Syndrome: When a Coma Is Not a Coma," *FindingDulcinea*, December 1, 2009, http://www.findingdulcinea.com/news/science/2009/dec/Locked-In-Syndrome-When-a-Coma-s-Not-a-Coma.html (accessed January 18, 2012). For

an early news report, see Kate Connelly, "Trapped in His Own Body for 23 Years—The Coma Victim Who Screamed Unheard," *The Guardian* [UK], November 23, 2009, http://www.guardian.co.uk/world/2009/nov/23/man-trapped-coma-23-years (accessed January 13, 2012).

41. Jill B. Taylor, *My Stroke of Insight: A Brain Scientist's Personal Journey* (New York: Viking, 2006).

42. Jeffrey P. Brosco, "More than the Names Have Changed: Exploring the Historical Epidemiology of Intellectual Disability in the US," in *Healing the World's Children: Comparative and Interdisciplinary Approaches to Child Health in the Twentieth Century*, ed. Cynthia Commachio, Janet Golden, and George Weisz (Montreal: McGill-Queens University Press, 2008), 205–234.

43. David C. Thomasma and Eric H. Lowey, "A Dialogue on Species-specific Rights: Humans and Animals in Bioethics," *Cambridge Quarterly of Healthcare Ethics* 6, no. 4 (1997): 435–444.

44. Michael Walzer, *Spheres of Justice: A Defence of Pluralism and Equality* (New York: Basic Books 1983), 31.

45. Singer, *Rethinking Life and Death*, 204.

46. Tom Koch, "Disabled Are Not Dogs: Commentary on the Robert Latimer case," *Vancouver Sun* (February 7, 2001), A15, http://www.chninternational.com/tomkoch.htm (accessed January 13, 2012).

47. As the lawyer Diane Coleman of the organization Not Dead Yet argues, it is the sense of pity and repugnancy that has influenced many court decisions, for example, *Bouvia v. Superior Court*. It's not just that "quality of life matters," but also that assumptions of life quality in relation to persons of difference are inherently incomplete, inaccurate, and prejudicial. See here Brian Liang and Laura Lin, "*Bouvia v. Superior Court*: Quality of Life Matters," *Virtual Mentor* 7, no. 2 (February 2005), http://virtualmentor.ama-assn.org/2005/02/hlaw1-0502.html (accessed July 7, 2011).

48. For the experiential argument on caring, see Tom Koch, *Mirrored Lives: Aging Children, Elderly Parents* (Westport, CT: Praeger Books, 1990); Tom Koch, *A Place in Time: Care Givers for Their Elderly* (Westport, CT: Praeger Books, 1993. Also see Kittay, *Love's Labour*.

49. Isaiah Berlin, *Four Essays on Liberty* (New York: Oxford University Press, 1969), 17.

50. Bruce Jennings, "Autonomy and Difference: The Travails of Liberalism in Bioethics," in *Bioethics and Society*, ed. Raymond Devries and Janardan Subedi (New York: Prentice Hall, 1998), 263.

51. Alan P. Fiske, "Human Sociality," *International Society for the Study of Personal Relationships Bulletin* 14, no. 2 (1998), 4–9. Published online as "The Inherent Sociability of *Homo sapiens*," http://www.sscnet.ucla.edu/anthro/faculty/fiske/relmodov.htm (accessed September 5, 2010).

52. Ibid. Also see Alan P. Fiske, "Relational Models Theory 2.0," in *Relational Models Theory: A Contemporary Overview*, ed. Nick Haslam (Mahwah, NJ: Erlbaum, 2004), 3–25.

53. Stephen J. Post, *The Moral Challenge of Alzheimer Disease* (Baltimore, MD: Johns Hopkins University Press, 1995), 179–181.

54. Steven H. Miles, “Informed Demand for ‘Non-beneficial Treatment,’” *New England Journal of Medicine* 325, no. 7 (1991): 512–515. For the court case itself, see *In re Conservatorship of Wanglie.*

55. Post, *Moral Challenge of Alzheimer Disease*, 106–107.

56. David B. McCurdy, “Alzheimer Disease, a Review of Stephen G. Post: The Moral Challenge of Alzheimer Disease,” *Making the Rounds in Health, Faith and Ethics* (March 5, 1996): 5.

57. Oliver Sacks, *Awakenings*, rev. ed. (London: Picador, 1982), 238. While read rarely by most, *Awakening*'s “Epilogue” and the proceeding short section “Accommodations” constitute a remarkable statement of a humanist science of medicine, and especially neurology in all its social complexity.

58. Ibid., 252–255.

59. Ibid., 240.

60. Kant's discussion of the beautiful is found in various texts, including his 1764 work, *Observation on the Feeling of the Beautiful and the Sublime*, and later in his 1790 *Critique of Judgment*. For a discussion, see Catherine Chalier, *What Ought I to Do?: Morality in Kant and Levinas* (Ithaca, NY: Cornell University Press, 2002), 16–17.

61. Ibid.

62. Singer, “Ethics and Disability,” 132.

63. Tom Koch, “The Canadian Question: What's So Great about Intelligence?” *Cambridge Quarterly on Healthcare Ethics* 5, no. 2 (1996): 307–210.

64. Froese's statement was included in a mailing of the Canadian Down Syndrome Society to its members.

65. Nicole Gerrand, “The Misuse of Kant in the Debate about a Market for Human Body Parts,” *Journal of Applied Philosophy* 16, no. 1 (1999): 60.

66. Post, *Moral Challenge of Alzheimer Disease*, 107.

67. *In the matter of Quinlan* (1976) 70 N.J. 10, 355 A. 2d. 647.

68. John M. Luce, “Making Decisions about the Forgoing of Life-sustaining Therapy,” *American Journal of Respiratory Critical Care* 156, no. 6 (1997): 1715.

69. Roy Porter, *The Greatest Benefit to Mankind: A Medical History of Humanity* (New York: W. W. Norton & Co), 1999.

8 Research and Genetics

1. James D. Watson, *The Double Helix: A Personal Account of the Discovery of the Structure of DNA*, ed. Gunther Stent (New York: Norton, 1980).

2. John Coggon, “Confrontations in ‘Genethics’: Rationalities, Challenges, and Methodological Responses,” *Cambridge Quarterly of Healthcare Ethics* 20, no. 1 (2011): 46.

3. It is easy to forget how important and indeed startling this discovery was. The 2000 review article by Avent and Reid provides a useful reminder. Neil D. Avent and Marion E. Reid, "The Rh Blood Group System: A Review," *Blood* 95, no. 2 (2000): 375–387.

4. Joseph S. Woo, "A Short History of Amniocentesis, Fetoscopy and Chorionic Villus Sampling," *A Short History of the Development of Ultrasound in Obstetrics and Gynecology* (2002), http://www.ob-ultrasound.net/amniocentesis.html (accessed June 21, 2011).

5. J. Langdon Down, "Observation on an Ethnic Classification of Idiots," *London Hospital Reports* 3 (1866): 259–262.

6. Edmund Pellegrino, *The Changing Moral Focus of Newborn Screening: An Ethical Analysis by the President's Council on Bioethics* (Washington, DC: Presidents Council on Bioethics, 2008), 6–7, http://www.bioethics.gov (accessed May 13, 2011).

7. All this took time, of course. For the pneumococcal prophylaxis of infants with sickle cell disease, for example, see Colin M. Sox et al., "Provision of Pneumococcal Prophylaxis for Publicly Insured Children with Sickle Cell Disease," *Journal of the American Medical Association* 290, no. 8 (2003): 1057–1061. The point is that the genetic investigation of disease was principally designed to promote treatment in the Hippocratic tradition of medicine into this period.

8. Henry L. Nadler and Albert B. Gerbie, "Role of Amniocentesis in the Intrauterine Diagnosis of Genetic Defects," *New England Journal of Medicine* 282, no. 11 (1970): 596–599.

9. J. M. G. Wilson and G. Junger, *Principles and Practice of Screening for Disease*, Public Health Papers No. 34 (Geneva, Switzerland: World Health Organization, 1968), http://whqlibdoc.who.int/php/WHO_PHP_34.pdf (accessed January 18, 2012).

10. Pellegrino, *Changing Moral Focus*, 2.

11. Wilson and Junger, *Principles and Practice.*

12. See, for example, Jeffrey R. Botkin et al., "Newborn Screening Technology: Proceed With Caution," *Pediatrics* 117, no. 5 (May 1, 2006): 1793–1799, http://pediatrics.aappublications.org/content/117/5/1793.full.pdf+html (accessed June 26, 2011).

13. Duane A. Alexander and Peter C. Van Dyck, "A Vision of the Future of Newborn Screening," *Pediatrics* 117, supp. 3 (May 1, 2006): S350–S354.

14. Paul Litton and F. G. Miller, "What Physician-Investigators Owe Patients Who Participate in Research," *Journal of the American Medical Association* 304, no. 13 (2010): 1492.

15. Cilia I. Kaye et al., "Assuring Clinical Genetic Services for Newborns Identified through U.S. Newborn Screening Programs," *Genetics in Medicine* 9, no. 8 (2007): 518–527; Pellegrino, *Changing Moral Focus*, 15–16.

16. Nicholas Wade, "Genes Show Limited Value in Predicting Diseases," *New York Times*, April 15, 2009, A1, http://www.nytimes.com/2009/04/

16/health/research/16gene.html (accessed July 4, 2011). This is also the point made elegantly, and clearly, in Richard Lewontin's 2011 review of Evelyn Fox Keller's book on the false debate between "nature" and nurture, "It's Even Less in Your Genes," *New York Review of Books*, May 26, 2011, http://www.nybooks.com/articles/archives/2011/may/26/its-even-less-your-genes (accessed June 20, 2011).

17. Therese M. Lysaught, "Docile Bodies: Transnational Research Ethics as Biopolitics," *Journal of Medicine and Philosophy* 34, no. 4 (2009): 397.

18. Gary Gutting, *Foucault: A Very Short Introduction* (New York: Oxford University Press, 2005), 82.

19. Rosamond Rhodes, "Rethinking Research Ethics," *American Journal of Bioethics* 5, no. 7 (2005): 7–28.

20. Lysaught, "Docile Bodies," 395.

21. Art Caplan, "Is There a Duty to Serve as a Subject in Biomedical Research?" *IRB Journal* 6, no. 5 (September 1984): 1–5; Art Caplan, "Is There an Obligation to Participate in Biomedical Research?," in *The Use of Human Beings in Research: With Special Reference to Clinical Trials*, ed. Stephen F. Spiker, Andre de Vries, and Llai Alon (Norwell, MA: Kluwer Academic Publishers, 1988), 229–248.

22. David Orentlicher, "Making Research a Requirement of Treatment: Why We Should Sometimes Let Doctors Pressure Patients to Participate in Research," *Hastings Center Report* (September–October 2005): 20–28.

23. Jeffrey P. Bishop, "Transhumanism, Metaphysics, and the Posthuman God," *Journal of Medicine and Philosophy* 35, no. 6 (2010): 711.

24. John Harris, *Enhancing Evolution: The Ethical Case for Making Better People* (Princeton, NJ: Princeton University Press, 2007), 194.

25. For a discussion, see Robert Andorno, "Human Dignity and Human Rights as a Common Ground for a Global Bioethics," *Journal of Medicine and Philosophy* 34, no. 3 (2009): 228.

26. Nicholas Wade, "Patient Dies during a Trial of Therapy Using Genes," *New York Times*, September 29, 1999, http://www.nytimes.com/1999/09/29/us/patient-dies-during-a-trial-of-therapy-using-genes.html (accessed June 21, 2011).

27. Julian Savulescu, "Harm, Ethics Committees, and the Gene Therapy Death," *Journal of Medical Ethics* 27, no. 3 (2001): 148–150.

28. Julian Savulescu and M. Spriggs, "The Hexamethonium Asthma Study and the Death of a Normal Volunteer in Research," *Journal of Medical Ethics* 28, no. 1 (2002): 3–4.

29. Gina Kolata, "NIH Shaken by Death of Research Volunteer," *Science* 209, no. 4455 (1980): 475–476.

30. See, for example, the 1984 report of the death of a patient in an arrhythmia treatment. Austin Darragh et al., "Sudden Death of a Volunteer," *Lancet* 325, no. 8420 (1985): 93–95.

31. Doris T. Zellen, "Gene Therapy in Crisis," *Trends in Genetics* 16, no. 6 (2000): 272–275.

32. Carl Elliott, "Pharma Buys a Conscience," *The American Prospect* 12, no. 16 (September 2001): 23, http://healthandpharma.awardspace.com/Week 6 Readings/Elliott Pharma Buys a Conscience.pdf (accessed September 20, 2010).

33. Carl Elliott, "Should Journals Publish Industry-funded Bioethics Articles?" *The Lancet* 366, no. 9483 (2005): 422–424.

34. Elliott, "Pharma Buys a Conscience," 2.

35. Nina Hallowell et al., "Healthcare Professionals' and Researchers' Understanding of Cancer Genetics Activities: A Qualitative Interview Study," *Journal of Medical Ethics* 35, no. 2 (2009): 113–119.

36. Stephen Joffee and Franklin G. Miller, "Bench to Bedside: Mapping the Moral Terrain of Clinical Research," *Hastings Center Report* 38, no. 2 (2008): 30–34. The secondary title of their paper gives their point of view: "A Clinical Trial Is Purely Science, Not Medical Care."

37. This is the point of Jill H. Fisher's *Medical Research for Hire: The Political Economy of Pharmaceutical Clinical Trials* (New Brunswick, NJ: Rutgers University Press, 2009), and to a great extent Catherine Waldby's and Robert Mitchell's *Tissue Economies: Blood, Organs and Cell Lines in Late Capitalism* (Durham, NC: Duke University Press), 2006.

38. Michael Walzer, *Spheres of Justice: A Defence of Pluralism and Equality* (New York: Basic Books, 1983), 86.

39. Fisher, *Medical Research for Hire*, 45.

40. Warren T. Reich, "How Bioethics Got Its Name," Special Supplement, *Hastings Center Report* 23, no. 6 (November–December 1993): S6–S7.

41. Nick Bostrom, "Dignity and Enhancement," commissioned for the President's Council on Bioethics, 2007, http://www.nickbostrom.com/ethics/dignity-enhancement.pdf (accessed May 15, 2011).

42. James Hughes, *Citizen Cyborg: Why Democratic Societies Must Respond to the Redesigned Human of the Future* (New York: Basic Books, 2004); James Hughes, "Virtue Engineering: Applications of Neurotechnology to Improve Moral Behavior," TransVision06 lecture, 2006, http://ieet.org/index.php/IEET/more/2035 (accessed January 18, 2012).

43. Nick Bostrom, "In Defense of Posthuman Dignity," *Bioethics* 19, no. 3 (2005): 202–203.

44. Ian Brasington, "Enhancing Evolution and *Enhancing* Evolution," *Bioethics* 24, no. 8 (2010): 395–402.

45. Matti Häyry, *Rationality and the Genetic Challenge: Making People Better?* (New York: Cambridge University Press, 2010), 2.

46. Stephen J. Gould, "The Smoking Gun of Eugenics," *Natural History* 12, no. 1 (1991): 8–17.

47. Julian Savulescu and Anders Sandberg, "Neuroenhancement of Love and Marriage: The Chemicals between Us," *Neuroethics* 1, no. 1 (2008): 33.

48. Yves Barral, "The Gates of Immortality," *The Scientist* 24, no. 10 (2010): 39, http://classic.the-scientist.com/article/display/57702 (accessed January 16, 2012).

49. Mark Witten, "Brainwashed: Rethinking Man's Genetic Makeup," *The Walrus* (November 2010): 20.

50. Lewontin, "It's Even Less in Your Genes."

51. A. Jacquard, *In Praise of Difference: Genetics and Human Affairs*, trans. M. M. Moriarty (New York: Columbia University Press, 1984).

52. Dennis Dutton, *The Art Instinct: Beauty, Pleasure, & Human Evolution* (New York: Bloomsbury Press 2009), 45.

53. A new book on altruism and the quest for its understanding appeared in 2010. Oren Harman, *The Price of Altruism: George Price and the Search for the Origins of Kindness* (New York: W. W. Norton & Co., 2010).

54. Ibid., 45.

55. Alla Katsnelson, "Odd Man Out: Do Fish Have Personalities?" *The Scientist* 24, no. 31 (2010): 34–39.

56. Gregor Wolbring, "Where Do We Draw the Line? Surviving Eugenics in a Technological World," in *Disability and the Life Course: Global Perspectives*, ed. Mark Priestly (Cambridge, UK: Cambridge University Press, 2001), 38–49.

57. Richard C. Lewontin, *Biology as Ideology: The Doctrine of DNA* (New York: HarperPerennial, 1994).

58. Geog Pfleiderer, Gabriela Brahier, and Klaus Lindpaintner, eds., *GenEthics and Religion* (New York: S. Karger Publishers), 2010.

59. Darlene Francis and Daniela Kaufer, "Beyond Nature vs. Nuture," *The Scientist* 25 (October 2011): 94, http://the-scientist.com/2011/10/01/beyond-nature-vs-nurture (accessed January 14, 2012).

60. Jeffrey P. Brosco, "More than the Names Have Changed: Exploring the Historical Epidemiology of Intellectual Disability in the US," in *Healing the World's Children: Comparative and Interdisciplinary Approaches to Child Health in the Twentieth Century*, ed. Cynthia Commachio, Janet Golden, and George Weisz (Montreal: McGill-Queens University Press), 216–217.

61. Phillip R. Reilly, *The Surgical Solution: A History of Involuntary Sterilization in the United States* (Baltimore, MD: Johns Hopkins University Press 1991), 86.

62. Reilly, *Surgical Solution*, 117.

63. Brosco, More than the Names Have Changed," 217–218.

64. This promise of human beneficence is presented on the MensaCanada website: The purpose of Mensa is "to identify and foster human intelligence for the benefit of humanity." From the organization's inception, this has been its general raison d'etre internationally. http://www.mensacanada.org/home.htm (accessed January 14, 2012).

65. Richard Dawkins, *The God Delusion* (New York: Houghton Mifflin Co., 2006), 299–301.

66. Michael J. White and John Griffin, *Stephen Hawking: A Life in Science* (New York: Penguin, 1992), 165.

67. Stephen Hawking, *Black Holes and Baby Universes, and Other Essays* (New York: Cambridge University Press, 1993), 167.

68. Bishop, "Transhumanism, Metaphysics," 703.

69. Craig J. Venter, "We Have Learned Nothing from the Genome," *Der Spiegel* online (July 29, 2010), 18, http://www.spiegel.de/international/world/0,1518, 709174-2,00.html (accessed May 29, 2011).

70. Paul A. Wade and Trevor K. Archer, "Epigenetics: Environmental Instructions for the Genome," *Environmental Health Perspectives* 114, no. 3 (March 2, 2006): A140–A141, http://www.ncbi.nlm.nih.gov/pmc/articles/PMC1392246 (accessed September 22, 2006).

71. The famous study of identical twins is often referenced in this context. Mario F. Fraga et al., "Epigenetic Differences Arise during the Lifetime of Monozygotic Twins," *Proceedings of the National Academy of Science* 102, no. 30 (2005): 10604–10609.

72. John Cloud, "Why Your DNA Isn't Your Destiny," *Time Magazine*, January 6, 2010, http://www.time.com/time/magazine/article/0,9171,1952313,00.html (accessed February 28, 2012).

73. Richard P. Grant, "Evolution, Tout de Suite," *The Scientist* (October 1, 2011): 27–29, http://the-scientist.com/2011/10/01/evolution-tout-de-suite/ (accessed October 18, 2011).

74. Lenny Moss, *What Genes Can't Do* (Cambridge, MA: MIT Press 2003), viii. Moss does a terrific job of untangling the conflicted histories of the gene as a simple deterministic blueprint and as agent in an interactive, epigenetic process.

75. Timo Vuorisalo and Olli Arjamaa, "Gene-culture Coevolution and Human Diet," *American Scientist* 98, no. 2 (2010): 140–142, http://www.americanscientist.org/issues/page2/2010/2/gene-culture-coevolution-and-human-diet (accessed September 22, 2010).

76. David Shenk, *The Genius in All of Us: Why Everything You've Been Told about Genetics, Talent, and IQ Is Wrong* (New York: Random House 2010).

77. Christopher Eppig, Corley L. Fisher, and Randy Thornhill, "Parasite Prevalence and the Worldwide Distribution of Cognitive Ability," *Proceedings of the Royal Society of Biological Sciences* 277 (2010): 3801–3808, http://yibudayi.com/wp-content/uploads/2010/07/ParasiteCognitive.pdf (accessed June 26, 2011).

78. Samuel S. Myers and Aaron Bernstein, "The Coming Health Crisis," *The Scientist* 25, no. 1 (2011): 32–37, http://classic.the-scientist.com/article/display/57882/ (accessed January 18, 2012).

79. Grant R. Steen, "This Is Not News," *The Scientist* (letters) 25, no. 1 (2011), 12, http://classic.the-scientist.com/2011/1/1/12/1/ (accessed January 18, 2011).

9 Choice, Freedom, and the Paternalism Thing

1. Kevin W. Wildes, "Moral Authority, Moral Standing, and Moral Controversy," *The Journal of Medicine and Philosophy* 18, no. 4 (1993): 347.

2. Ronald Dworkin, *Taking Rights Seriously* (Cambridge, MA: Harvard University Press, 1977), 20.

3. *Cruzan v. Director, Missouri Department of Health* (1990) 497 U.S. 261, http://www.law.cornell.edu/supct/html/historics/USSC_CR_0497_0261_ZO.html (accessed February 21, 2012).

4. Robert Bartz, "Remembering the Hippocratics: Practice and Ethos of Ancient Greek Physician-Healers," in *Bioethics: Ancient Themes in Contemporary Issues*, ed. Mark G. Kuczewski and Ronald Polansky (Cambridge, MA: MIT Press, 2000), 12.

5. The details are both in the court files (*Cruzan v. Director, Missouri Department of Health*) and the many articles commenting on the case. It is useful to note, however, that interpretations differ wildly about the meaning of the case and its arguments depending on authorial perspectives.

6. *Cruzan v. Director, Missouri Department of Health*, 262. See the more general argument.

7. This is from blog of the Center for Practical Ethics, "Legacy of Nancy Cruzan: 20 Years Later, Are We Any Better at Healthcare?" *Practical Bioethics*, September 15, 2010, http://practicalbioethics.blogspot.com/2010/09/legacy-of-nancy-cruzan-20-years-later.html (accessed January 15, 2012).

8. The question of what people know in health about states of physical limit was the subject of Tom Koch, "Life Quality versus the 'Quality of Life': Assumptions Underlying Prospective Quality of Life Instruments in Health Care Planning," *Social Science & Medicine* 51 (3): 419–428.

9. Dismissing communitarianism as "utilitarianism with a happy face" is my judgment and one that Callahan would hotly dispute. See Tom Koch, *Scarce Goods: Justice, Fairness, and Organ Transplantation* (Westport, CT: Praeger Books, 2002), 181.

10. Franklin G. Miller and Robert D. Truog, "Rethinking the Ethics of Vital Organ Donations," *Hastings Center Report* 38, no. 6 (2008): 42. http://www.maceyleigh.net/articles/ethics_of_vital_organ_donations.pdf (accessed June 20, 2011).

11. Miller and Truog, "Rethinking the Ethics."

12. Lewis M. Cohen, *No Good Deed: A Story of Medicine, Murder Accusations, and the Debate over How We Die* (New York: Harper Collins Publishers 2010), 91–92.

13. Robert Cribb, "Lawsuit Could Set Precedent about End-of-Life Decisions," *Toronto Star*, September 4, 2010, http://www.thestar.com/news/gta/article/856741--lawsuit-could-set-precedent-about-end-of-life-decisions (accessed September11, 2010).

14. Kenneth Arrow, "Uncertainty and the Welfare Economics of Medical Care," *The American Economic Review* 53, no. 5 (1963): 941–973.

15. Michael Specter, "A Deadly Misdiagnosis," *New Yorker* (November 15, 2010): 48–53.

16. Kenneth Arrow, "Uncertainty and the Welfare Economics of Medical Care," *American Economic Review* 53, no. 5 (1963): 949, http://stevereads.com/papers

_to_read/uncertainty_and_the_welfare_economics_of_medical_care.pdf (accessed February 21, 2012).

17. Ibid., 952.

18. Trisha Phillips, "From the Ideal Market to the Ideal Clinic: Constructing a Normative Standard of Fairness for Human Subjects Research," *Journal of Medicine and Philosophy* 36, no. 1 (2011): 81.

19. This distinction comes from the World Records Academy, "Most Expensive Medicine—World Record Set by Soliris," February 23, 2010, http://www.worldrecordsacademy.org/business/most_expensive_medicine_world_record_set_by_Soliris_101573.htm (accessed February 2, 2011). By the time this book is published, a new drug may have won the title of most expensive drug, beating Soliris's cost of $500,000 a year.

20. The Global Forum in Health Research produces a yearly report on money flows in global health and research. Its 2008 report estimated the $80 million spent by private companies on research and development represented 51 percent of all research monies. That breakdown did not, however, include federal support in various countries to train researchers through the funding of education or of hospitals where patients are treated in new trials. Nor did the ratio adequately reflect the cost to governments of monitoring new drugs and procedures and assessing their safety. For a discussion of the report see Wendy Rogers and Angela Ballantyne, "Justice in Health Research: What is the Role of Evidence-based Medicine?" *Perspectives in Biology and Medicine* 52, no. 2 (2009): 188–202.

21. Tom L. Beauchamp, "History and Theory in 'Applied Ethics,'" *Kennedy Institute of Ethics Journal* 17, no. 1 (2007): 60.

22. Isaiah Berlin, *Four Essays on Liberty* (New York: Oxford University Press, 1969), 175.

23. Ibid., 121–122.

24. Peter Singer, *Hegel: A Very Short Introduction* (New York: Oxford University Press, 1983), 34.

25. Ibid.

26. John S. Mill, *On Liberty* (Indianapolis: Bobbs Merrill, 1956), 13.

27. Berlin, *Four Essays*, 157.

28. Ibid., 139.

29. Ibid., 122.

30. Carl Elliott, "The Deadly Corruption of Clinical Trials," *Mother Jones* (September/October 2010): 6, http://motherjones.com/environment/2010/09/dan-markingson-drug-trial-astrazeneca (accessed November 25, 2010). Of course, Carol Elliott is polite in his use of the conditional "if . . . then" proposition.

31. This is the reality faced by all those with, for example, spinal cord injuries or types of stroke. For an interesting masters thesis on the issues that arise in these situations, see Jenny Young, "Choosing Self-termination in a Rehabilitation Setting following High Lesion Spinal Cord Injury," M.A. thesis, Medical College of Wisconsin Graduate School of Bioethics, Milwaukee, 2004.

32. Marie-Aurèlie Bruno et al., "A Survey on Self-assessed Well-being in a Cohort of Chronic Locked-in Syndrome Patients: Happy Majority, Miserable Minority," *British Medical Journal Open Access* (February 24), http://www.coma.ulg.ac.be/papers/vs/LIS_BMJ_2011.pdf (accessed January 17, 2012).

33. See also, here, Tom Koch, "Future States: Testing the Axioms Underlying Prospective, Future-oriented, Health Planning Instruments," *Social Science & Medicine* 52, no. 3 (2001): 453–466.

34. This was the argument I (and others) have made, both generally, for example, in Tom Koch, "Living vs. Dying 'with Dignity'": A New Perspective on the Euthanasia Debate," *Cambridge Quaterly of Healthcare Ethics* 5, no. 1 (1996): 50–60, and specifically in terms of "assisted suicide" (or euthanasia, or physician-assisted suicide, etc.). Thus see here my 1998 forensic retrospective analysis of Dr. Jack Kevorkian's first eighty-five deaths: Tom Koch, "On the Subject(s) of Jack Kevorkian, MD: A Retrospective Analysis," *Cambridge Quarterly of Healthcare Ethics* 7, no. 4 (1998): 436–441.

35. Bruce Jennings, "Public Health and Liberty: Beyond the Millian Paradigm," *Public Health Ethics* 2, no. 2 (2009): 123–134.

36. Bjug Borgundvaag et al., "SARS Outbreak in the Greater Toronto Area: The Emergency Department Experience," *Journal of the Canadian Medical Association* 171, no. 11 (2004): 1342–1344, http://www.cmaj.ca/content/171/11/1342.full (accessed January 16, 2012).

37. *Jacobson v. Commonwealth of Massachusetts* 197 U.S. 11 (1905).

38. Shigehiro Oishi and Jessie Graham, "Social Ecology: Lost and Found in Psychological Science," *Perspectives on Psychological Science* 5, no. 4 (2010): 356.

39. This is my own, admittedly free translation of Mencius (Mung Tzu), *The Chinese Classics, Vol. 2*, trans. James Legge (Oxford, UK: Oxford University Press, 1895/1935), chap. 28, http://www.sacred-texts.com/cfu/menc/index.htm (accessed May 20, 2011).

10 Complex Ethics

1. Richard Ashcroft, "Editorial: Future for Bioethics?" *Bioethics* 24, no. 5 (2010): ii.

2. Angus Dawson, "The Future of Bioethics: Three Dogmas and a Cup of Hemlock," *Bioethics* 24 no. 5 (2010): 218–225.

3. Miran Epstein, "How Will the Economic Downturn Affect Academic Bioethics?" *Bioethics* 24, no. 5 (2010): 226–233.

4. Rita Macklin, "The Death of Bioethics (As We Once Knew It)," *Bioethics* 24, no. 5 (June 2010): pp. 211–217.

5. Jeffrey P. Bishop, *The Anticipatory Corpse: Medicine, Power, and the Care of the Dying* (Notre Dame, IN: University of Notre Dame Press, 2011).

6. See, for example Carnevale and Weinstock's essay introducing a special issue of the *Journal of Medicine and Philosophy* on the relevance of Charles Taylor to

medical ethics. Franco A. Carnevale and Daniel M. Weinstock, "Questions in Contemporary Medicine and the Philosophy of Charles Taylor: An Introduction," *Journal of Medicine and Philosophy* 36, no. 4 (2011): 329–344.

7. Winston Chiong, "The Real Problem with Equipoise," *American Journal of Bioethics* 6, no. 4 (2006): 37–47.

8. Howard Brody, "Are There Three or Four Distinct Types of Medical Practice?" *American Journal of Bioethics* 6, no. 4 (2006): 51–53.

9. H. Tristram Engelhardt Jr., "Confronting Moral Pluralism in Posttraditional Western Societies: Bioethics Critically Reassessed," *Journal of Medicine and Philosophy* 36, no. 2 (April 2011): 244.

10. Daniel E. Hall, "The Guild of Surgeons as a Tradition of Moral Enquiry," *Journal of Medicine and Philosophy* 36, no. 2 (2011): 124.

11. Mark G. Kuczewski, "Disability: An Agenda for Bioethics," *American Journal of Bioethics* 1, no. 3 (2001): 37.

12. Stephan A. Erickson, "The Wrong of Rights: The Moral Authority of the Family," *Journal of Medicine and Philosophy* 35, no. 5 (2010): 606.

13. Kuczewski, "Disability," 36.

14. Tom Koch and Sarah Jones, "The Ethical Professional as Endangered Person: Blog Notes on Doctor-Patient Relationships," *Journal of Medical Ethics* 36, no. 6 (2010): 371–374.

15. Alasdair MacIntyre, *After Virtue: A Study in Moral Theory*, 2nd ed. (Notre Dame, IN: University of Notre Dame Press, 1984), 263.

16. Beauchamp cites Davenport as author of of the first tract on "practical ethics." See Tom L. Beauchamp, "History and Theory in 'Applied Ethics,'" *Kennedy Institute of Ethics Journal* 17, no. 1 (2007): 58–59.

17. Alasdair MacIntyre, *Whose Justice? Which Rationality*? (Notre Dame, IN: University of Notre Dame Press, 1988), 263.

18. Catherine Belsey, *Poststructuralism: A Very Short Introduction* (New York: Oxford University Press, 2002), 90.

19. Immanuel Kant, *Groundwork for the Metaphysics of Morals*, ed. Lara Denis, trans. Thomas K. Abbott (Orchard Park, NY: Broadview Press Ltd., 1785/2005), 87.

20. S. Bakewell, *How to Live: A Life of Montaigne in One Question and Twenty Attempts at an Answer* (New York: Vintage, 2010), 326.

Bibliography

Ad Hoc Committee of the Harvard Medical School. 1968. "A Definition of Irreversible Coma: Report of the Ad Hoc Committee of the Harvard Medical School to Examine the Definition of Brain Death." *Journal of the American Medical Association* 205 (6): 85–88.

Adler, Howard, and John A. Francis. 1991. "Proximate Cause: A Growing Limitation on Civil RICO Actions." 13 *Rico Law Reporter* 1443. http://www.dgslaw.com/documents/articles/273380.pdf (accessed July 21, 2010).

AdvaMed. 2004. "The Medical Technology Industry at a Glance." Advanced Medical Technology Association. http://www.omnex.com/training/iso13485/articles/ADVAMED-Medical-Device-Industry-Facts.pdf (accessed December 2, 2008).

Albrecht, Gary L., and Patrick J. Devlieger. 1998. "The Disability Paradox: High Quality of Life Against All Odds." *Social Science & Medicine* 48 (8): 977–988.

Alexander, Duane A., and Peter C. Van Dyck. 2006. "A Vision of the Future of Newborn Screening." *Pediatrics* 117 (supp. 3) (May 1): S350–S354.

Alexander, Shana. 1962. "They Decide Who Lives, Who Dies." *Life Magazine* 53: 102–125.

Alexander, Shana. 1993. "Thirty Years Ago. The Birth of Bioethics: Hastings Centre Report," Special Supplement. *Hastings Center Report* 23 (6) (November–December): S5.

American Heritage Dictionary of the English Language. 1973. New York: Houghton Mifflin Co.

American Medical Association. 1957. *Principles of Medical Ethics*. http://www.ama-assn.org/resources/doc/ethics/1957_principles.pdf (accessed June 27, 2011).

Anderson, James A. 2010. "Clinical Research in Practice: Reexamining the Distinction between Research and Practice." *Journal of Medicine and Philosophy* 35 (1): 46–63.

Andorno, Robert. 2009. "Human Dignity and Human Rights as a Common Ground for a Global Bioethics." *Journal of Medicine and Philosophy* 34 (3): 223–240.

Andre, Judith. 2002. *Bioethics as Practice*. Chapel Hill: University of North Carolina Press.

Andrews, Keith, Leslie Murphy, Ros Munday, and Claire Littlewood. 1996. "Misdiagnosis of the Vegetative State: Retrospective Study in a Rehabilitation Unit." *British Medical Journal* 313 (36): 13–16.

Applebaum, Paul S., Loren H. Roth, and Charles W. Lidz. 1982. "The Therapeutic Misconception: Informed Consent in Psychiatric Research." *International Journal of Law and Psychiatry* 5 (3–4): 319–329.

AP. 2000. "Accusations in Gene Therapy Death." February 2. http://www.netlink.de/gen/Zeitung/2000/000203b.html (accessed July 2, 2011).

AP. 1984. "Gov. Lamm Asserts Elderly, If Very Ill, Have 'Duty to Die.'" *New York Times*, March 29, 16. http://www.nytimes.com/1984/03/29/us/gov-lamm-asserts-elderly-if-very-ill-have-duty-to-die.html (accessed December 26, 2009).

Arndt, Hannah. 1963. *Eichman in Jerusalem: A Report on the Banality of Evil*. New York: Viking Press.

Arras, John D. 2009. "The Hedgehog and the Borg: Common Morality in Bioethics." *Theoretical Medicine and Bioethics* 30 (1): 13–30. http://pages.shanti.virginia.edu/jda3a/files/2009/11/Common-Morality-PDF1.pdf (accessed June 27, 2011).

Arrow, Kenneth. 1963. "Uncertainty and the Welfare Economics of Medical Care." *American Economic Review* 53 (5): 941–973, http://stevereads.com/papers_to_read/uncertainty_and_the_welfare_economics_of_medical_care.pdf (accessed February 21, 2012).

ASBH. 2009. Lifetime Achievement Award. Translating Bioethics and Humanities: American Society for Bioethics and the Humanities Annual Meeting. Hyatt Regency Hotel, Washington, DC. October 17.

Ashcroft, Richard. 2010. "Editorial: Future for Bioethics?" *Bioethics* 24 (5): ii.

Asimov, Isaac. 1950. *I, Robot*. New York: Gnome Press.

Avent, Neil D., and Marion E. Reid. 2000. "The Rh Blood Group System: A Review." *Blood* 95 (2): 375–387. http://bloodjournal.hematologylibrary.org/content/95/2/375.full.pdf+html (accessed June 26, 2011).

Baker, Robert, and Lawrence B. McCullough. 2007. "Medical Ethics' Appropriation of Moral Philosophy: The Case of the Sympathetic and Unsympathetic Physician." *Kennedy Institute of Ethics Journal* 17 (1): 3–22.

Bakewell, S. 2010. *How to Live: A Life of Montaigne in One Question and Twenty Attempts at an Answer*. New York: Vintage.

Barral, Yves. 2010. "The Gates of Immortality." *The Scientist* 24 (10): 39–43. http://classic.the-scientist.com/article/display/57702/ (accessed January 16, 2012).

Bartz, Robert. 2000. Remembering the Hippocratics: Practice and Ethos of Ancient Greek Physician-Healers. In *Bioethics: Ancient Themes in Contemporary Issues*, ed. Mark G. Kuczewski and Ronald Polansky, 3–29. Cambridge, MA: MIT Press.

Beauchamp, Tom L. 2007. "History and Theory in 'Applied Ethics.'" *Kennedy Institute of Ethics Journal* 17 (1): 55–64.

Beauchamp, Tom L., and James F. Childress. 2001. *Principles of Biomedical Ethics*. 5th ed. New York: Oxford University Press.

Beecher, Henry K. 1966. "Ethics and Clinical Research." *New England Journal of Medicine* 274 (24): 1354–1360.

Beecher, Henry K., and Henry I. Dorr. 1971. "The New Definition of Death: Some Opposing Views." *International Journal of Clinical Pharmacology, Therapy and Toxicology* 5 (2): 120–124.

Belling, Catherine. 2009. "Graphic Brain-Imaging." *Atrium* 6 (Winter): 2–7. http://bioethics.northwestern.edu/atrium/pdf/atrium-issue6.pdf (accessed June 22, 2011).

Belsey, Catherine. 2002. *Poststructuralism: A Very Short Introduction*. New York: Oxford University Press.

Berlin, Isaiah. 1959. Two Concepts of Liberty. In *Four Essays on Liberty*, 1–32. Oxford, UK: Oxford University Press.

Berlin, Isaiah. 1969. *Four Essays on Liberty*. New York: Oxford University Press.

Binding, Karl, and Alfred Hoche. 1920. *Permitting the Destruction of Unworthy Life*. Leipzig: Verlag von Felix Meiner.

Binding, Karl, and Alfred Hoche. 1992. "Permitting the Destruction of Unworthy Life." Trans. Walter Wright, Patrick G. Derr, and Robert Solomon. *Issues in Law and Medicine* 8 (2): 231–265.

Binney, Elizabeth A., and Carroll L. Estes. 1988. "The Retreat of the State and Its Transfer of Responsibility: The Intergenerational War." *International Journal of Health Services* 18 (1): 83–96.

Binstock, Robert H. 1992. "Another Form of 'Elderly Bashing.'" *Journal of Health Politics, Policy and Law* 17 (2): 269–272.

Binstock, Robert H., and Stephen G. Post. 1991. *Too Old for Health Care? Controversies in Medicine, Law, Economics, and Ethics*. Baltimore, MD: Johns Hopkins University Press.

Bishop, Jeffrey P. 2010. "Transhumanism, Metaphysics, and the Posthuman God." *Journal of Medicine and Philosophy* 35 (6): 700–720.

Bishop, Jeffrey P. 2011. *The Anticipatory Corpse: Medicine, Power, and the Care of the Dying*. Notre Dame, IN: University of Notre Dame Press.

Bliss, Michael. 1999. *William Osler: A Life in Medicine*. New York: Oxford University Press.

Blayney, Keith. 2005. "The Caduceus vs the Staff of Asclepius." http://drblayney.com/Asclepius.html#hygiene (accessed June 27, 2011).

Borgundvaag, Bjug, et al. 2004. "SARS Outbreak in the Greater Toronto Area: The Emergency Department Experience." *Journal of the Canadian Medical Association* 171 (11): 1342–1344. http://www.cmaj.ca/cgi/content/full/171/11/1342 (accessed January 16, 2012).

Bosk, Charles L. 1999. "Professional Ethicist Available: Logical, Secular, Friendly." *Daedalus* 128 (4): 47–68.

Bostrom, Nick. 2005. "In Defense of Posthuman Dignity," *Bioethics* 19 (3): 3202–3214. http://www.nickbostrom.com/ethics/dignity.html (accessed January 17, 2012).

Bostrom, Nick. 2007. "Dignity and Enhancement." Commissioned for the President's Council on Bioethics. http://www.nickbostrom.com/ethics/dignity-enhancement.pdf (accessed May 15, 2011).

Botkin, Jeffrey R., Ellen W. Clayton, Norman C. Fost, Burke Wylie, Thomas H. Murray, Mary Ann Baily, Benjamin Wilfond, Alfred Berg, and Lainie Friedman Ross. 2006. "Newborn Screening Technology: Proceed with Caution." *Pediatrics* 117 (5) (May 1): 1793–1799. http://pediatrics.aappublications.org/content/117/5/1793.full.pdf+html (accessed June 26, 2011).

Bradshaw, Heather G., and Ruud Ter Meulen. 2010. "A Transhumanist Fault Line around Disability: Morphological Freedom and the Obligation to Enhance." *Journal of Medicine and Philosophy* 35 (6): 670–684.

Brasington, Ian. 2010. "Enhancing Evolution and *Enhancing* Evolution." *Bioethics* 24 (8): 395–402.

Brody, Howard. 1992. *The Healer's Power*. New Haven, CT: Yale University Press.

Brody, Howard. 2006. "Are There Three or Four Distinct Types of Medical Practice?" *American Journal of Bioethics* 6 (4): 51–53.

Brody, Howard. 2009. *The Future of Bioethics*. New York: Oxford University Press.

Brothers, Kyle B. 2011. "Dependent Rational Providers." *Journal of Medicine and Philosophy* 36 (2) (April): 133–147.

Broyde, Michael J. 2001. "The Diagnosis of Brain Death: Correspondence." *New England Journal of Medicine* 345 (8): 617. http://www.nejm.org/doi/full/10.1056/NEJM200108233450813 (accessed June 20, 2011).

Brosco, Jeffrey P. 2008. More than the Names Have Changed: Exploring the Historical Epidemiology of Intellectual Disability in the US. In *Healing the World's Children: Comparative and Interdisciplinary Approaches to Child Health in the Twentieth Century*, ed. Cynthia Commachio, Janet Golden, and George Weisz, 205–234. Montreal: McGill-Queens University Press.

Bruno, Marie-Aurèlie, Jan L. Bernheim, Didier Ledoux, Pellas Frèderic, Athena Demertzi, and Steven Laureys. 2011. "A Survey on Self-assessed Well-being in a Cohort of Chronic Locked-in Syndrome Patients: Happy Majority, Miserable Minority." *British Medical Journal Open Access* (February 24). http://www.coma.ulg.ac.be/papers/vs/LIS_BMJ_2011.pdf (accessed January 17, 2012).

Buchanan, Allen, Dan W. Brock, Norman Daniels, and Daniel Wikler. 2000. *From Chance to Choice: Genetics and Justice*. Cambridge, UK: Cambridge University Press.

Butler, Robert N. 1975. *Why Survive? Being Old in America*. New York: Harper & Row.

Bytheway, Bill. 2009. "Unequal Aging: The Untold Story of Exclusion in Old Age." *Sociology of Health and Illness* 32 (6) (September 10): 967–968.

Callahan, Daniel. 1987. *Setting Limits: Medical Goals in an Aging Society*. New York: Simon and Schuster.

Callahan, Daniel. 1990. *What Kind of Life? The Limits of Medical Progress*. Washington, DC: Georgetown University Press.

Callahan, Daniel. 1992. "Why America Accepted Bioethics." *Hastings Center Report* 23 (6): S8–S9.

Callahan, Daniel. 2003. "Individual Good and Common Good: A Communitarian Approach to Bioethics." *Perspectives in Biology and Medicine* 46 (4): 496–507.

Callahan, Daniel. 2003. "Principlism and Communitarianism." *Journal of Medical Ethics* 29 (5): 287–291.

Callahan, Daniel. 2008. "The Economic Woes of Medicare." *New York Times* blog, November 13. http://newoldage.blogs.nytimes.com/2008/11/13/heart-surgery-how-old-is-too-old/?scp=2&sq=DanielCallahan&st=cse (accessed December 28, 2009).

Camosy, Charles C. 2008. "Common Ground on Surgical Abortion?—Engaging Peter Singer on the Moral Status of Potential Persons." *Journal of Medicine and Philosophy* 33 (6): 577–593.

Campbell, Tom. 2009. "U.S. Has Much to Learn from Our Health Care." *Toronto Star* 19 (July): A15. http://www.thestar.com/article/668161 (accessed June 20, 2011).

Caplan, Arthur L. 1984. "Is There a Duty to Serve as a Subject in Biomedical Research?" *IRB Journal* 6 (5) (September): 1–5.

Caplan, Arthur L. 1988. Is There an Obligation to Participate in Biomedical Research? In *The Use of Human Beings in Research: With Special Reference to Clinical Trials*, ed. Stephen F. Spiker, Andre de Vries, and Llai Alon, 229–248. Norwell, MA: Kluwer Academic Publishers.

Caplan, Arthur L. 2005. "Misusing the Nazi Analogy." *Science* 309 (5734) (July 22): 535.

Capron, Alexander M. 1987. "Anencephalic Donors: Separate the Dead from the Dying." *Hastings Center Report* 17 (1): 7–9.

Carel, Havi. 2008. *Illness: The Cry of the Flesh*. Durham, UK: Acumen.

Carnevale, Franco A., and Daniel M. Weinstock. 2011. "Questions in Contemporary Medicine and the Philosophy of Charles Taylor: An Introduction." *Journal of Medicine and Philosophy* 36 (4): 329–344.

Cassedy, James H. 1984. *American Medicine and Statistical Thinking, 1800–1860*. Cambridge, MA: Harvard University Press.

Center for Practical Ethics. 2010. "Legacy of Nancy Cruzan: 20 Years Later, Are We Any Better at Healthcare?" *Practical Ethics*, September 15, 2010, http://practicalbioethics.blogspot.com/2010/09/legacy-of-nancy-cruzan-20-years-later.html (accessed January 15, 2012)

Chalier, Catherine. 1998. *What Ought I to Do? Morality in Kant and Levinas*. Trans. J. M. Todd. Ithaca, NY: Cornell University Press.

Chase, Owen. 1965. *The Wreck of the Whaleship Essex: A Narrative Account by Owen Chase, First Mate*. Ed. J. Haverstick and B. Shepard. New York: Harcourt Brace & Co.

Childs, Nancy L., Walter N. Mercer, and Helen W. Childs. 1993. "Accuracy of Diagnosis of Persistent Vegetative State." *Neurology* 43 (8): 1465–1467.

Chiong, Winston. 2006. "The Real Problem with Equipoise." *American Journal of Bioethics* 6 (4): 37–47.

Churchill, Larry R. 1999. "Are We Professionals? A Critical Look at the Social Role of Bioethicists." *Daedalus* 128 (4): 253–274.

Clark, T. J. 1999. *Farewell to an Idea: Episodes from a History of Modernism*. New Haven, CT: Yale University Press.

Cloud, John. 2010. "Why Your DNA Isn't Your Destiny." *Time Magazine*, January 6, 2010. http://www.time.com/time/magazine/article/0,9171,1952313,00.html (accessed February 28, 2012).

Coggon, John. 2011. "Confrontations in 'Genethics': Rationalities, Challenges, and Methodological Responses." *Cambridge Quarterly of Healthcare Ethics* 20 (1): 46–55.

Cohen, G. A. 2009. *Why Not Socialism?* Princeton, NJ: Princeton University Press.

Cohen, Lewis M. 2010. *No Good Deed: A Story of Medicine, Murder Accusations, and the Debate over How We Die*. New York: Harper Collins Publishers.

Collins, Mike. 2010. "Reevaluating the Dead Donor Rule." *Journal of Medicine and Philosophy* 35 (2): 154–179.

Confucius. 1935. *The Chinese Classics—Vol. 1: Confucian Analects*. Trans. James Legge. Oxford, UK: Oxford University Press. http://www.gutenberg.org/ebooks/4094 (accessed May 15, 2011).

Congressional Record. 1972. 118th Congress, September 30: 33, 004-33.

Connelly, Kate. 2009. "Trapped in His Own Body for 23 Years—The Coma Victim Who Screamed Unheard." *The Guardian* [UK], November 23. http://www.guardian.co.uk/world/2009/nov/23/man-trapped-coma-23-years (accessed January 13, 2012).

Cranston, Robert E. 2001. "The Diagnosis of Brain Death." *New England Journal of Medicine* 345 (8): 616. http://www.nejm.org/doi/full/10.1056/NEJM200108233450813 (accessed January 16, 2012)

Cribb, Robert. 2010. "Lawsuit Could Set Precedent about End-of-life Decisions." *Toronto Star*, September 4. http://www.thestar.com/news/gta/article/856741--lawsuit-could-set-precedent-about-end-of-life-decisions (accessed September 11, 2010).

Crisp, Roger, Tony Hope, and David Ebbes. 1996. "The Asbury Draft Policy on Ethical Use of Resources." *British Medical Journal* 312 (7045): 1528–1533.

Daniels, Norman. 2008. *Just Health*. New York: Cambridge University Press.

Darragh, Austin, Ronan Lambe, Marie Kenny, and Ian Brick. 1985. "Sudden Death of a Volunteer." *Lancet* 325 (8420) (Jan 12): 93–95.

Davenant, Charles. 1697. *Two Discourses on the Public Revenues and Trade of England*. London. http://www.archive.org/stream/politicalandcom00davegoog #page/n5/mode/2up (accessed January 16, 2012).

Davis, John K. 2008 "Futility, Conscientious Refusal, and Who Gets to Decide." *Journal of Medicine and Philosophy* 33 (4): 356–374.

Dawkins, Richard. 2006. *The God Delusion*. New York: Houghton Mifflin Co.

Dawson, Angus. 2010. "The Future of Bioethics: Three Dogmas and a Cup of Hemlock." *Bioethics* 24 (5): 218–225.

de Melo-Martin, Imaculata, and Ann Ho. 2008. "Beyond Informed Consent: The Therapeutic Misconception and Trust." *Journal of Medical Ethics* 34 (3): 202–205.

Dingwall, Robert. 2010. "Public Health Ethics and Practice." *Sociology of Health and Illness* 32 (6): 969–970.

Dingwall, Robert, and Vienna Rozelle. 2011. "The Ethical Governance of German Physicians 1890–1939: Are There Lessons from History?" *Journal of Policy History* 23 (1): 29–52.

Down, J. Langdon. 1866. "Observation on an Ethnic Classification of Idiots." *London Hospital Reports* 3: 259–262. http://www.neonatology.org/classics/down.html (accessed April 4, 2010).

Drake, Stephen. 2009. "Peter Singer's "Tribute" to Harriet McBride Johnson—and Paul Longmore's Response." *Not Dead Yet* news commentary, January 13. http://notdeadyetnewscommentary.blogspot.com/2009/01/peter-singers-tribute-to-harriet.html (accessed January 13, 2012).

Dutton, Dennis. 2009. *The Art Instinct: Beauty, Pleasure, & Human Evolution*. New York: Bloomsbury Press.

Dworkin, Gerald. 1987. Paternalism. In *Paternalism*, ed. Rolf Sartorius, 19–35. Minneapolis: University of Minnesota Press.

Dworkin, Ronald. 1977. *Taking Rights Seriously*. Cambridge, MA: Harvard University Press.

Editors' Note. 1993. *New York Times*, November 23. http://www.nytimes.com/1993/11/23/nyregion/editors-note-031193.html?ref=richarddlamm (accessed January 20, 2012).

Elliott, Carl. 2001. "Pharma Buys a Conscience." *American Prospect* 12 (16) (September): 23. http://healthandpharma.awardspace.com/Week 6 Readings/Elliott Pharma Buys a Conscience.pdf (accessed September 20, 2010).

Elliott, Carl. 2005. "Should Journals Publish Industry-funded Bioethics Articles?" *Lancet* 366 (9483): 422–424. http://www.geneticsandsociety.org/article.php?id=1681 (accessed September 20, 2010).

Elliott, Carl. 2010. "The Deadly Corruption of Clinical Trials." *Mother Jones* (September/October): 55–63. http://motherjones.com/environment/2010/09/dan-markingson-drug-trial-astrazeneca (accessed November 25, 2010).

Emanuel, Ezekiel J. 2009. "Welcome and Plenary Lecture." Annual meeting of the American Association of Bioethics and the Humanities. Hyatt Regency Hotel, Washington, DC. October 15.

Engelhardt, H. Tristram, Jr. 1986. *The Foundations of Bioethics*. 2nd ed. New York: Oxford University Press.

Engelhardt, H. Tristram, Jr. 2003. Managed Care and the Deprofessionalization of Medicine. In *The Ethics of Managed Care: Professional Integrity and Patient Rights*, ed. William B. Bondeson and James W. Jones, 93–107. Dordrecht: Kluwer Academic Publishers.

Engelhardt, H. Tristram, Jr. 2011. "Confronting Moral Pluralism in Posttraditional Western Societies: Bioethics Critically Reassessed." *Journal of Medicine and Philosophy* 36 (2) (April): 243–260.

Eppig, Christopher, Corley L. Fisher, and Randy Thornhill. 2010. "Parasite Prevalence and the Worldwide Distribution of Cognitive Ability." *Proceedings of the Royal Society of Biological Sciences* 277: 3801–3808. http://yibudayi.com/wp-content/uploads/2010/07/ParasiteCognitive.pdf (accessed June 26, 2011).

Epstein, Miran. 2009. "The Political Economy of Death and the History of its Criteria." *Reviews in the Neurosciences* 20 (3–4): 293–297.

Epstein, Miran. 2010. "How Will the Economic Downturn Affect Academic Bioethics?" *Bioethics* 24 (5): 226–233.

Epstein, Miran, and Mark Wilson. 2011. "Consent in Emergency Care Research." *Lancet* 373 (9785) (July): 26.

Erickson, Stephen A. 2010. "The Wrong of Rights: The Moral Authority of the Family." *Journal of Medicine and Philosophy* 35 (5): 600–616.

Ernst & Young. 2010. *The Economic Contributions of the Biotechnology Industry to the U.S. Economy*. Biotechnology Organization, 2000. http://www.bio.org/articles/economic-contributions-biotechnology-industry (accessed January 15, 2012).

Evans, Bob, and Marko Vujicic. 2005. Political Wolves and Economic Sheep: The Sustainability of Public Health Insurance in Canada. In *Public-Private Mix for Health*, ed. Allan Maynard, 117–140. Oxford, UK: Radcliff Publishing Ltd.

Evans, John H. 2002. *Playing God: Human Genetic Engineering and the Rationalization of Public Bioethical Debate*. Chicago: University of Chicago Press.

Fairlie, Henry. 1988. "Talking 'bout My Generation." *New Republic* 28 (March): 19–22.

Farmer, Paul, and Nicole Gastineau Campos. 2006. Rethinking Medical Ethics: A View from Below. In *Ethics and Infectious Disease*, ed. Michel J. Selgelid, Margaret P. Battin, and Charles B. Smith, 261–284. Malden, MA: Blackwell Publishing.

Fins, Joseph J. 2008. "A Leg to Stand On: Sir William Osler and Wilder Penfield's 'Neuroethics.'" *American Journal of Bioethics* 8 (1): 37–46.

Fins, Joseph J. 2008. "Neuroethics and Neuroimaging: Moving toward Transparency." *American Journal of Bioethics* 8 (9): 46–52.

Fins, Joseph J., Judith Illes, James L. Bernat, Joy Hirsch, Steven Laureys, and Emily Murphy. 2008. "Neuroimaging and Disorders of Consciousness: Envisioning an Ethical Research Agenda." *American Journal of Bioethics-Neuroscience* 8 (9): 3–12.

Firth, Shanon. 2009. "Locked-in Syndrome: When a Coma Is Not a Coma." *FindingDulcinea*, December 1. http://www.findingdulcinea.com/news/science/2009/dec/Locked-In-Syndrome-When-a-Coma-s-Not-a-Coma.html (accessed January 18, 2012).

Fisher, Jill H. 2009. *Medical Research for Hire: The Political Economy of Pharmaceutical Clinical Trials*. New Brunswick, NJ: Rutgers University Press.

Fischer, Josie. 1999. "Re-examining Death: Against a Higher Brain Criterion." *Journal of Medical Ethics* 225 (6): 473–476.

Fiske, Alan P. 1998. "Human Sociality." *International Society for the Study of Personal Relationships Bulletin* 14 (2): 4–9. Published online as "The Inherent Sociability of *Homo sapiens*." http://www.sscnet.ucla.edu/anthro/faculty/fiske/relmodov.htm (accessed September 5, 2010).

Fiske, Alan P. 2004. Relational Models Theory 2.0. In *Relational Models Theory: A Contemporary Overview*, ed. Nick Haslam, 3–25. Mahwah, NJ: Erlbaum.

Foucault, Michel. 1978. *The History of Sexuality*. Vol. 1: *An Introduction*. Trans. Robert Hurley New York: Random House.

Foucault, Michel. 1970. *The Order of Things: An Archaeology of the Human Sciences (Les motes et les choses)*. London: Tavistock.

Fox, Renée C. 1999. "Is Medical Education Asking Too Much of Bioethics?" *Daedalus* 128 (4): 1–25.

Fox, Renée C., and Judith P. Swazey. 2008. *Observing Bioethics*. New York: Oxford University Press.

Fraga, Mario F., et al. 2005. "Epigenetic Differences Arise during the Lifetime of Monozygotic Twins." *Proceedings of the National Academy of Sciences of the United States of America* 102 (30): 10604–10609.

Francis, Darlene, and Daniela Kaufer. 2011. "Beyond Nature vs. Nuture." *Scientist* 25 (October 1): 94. http://the-scientist.com/2011/10/01/beyond-nature-vs-nurture (accessed January 14, 2012).

Froese, D. 2010. "It's Good to Be Me." Canadian Down Syndrome Society. Calgary, Alberta. September 2010.

Fost, Norman. 1992 "Ethical Implications of Screening Asymptomatic Individuals." *FASEB Journal* [Federation of American Societies for Experimental Biology] 6: 2813–2817. http://www.fasebj.org/content/6/10/2813.full.pdf (accessed June 21, 2011).

Gall, Franz. 1810. *J. Anatomie et physiologie du système nerveux en général, et du cerveau en particulier, avec des observations sur la possibilité de reconnoitre plusieurs dispositions intellectuelles et morales de l'homme et des animaux, par la configuration de leurs têtes*. Paris: Schoell.

Gee, Ellen M., and Gloria M. Gutman. 2000. *The Overselling of Population Aging: Apocalyptic Demography, Intergenerational Challenges, and Social Policy*. New York: Oxford University Press.

Gerrand, Nicole. 1999. "The Misuse of Kant in the Debate about a Market for Human Body Parts." *Journal of Applied Philosophy* 16 (1): 59–67.

Gert, Bernard, Charles M. Culver, and K. D. Culber. 2006. *Bioethics: A Systematic Approach*. New York: Oxford University Press.

Geuss, Raymond. 2008. *Philosophy and Real Politics*. Princeton, NJ: Princeton University Press.

Gilligan, Carol. 1982. *In a Different Voice: Psychological Theory and Women's Development*. Cambridge, MA: Harvard University Press.

Gillon, Raanan. 1986. *Philosophical Medical Ethics*. Chichester, NH: Wiley.

Gillon, Raanan. 1996. Transplantation and Ethics. In *Birth to Death: Science and Bioethics*, ed. David C. Thomas and Tommi Kushner, 106–118. New York: Cambridge University Press.

Glover, Jonathan. 2006. *Choosing Children: The Ethical Dilemmas of Genetic Intervention*. New York: Oxford University Press.

Glover, Jonathan. 2008. *Choosing Children: Genetics, Disability, and Design*. Oxford, UK: Clarendon Press.

Gluckman, L. 1988. "The Caduceus—A Further Interpretation." *New Zealand Medical Journal* 111 (1070): 281–282.

Goffman, Erving. 1989. *Presentation of Self in Everyday Life*. New York: Doubleday Anchor Books.

Gould, Stephen J. 1981. *The Mismeasure of Man*. New York: W. W. Norton.

Gould, Stephen J. 1991. "The Smoking Gun of Eugenics." *Natural History* 12 (1): 8–17.

"Gov. Lamm Asserts Elderly, If Very Ill, Have 'Duty to Die.'" 1984. *New York Times*, March 29, A16, http://www.nytimes.com/1984/03/29/us/gov-lamm-asserts-elderly-if-very-ill-have-duty-to-die.html (accessed February 22, 2012).

Grant, Richard P. 2011. "Evolution, Tout de Suite," *The Scientist* (October 1): 27–29. http://the-scientist.com/2011/10/01/evolution-tout-de-suite (accessed October 18, 2011).

Green, Sarah. 2010. "Innovations 'R' Us." *Scientist* 24 (12): 13. http://classic.the-scientist.com/article/display/57823/ (accessed February 28, 2012).

Guillet, Edwin C. 1963. *The Great Migration: The Atlantic Crossing by Sailing-Ship Since 1770*. 2nd ed. Toronto: University of Toronto Press.

Gutting, Gary. 2005. *Foucault: A Very Short Introduction*. New York: Oxford University Press.

Hacking, Ian. 2005. "Why Race Still Matters." *Daedulus* 134 (1): 102–116.

Hall, Daniel E. 2011. "The Guild of Surgeons as a Tradition of Moral Enquiry." *Journal of Medicine and Philosophy* 36 (2): 114–132.

Hallowell, Nina, Cook Samuel, Michael Parker, and Anneke Lucassen. 2009. "Healthcare Professionals' and Researchers' Understanding of Cancer Genetics Activities: A Qualitative Interview Study." *Journal of Medical Ethics* 35 (2): 113–119.

Harman, Oren. 2010. *The Price of Altruism: George Price and the Search for the Origins of Kindness*. New York: W. W. Norton & Co.

Harris, John. 2007. *Enhancing Evolution: The Ethical Case for Making Better People*. Princeton, NJ: Princeton University Press.

Harsanyi, John C. 1975. "Can the Maximin Principle Serve as a Basis for Morality? A Critique of John Rawls's Theory." *American Political Science Review* 69 (2): 594–606.

Harvey, David. 1973. *Social Justice and the City*. Cambridge, MA: Basil Blackwell Press.

Harvey, David. 1974. "Population, Resources, and the Ideology of Science." *Economic Geography* 40 (3): 256–277.

Hastings Center. 2010. "About Us." http://www.thehastingscenter.org/About/Default.aspx (accessed January 5, 2010).

Hawking, Stephen. 1993. *Black Holes and Baby Universes, and Other Essays*. New York: Cambridge University Press.

Häyry, Matti. 2010. *Rationality and the Genetic Challenge: Making People Better?* New York: Cambridge University Press.

Heidegger, M. 1962. *Being and Time*. Trans. John Macquarrie and Edward Robinson. Malden, MA: Blackwell Publishing.

Helvesi, Allan G., and Kenneth B. Bleiwas. 2005. "The Economic Impact of the Biotechnology and Pharmaceutical Industries in New York State," Office of the Comptroller Report 11–205 (Albany, NY: Office of the Comptroller). http://www.docstoc.com/docs/69310177/The-Economic-Impact-of-the-Biotechnology-and-Pharmaceutical (accessed August 22, 2011).

Hess, John L. 1990. "Social Security Wars: Confessions of a Greedy Geezer." *Nation* 250 (April 2): 437–439.

Hippocrates. 1849. *The Genuine Words of Hippocrates translated from the Greek by Francis Adams, Surgeon*. Vol. 2. London: Sydenham Society.

Hippocratic Oath. http://classics.mit.edu/Hippocrates/hippooath.html (accessed June 27, 2011).

Höchsmann, Hyun. 2002. *On Peter Singer*. Belmont, CA: Wadsworth/Thompson Learning.

Howe, G. M. 1963. *National Atlas of Disease Mortality in the United Kingdom*. 2nd ed. London: Thomas Nelson and Sons, Ltd.

Huber, Mathew T. 2011. "Enforcing Scarcity: Oil, Violence, and the Making of the Market." *Annals of the Association of American Geographers* 101 (4): 816–826.

Hughes, James. 2004. *Citizen Cyborg: Why Democratic Societies Must Respond to the Redesigned Human of the Future*. New York: Basic Books.

Hughes, James. 2006. "Virtue Engineering: Applications of Neurotechnology to Improve Moral Behavior." TransVision06 lecture. http://ieet.org/index.php/IEET/more/2035 (accessed January 18, 2012).

Hume, Leonard J. 1974. "Charles Davenant on Financial Administration." *History of Political Economy* 6 (4): 463–477.

Husserl, Edmund. 1913. *Ideas Pertaining to a Pure Phenomenology and to a Phenomenological Philosophy—First Book: General Introduction to a Pure Phenomenology*. Trans. F. Kersten. Norwell, MA: Kluwer Academic Publishers.

Huxley, J. 1942. *Evolution: The Modern Synthesis*. London: Allen & Unwin.

Ignatieff, Michael. 2000. *A Life of Isaiah Berlin*. New York: Penguin Books.

Jacob, Joseph M. 1988. *Doctors and Rules: A Sociology of Professional Values*. London: Routledge.

James, Timothy. 2008. "The Appeal to Law to Provide Public Answers to Bioethical Questions: It All Depends on What Sort of Answers You Want." *Health Care Analysis* 16 (1): 65–76.

Jameson, James. 1819. *Report on the epidemick cholera morbus, as it visited the territories subject to the Presidency of Bengal, in the years 1817, 1818 and 1819. Drawn up by order of the Government, under the superintendence of the Medical Board*. Calcutta: Government Gazette Press, by A. G. Balfour. http://pds.lib.harvard.edu/pds/view/7095430 (accessed February 21, 2012).

Jacquard, A. 1984. *In Praise of Difference: Genetics and Human Affairs*. Trans. M. M. Moriarty. New York: Columbia University Press.

Jaworska, Agnieszka. 1999. "Respecting the Margins of Agency: Alzheimer's Patients and the Capacity to Value." *Philosophy & Public Affairs* 28 (2): 105–138.

Jennings, Bruce. 1998. Autonomy and Difference: The Travails of Liberalism in Bioethics. In *Bioethics and Society*, ed. Raymond Devries and Janardan Subedi, 258–269. New York: Prentice Hall.

Jennings, Bruce. 2001. "From the Urban to the Civic: The Moral Possibilities of the City." *Journal of Urban Health: Bulletin of the New York Academy of Medicine* 78 (1): 88–103.

Jennings, Bruce. 2009. "Public Health and Liberty: Beyond the Millian Paradigm." *Public Health Ethics* 2 (2): 123–134.

Joffee, Stephen, and Franklin G. Miller. 2008. "Bench to Bedside: Mapping the Moral Terrain of Clinical Research." *Hastings Center Report* 38 (2): 30–42.

Johnson, Harriet McBryde. 2003. "Unspeakable Conversations." *New York Times Sunday Magazine*, February 16. http://www.racematters.org/harrietmcbrydejohnson.htm (accessed January 18, 2008).

Johnson, Harriet McBryde. N.d. "When Is a Life Worth Living?" http://www.scpronet.com/point/0104/p07.html (accessed September 5, 2010).

Johnson, Mark. 1993. *Moral Imagination: Implications of Cognitive Science for Ethics*. Chicago: University of Chicago Press.

Jonsen, Albert R. 1993. "The Birth of Bioethics," Special Supplement. *Hastings* Center *Report* 23 (6) (November–December): S1–S4.

Jonsen, Albert R. 1997. "The Birth of Bioethics: The Origins and Evolution of a Demi-discipline." *Medical Humanities Review* 11 (1): 9–21.

Jonsen, Albert R. 1998. *The Birth of Bioethics*. New York: Oxford University Press.

Jordan, Mathew A. 2010. "Bioethics and 'Human Dignity.'" *Journal of Medicine and Philosophy* 35 (1): 180–196.

Jotterand, Fabrice. 2005. "The Hippocratic Oath and Contemporary Medicine: Dialectic between Past Ideals and Present Reality." *Journal of Medicine and Philosophy* 30 (1): 107–128.

Jotterand, Fabrice. 2010. "Human Dignity and Transhumanism: Do Anthro-Technological Devices Have Moral Status?" *American Journal of Bioethics* 10 (7): 45–52.

Kahane, Guy, and Julien Savulescu. 2009. "Brain Damage and the Moral Significance of Consciousness." *Journal of Medicine and Philosophy* 34 (1): 6–26.

Kant, Immanuel. 1781/2005. *A Critique of Practical Reason*. Trans. J. M. Meiklejohn. New York: Dover Publication.

Kant, Immanuel. 1785/1948. *Groundwork of the Metaphysic of Morals*. Trans. H. J. Patton. New York: HarperCollins Publisher.

Kant, Immanuel. 1785/1959. *Foundations of the Metaphysics of Morals (Grundlegung zu Metaphysik der Sitten)*. Trans. Lewis W. Beck. New York: Macmillan Publishing Co.

Kant, Immanuel. 1785/2005. *Groundwork for the Metaphysics of Morals*. Ed. Lara Denis. Trans. Thomas K. Abbott. Orchard Park, NY: Broadview Press Ltd.

Kant, Immanuel. 1790/2010. *The Critique of Judgment*. Trans. J. H. Bernard. Adelaide, South Australia: University of Adelaide. http://ebooks.adelaide.edu.au/k/kant/immanuel/k16ju/ (accessed September 6, 2010).

Katsnelson, Alla. 2010. "Odd Man Out: Do Fish Have Personalities?" *Scientist* 24 (31): 34–39.

Katz, Stephen. 1996. *Disciplining Old Age: The Formation of Gerontological Knowledge*. Charlottesville: The University Press of Virginia.

Kaufert, Joseph, Rebecca Wiebe, Karen Schwartz, Lisa Labane, Zana M. Lutfiyya, and Catherine Pearse. 2010. "End-of-Life Ethics and Disability: Differing Perspectives on Case-based Teaching." *Medicine, Health Care, and Philosophy* 13, no. 2: 115–126.

Kaye, Cilia I., Judith Livingston, Mark A. Canfield, Marie Y. Mann, Michele A. Lloyd-Puryear, and Bradford L. Therrell Jr. 2007. "Assuring Clinical Genetic Services for Newborns Identified through U.S. Newborn Screening Programs." *Genetics in Medicine* 9 (8): 518–527.

Kellehear, Allan. 2008. "Dying as a Social Relationship: A Sociological Review of Debates on the Determination of Death." *Social Science & Medicine* 66 (7): 1533–1544.

Keller, Evelyn F. 2011. *The Mirage of a Space between Nature and Nurture*. Durham, NC: Duke University Press.

Kevles, Bettyann H. 1997. *Naked to the Bone: Medical Imaging in the Twentieth Century*. New Brunswick, NJ: Rutgers University Press.

Kilner, John F. 1990. *Who Lives? Who Dies? Ethical Criteria in Patient Selection*. New Haven, CT: Yale University Press.

Kimball, R. F. 1943. "The Great Biological Generalization." *Quarterly Review of Biology* 18 (4): 364–367.

Kittay, Eva. F. 1999. *Love's Labour: Essays on Women, Equality, and Dependency*. New York: Routledge.

Kobayashi, Audrey. 2011. "Paradoxes of Our Time." *AAG Newsletter* 46 (2): 3.

Koch, Tom. 1990. *Mirrored Lives: Aging Children, Elderly Parents*. Westport, CT: Praeger Books.

Koch, Tom. 1990. *The News as Myth: Fact and Context in Journalism*. Westport, CT: Praeger Books.

Koch, Tom. 1993. *A Place in Time: Care Givers for their Elderly*. Westport, CT: Praeger Books.

Koch, Tom. 1994. Showtime. In *Watersheds: Stories of Crisis and Renewal in Our Everyday Lives*, 13–49. Toronto: Lester Publishing.

Koch, Tom. 1996. "The Canadian Question: What's So Great about Intelligence?" *Cambridge Quarterly of Healthcare Ethics* 5 (2): 307–310.

Koch, Tom. 1996. "Living vs. Dying 'with Dignity': A New Perspective on the Euthanasia Debate." *Cambridge Quarterly of Healthcare Ethics* 5 (1): 50–60.

Koch, Tom. 1998. "On the Subject(s) of Jack Kevorkian, MD: A Retrospective Analysis." *Cambridge Quarterly of Healthcare Ethics* 7 (4): 436–441.

Koch, Tom. 1999. "They Might as Well Be in Bolivia: Race, Ethnicity and the Problem of Solid Organ Donation." *Theoretical Medicine and Bioethics* 20 (6): 563–575.

Koch, Tom. 2000. "The Illusion of Paradox: Commentary on Albrecht, G. L. and Develiger, P. J. (1998): 'The Disability Paradox: High Quality against All Odds.'" *Social Science & Medicine* 50 (6): 757–759.

Koch, Tom. 2000. "Life Quality versus the 'Quality of Life': Assumptions Underlying Prospective Quality of Life Instruments in Health Care Planning." *Social Science & Medicine* 51 (3): 419–428.

Koch, Tom. 2001. "Disabled Are Not Dogs: Commentary on the Robert Latimer Case." *Vancouver Sun*, February 7, A15. http://www.chninternational.com/tomkoch.htm (accessed January 26, 2010).

Koch, Tom. 2001. "Future States: Testing the Axioms Underlying Prospective, Future-oriented, Health Planning Instruments." *Social Science & Medicine* 52 (3): 453–466.

Koch, Tom. 2002. *Scarce Goods: Justice, Fairness, and Organ Transplantation*. Westport, CT: Praeger Books.

Koch, Tom. 2004. *The Wreck of the William Brown*. Camden, ME: McGraw-Hill Marine.

Koch, Tom. 2005. *Cartographies of Disease: Maps, Mapping, and Medicine*. Redlands, CA: ESRI Press.

Koch, Tom. 2005. "The Challenge of Terri Schiavo: Lessons for Bioethics." *Journal of Medical Ethics* 31 (7): 376–378.

Koch, Tom. 2005. "The Ideology of Normalcy: The Ethics of Difference." *Journal of Disability Policy Studies* 16 (2): 123–129.

Koch, Tom. 2005. "Mapping the Miasma: Air, Health, and Place in Early Medical Mapping." *Cartographic Perspectives* 52 (4): 4–27.

Koch, Tom. 2006. "'False Truths': Ethics and Mapping as a Profession." *Cartographic Perspectives* 54: 4–15.

Koch, Tom. 2008. "Were Polio to Return, Today . . ." *Journal of the Canadian Medical Association* 178 (9): 1244. http://www.cmaj.ca/content/178/9/1244.full.pdf+html (accessed December 12, 2011).

Koch, Tom. 2009. "End of Life, Year, after Year, after Year." *Journal of the Canadian Medical Association* 181 (11): 868.

Koch, Tom. 2010. "Enhancing Who? Enhancing What? Ethics, Bioethics, and Transhumanism." *Journal of Medicine and Philosophy* 35 (6): 685–699.

Koch, Tom. 2011. *Disease Maps: Epidemics on the Ground*. Chicago: University of Chicago Press.

Koch, Tom. 2011. "Eugenics and the 'Genetic Challenge,' Again: All Dressed Up and Just Everywhere to Go." Special Issue: Review of Matty Häyry's *Rationality and the Genetic Challenge, Cambridge Quarterly of Healthcare Ethics* 20 (2) (April): 1–13.

Koch, Tom. 2012. Images of Uncertainty: Two Cases of Neuroimaging and What They Cannot Say. In *Advances in Neurotechnology: Ethical, Legal and Social Issues*. Vol. 1: *Philosophical Premises in Application*, ed. James Giordano, 45–55. Boca Raton, FL: CRC Press.

Koch, Tom, and Sarah Jones. 2010. "The Ethical Professional as Endangered Person: Blog Notes on Doctor-Patient Relationships." *Journal of Medical Ethics* 36 (6): 371–374.

Kohlberg, Lawrence. 1973. "The Claim to Moral Adequacy of a Highest Stage of Moral Judgment." *Journal of Philosophy* 70 (18): 630–646.

Kolata, Gina. 1980. "NIH Shaken by Death of Research Volunteer." *Science* 209 (4455): 475–476; 478–479.

Koppel, T. 1996. *Who Lives? Who Dies? Who Decides?* San Francisco: California Medical Centre.

Krause, Elliott A. 1996. *Death of the Guilds: Professions, States, and the Advance of Capitalism, 1930 to the Present*. New Haven, CT: Yale University Press.

Kruger, Justin, and David Dunning. 1999. "Unskilled and Unaware of It: How Difficulties of Recognizing One's Own Incompetence Lead to Inflated Self-assessments." *Journal of Personality and Social Psychology* 77 (6): 1121–1134.

Kuczewski, Mark G. 2001. "Disability: An Agenda for Bioethics." *American Journal of Bioethics* 1 (3): 36–44.

Kuczewski, Mark G. 2010. "Taking It Personally: Reflections on Living Bioethics and Medical Humanities." *ASBH Reader* (Summer–Autumn): 3–9.

Laing, R. D. 1961. *Self and Others*. London: Tavistock Publications.

Lakoff, George, and Mark Johnson. 1980. *Metaphors We Live By*. Chicago: University of Chicago Press.

Lamm, Richard D. 1989. "Columbus and Copernicus: New Wine in Old Wineskins." *Mount Sinai Journal of Medicine* 56 (1): 1–10.

Lamm, Richard D. 1989. "Saving a Few—Sacrificing Many, at Great Cost." *New York Times*, August 2, 23. http://www.nytimes.com/1989/08/02/opinion/saving-a-few-sacrificing-maNY-at-great-cost.html (accessed December 26, 2009).

Lamm, Richard D. 1993. "New World of Medical Ethics: Our Duty Lies Both to the Individual and the Population." *Vital Speeches of the Day* 59 (July 1): 549–553.

Lamm, Richard D. 2006. "Copernican Health Ethics." Annual Meeting of the American Society of Bioethics and the Humanities. Marriott Denver City Center, Denver, CO. October 26.

Lamm, Richard D. 2006. Doctors Have Patients, Governors Have Citizens. In *Narrative Matters: The Power of the Personal Essay in Health Policy*, ed. Fitzhugh Mullan, Ellen Ficklen, and Kyna Rubin, 34–41. Baltimore, MD: Johns Hopkins University Press.

Lancet. 1831. "History of the Rise, Progress, Ravages, Etc. of the Blue Cholera of India." *Lancet* 17: 241–284.

Lasagna, Louis. 1991. "Mortal Decisions: The Search for an Ethical Policy on Allocating Health Care." *Science* 43: 43–44.

Lasagna, Louis, and J. M. Von Felsinger. 1954. "The Volunteer Subject in Research." *Science* 120 (3114): 359–361.

Latour, Bruno. 1993. *We Have Never Been Modern*. Trans. Catherine Porter. Cambridge, MA: Harvard University Press.

Law, John. 2004. *After Method: Mess in Social Science Research*. New York: Routledge.

Law, John, and Annemarie Mol. 2002. Complexities: An Introduction. In *Complexities: Social Studies of Knowledge Practices*, ed. John Law and Annamarie Mol, 1–22. Durham, NC: Duke University Press.

Lawrence, Dana J. 2007. "The Four Principles of Biomedical Ethics: A Foundation for Current Bioethical Debate." *Journal of Chiropractic Humanities* 14: 34–40.

"The Legacy of Nancy Cruzan: 20 Years Later, Are We Any Better at Healthcare?" 2011. A National Conference on the Past, Present and Future of the PSDA, Nutrition-Hydration, and Palliative Care, Kansas City, MO. November 12–13. https://pmr.uchicago.edu/events/2010-11-12/legacy-nancy-cruzan-20-years-later-are-we-any-better-healthcare (accessed January 18, 2012).

Lejeune, Jerome, Marthe Gautier, and Raymond R. Turpin. 1959. "Etude des chromosomes somatiques de neuf enfants mongoliens." *Comptes Rendus Hebdomadaires des Séances de l'Académie des Sciences* 248 (11): 1721–1722. http://gallica.bnf.fr/ark:/12148/bpt6k32002/f1759.chemindefer (accessed June 8, 2011).

Lepore, Jill. 2010. Fixed: The Rise of Marriage Therapy, and Other Dreams of Human Betterment. *New Yorker* (March 29): 93–97. http://www.newyorker.com/arts/critics/atlarge/2010/03/29/100329crat_atlarge_lepore (accessed January 17, 2013).

Lewontin, Richard C. 1994. *Biology as Ideology: The Doctrine of DNA*. New York: HarperPerennial.

Lewonton, Richard C. 2011. "It's Even Less in Your Genes." *New York Review of Books* (May 26): 26. http://www.nybooks.com/articles/archives/2011/may/26/its-even-less-your-genes (accessed January 18, 2012).

Liang, Bryan A., and Laura Lin. 2005. "*Bouvia v. Superior Court*: Quality of Life Matters." *Virtual Mentor* 7 (2) (February). http://virtualmentor.ama-assn.org/2005/02/hlaw1-0502.html (accessed July 7, 2011).

Lindemann, Hilde. 2009. "President's Letter." *ASBH Reader* 2–3: 35.

Lindemann, Hilde. 2010. "Speaking Truth to Power." *Hastings Center Report* 40 (1): 44–45.

Litton, Paul, and F. G. Miller. 2010. "What Physician-Investigators Owe Patients Who Participate in Research." *Journal of the American Medical Association* 304 (13): 1391–1493.

Luce, John M. 1997. "Making Decisions about the Forgoing of Life-sustaining Therapy." *American Journal of Respiratory Critical Care* 156 (6): 1715–1718.

Luiggi, Cristina. 2010. "The Philadelphia Chromosome, circa 1960." *The Scientist* 24 (12): 84. http://classic.the-scientist.com/article/display/57846/ (accessed January 18, 2012).

Lysaught, Therese M. 2004. "Respect: Or, How Respect for Persons Became Respect for Autonomy." *Journal of Medicine and Philosophy* 29 (6): 665–680.

Lysaught, Therese M. 2009. "Docile Bodies: Transnational Research Ethics as Biopolitics." *Journal of Medicine and Philosophy* 34 (4): 384–408.

Machado, Calixto, Julius Kerein, Jasmina Ferrer, Liana Portela, Maria de la Gracia, and José M. Manero. 1997. "The Concept of Brain Death Did Not Evolve to Benefit Organ Transplants." *Journal of Medical Ethics* 33 (4): 197–200.

MacIntyre, Alasdair. 1984. *After Virtue: A Study in Moral Theory*. 2nd ed. Notre Dame, IN: University of Notre Dame Press.

MacIntyre, Alasdair. 1988. *Whose Justice? Which Rationality?* Notre Dame, IN: University of Notre Dame Press.

Macklin, Rita. 2010. "The Death of Bioethics (As We Once Knew It)." *Bioethics* 24 (5) (June): 211–217.

Malthus, Thomas R. 1798. *An Essay on the Principle of Population, as It Affects the Future Improvement of Society*. London: J. Johnson, in St. Paul's Church-Yard. http://www.esp.org/books/malthus/population/malthus.pdf (accessed July 19, 2010).

Markert, John. 2005. "The Malthusian Fallacy: Prophecies of Doom and the Crisis of Social Security." *Social Science Journal* 42 (4): 555–568.

Marks, Geoffrey, and William K. Beatty. 1976. *Epidemics*. New York: Charles Scribner's Sons.

McCullough, Lawrence B. 1983. "Introduction." *Theoretical Medicine* 4 (2): 227–229.

McCurdy, David B. 1996. "Alzheimer Disease, a Review of Stephen G. Post: The Moral Challenge of Alzheimer Disease." *Making the Rounds in Health, Faith, & Ethics* (March 5): 5–6.

Mencius (Mung Tzu). 1895/1935. *The Chinese Classics, Vol. 2*. Trans. James Legge. Oxford, UK: Oxford University Press. http://www.sacred-texts.com/cfu/menc/index.htm (accessed May 20, 2011).

Mensa Canada. http://www.mensacanada.org/home.htm (accessed January 14, 2012).

Menzel, Paul T. 1990. *Strong Medicine: The Ethical Rationing of Health Care*. New York: Oxford University Press.

Merle, Jean-Christophe. 2000. "A Kantian Argument for a Duty to Donate One's Own Organs. A Reply to Nicole Gerand." *Journal of Applied Philosophy* 17 (1): 93–101.

Michel, Andrew A. 2011. "Psychiatry after Virtue: A Modern Practice in the Ruins." *Journal of Medicine and Philosophy* 36 (2): 186–211.

Miles, Steven H. 1991. "Informed Demand for 'Non-beneficial Medical Treatment.'" *New England Journal of Medicine* 325 (7): 512–515.

Mill, John S. 1956. *On Liberty*. Indianapolis: Bobbs Merrill.

Mill, John S. 2008. *On Liberty and Other Essays*. Ed. John Gray. New York: Oxford University Press.

Miller, Franklin G., and Robert D. Truog. 2008. "Rethinking the Ethics of Vital Organ Donations." *Hastings Center Report* 38 (6): 38–46. http://www.maceyleigh.net/articles/ethics_of_vital_organ_donations.pdf (accessed June 20, 2011).

Mitman, Gregg, and Ronald L. Numbers. 1993. "From Miasma to Asthma: The Changing Fortunes of Medical Geography in America." *History and Philosophy of the Life Sciences* 25 (3): 391–412.

Morris, Errol. 2010. "The Anosognosic's Dilemma: Something's Wrong but You'll Never Know What It Is (Part 5)." *New York Times*, June 24. http://opinionator.blogs.nytimes.com/tag/anosognosiah (accessed December 23, 2010).

Morris, R. J. 1976. *Cholera 1832: Social Response to an Epidemic*. London: Croom Helm.

Montgomery, Jonathan. 2006. Law and the Demoralization of Medicine. *Legal Studies* 26 (2): 185–210.

Morris, Robert J. 1976. *Cholera in 1832: The Social Response to an Epidemic*. London: Croom Helm.

Moss, Lenny. 2003. *What Genes Can't Do*. Cambridge, MA: MIT Press.

Müller-Hill, Benno. 2006. Lessons from a Dark and Distant Past. In *Bioethics: An Anthology*. 2nd ed., ed. Helga Khuse and Peter Singer, 231–245. Malden, MA: Blackwell Publishing.

Murrow, Edward R. 1960. "Harvest of Shame." *CBS Reports*. November 26.

Myers, Samuel S., and Aaron Bernstein. 2011. "The Coming Health Crisis." *The Scientist* 25 (1): 32–37. (accessed January 18, 2012).

Nadler, Henry L., and Albert B. Gerbie. 1970. "Role of Amniocentesis in the Intra-uterine Diagnosis of Genetic Defects." *New England Journal of Medicine* 282 (11): 596–599.

Napier, Stephen. 2009. "A Regulatory Argument against Human Embryonic Stem Cell Research." *Journal of Medicine and Philosophy* 34 (5): 496–508.

National Commission for the Protection of Human Subjects of Biomedical and Behavioral Research. 1979. *The Belmont Report: Ethical Principles and Guidelines for the Protection of Human Subjects of Research*. Washington, DC: U.S. Government Printing Office. http://ohsr.od.nih.gov/guidelines/belmont.html (accessed January 8, 2009).

Nozick, Robert. 1974. *Anarchy, State, and Utopia*. New York: Basic Books.

Nuland, Sherwin B. 1988. *Doctors: The Biography of Medicine*. New York: Alfred A. Knopf, Inc.

Nuremberg Military Tribunal. 1949. *Trials of War Criminals before the Nuremberg Military Tribunals under Control Council Law*. Washington, DC: Government Printing Office, 181–182.

Nussbaum, Margaret C. 2006. *Frontiers of Justice: Disability, Nationality, Species Membership*. Cambridge, MA: Belknap Press.

Ogilvie, Richard I. 2001. "The Death of a Volunteer Research Subject. Lessons to Be Relearned." *Journal of the Canadian Medical Association* 165 (10): 1335–1357.

Oishi, Shigehiro, and Jessie Graham. 2010. "Social Ecology: Lost and Found in Psychological Science." *Perspectives on Psychological Science* 5 (4): 356–377.

Orentlicher, David. 2005. "Making Research a Requirement of Treatment: Why We Should Sometimes Let Doctors Pressure Patients to Participate in Research." *Hastings Center Report* (September–October): 20–28.

Oxford Online Etymology Dictionary. 2001. *Paternalism*. Oxford, UK: Oxford University Press. http://www.etymonline.com/ (accessed January 16, 2010).

Parsons, Talcott. 1951. *The Social System*. London: Routledge & Kegan Paul Ltd.

Pellegrino, Edmund. 1993. "The Metamorphosis of Medical Ethics: A 30-Year Perspective." *Journal of the American Medical Association* 269 (9): 1158–1162.

Pellegrino, Edmund. 2008. *The Changing Moral Focus of Newborn Screening: An Ethical Analysis by the President's Council on Bioethics*. Washington, DC: The President's Council on Bioethics. http://www.bioethics.gov (accessed May 13, 2011).

Percival, Thomas. 1794. *Medical Jurisprudence, or a Code of Ethics and Institutes Adopted to the Professions of Physic and Surgery*. Manchester, UK

Perkin, Harold J. 1989. *The Rise of Professional Society: England since 1880*. London: Routledge.

Perkin, Harold J. 1996. *The Third Revolution: Professional Elites in the Modern World*. London: Routledge.

Pernick, Martin S. 1996. *The Black Stork: Eugenics and the Death of "Defective" Babies in American Medicine and Motion Pictures since 1915*. New York: Oxford University Press.

Persad, Govind, Alan Wertheimer, and Ezekiel J. Emanuel. 2009. "Principles for Allocation of Scarce Medical Interventions." *Lancet* 373 (9661): 423–431.

Peters, Charles. 1983. "A Neoliberal's Manifesto." *Washington Monthly* 15, no. 3 (May): 8–18. http://www.washingtonmonthly.com/features/1983/8305_Neoliberalism.pdf (accessed January 18, 2012).

Pfleiderer, Geog, Gabriela Brahier, and Klaus Lindpaintner, eds. 2010. *GenEthics and Religion*. New York: S. Karger Publishers.

Philbrick, Nathaniel. 2000. *In the Heart of the Sea: The Tragedy of the Whaleship Essex*. New York: Viking.

Phillips, Trisha. 2011."From the Ideal Market to the Ideal Clinic: Constructing a Normative Standard of Fairness for Human Subjects Research." *Journal of Medicine and Philosophy* 36 (1): 79–106.

Pickering, Andrew. 1995. *The Mangle of Practice: Time, Agency, and Science*. Chicago: University of Chicago Press.

Porter, Roy. 1999. *The Greatest Benefit to Mankind: A Medical History of Humanity*. New York: W. W. Norton & Co.

Porter, Stephen. 2005. *Lord Have Mercy Upon Us: London's Plague Years*. Stroud, Gloucestershire: Tempus Publishing.

Post, Stephen G. 1995. *The Moral Challenge of Alzheimer Disease*. Baltimore, MD: Johns Hopkins University Press.

Privy Council. 1832. Instructions and Regulations Regarding Cholera, Issued under the Authority of the Privy Council. In *Annual Register or a View of the History, Politics, and Literature of the Year 1831*, 357–360. London: Baldwin and Cradock.

Quill, Timothy E. 1991. "Death and Dignity: A Case of Individualized Decision Making." *New England Journal of Medicine* 324 (10): 691–694. http://web.missouri.edu/~bondesonw/Quill.HTM (accessed December 9 2009).

Quill, Timothy E. 2005. "Terri Schiavo—A Tragedy Compounded." *New England Journal of Medicine* 352 (16): 1630–1633.

Quill, Timothy E., and Margaret P. Battin. 2004. *Physician-assisted Dying: The Case for Palliative Care and Patient Choice*. Baltimore, MD: Johns Hopkins University Press.

Rabinbach, Anson. 1990. *The Human Motor: Energy, Fatigue, and the Origins of Modernity*. New York: Basic Books.

Rachlis, Michael. 2010. "Medicare Attack Dogs Barking up Wrong Tree." *Toronto Star* (February 4): A21.

Ramos, Kenneth S. 2005. "A Vision That Challenges Dogma Gives Rise to a New Era in the Environmental Health Sciences." *Environmental Health Perspectives* 113: 162–167. http://findarticles.com/p/articles/mi_m0CYP/is_8-1_113/ai_n27867600/?tag=content;col1 (accessed January 15, 2012).

Rauprich, Oliver, and Jochen Vollman. 2011. "30 Years *Principles of Biomedical Ethics*: Introduction to a Symposium on the 6th Edition of Tom L. Beauchamp and James F. Childress' Seminal Work." *Journal of Medical Ethics* 37 (8): 582–583.

Rawls, John. 1971. *A Theory of Justice*. Cambridge, MA: Belknap Press.

Rawls, John. 2003. *Justice as Fairness: A Restatement*. Cambridge, MA: Belknap Press.

Reich, Warren T. 1993. "How Bioethics Got Its Name," Special Supplement. *Hastings Center Report* 23 (6) (November–December): S6–S7.

Reichel, William. 1999. "Physician Know Thyself." *Journal of the American Board of Family Practice* 12 (3): 258–259.

Reilly, Phillip R. 1991. *The Surgical Solution: A History of Involuntary Sterilization in the United States*. Baltimore, MD: Johns Hopkins University Press.

Rhodes, Rosamond. 2005. "Rethinking Research Ethics." *American Journal of Bioethics* 5 (7): 7–28.

Richardson, Ruth. 2008. *The Making of Mr. Gray's Anatomy: Bodies, Books, Fortune, Fame*. New York: Oxford University Press.

Roberts, Ian, David Prieto-Marino, Haleema Shakur, Ian Chalmers, and Jon Nicoll. 2011. "Effect of Consent Rituals on Mortality in Emergency Care Research." *Lancet* 377 (9771) (March 26): 1071–1072. http://www.thelancet.com/journals/lancet/article/PIIS0140-6736(11)60317-6/fulltext (accessed July 7, 2011).

Rogers, Naomi. 1996. *Dirt and Disease: Polio before FDR*. New Brunswick, NJ: Rutgers University Press.

Rogers, Wendy, and Angela Ballantyne. 2009. "Justice in Health Research: What Is the Role of Evidence-based Medicine." *Perspectives in Biology and Medicine* 52 (2): 188–202.

Rosen, George. 1993. *A History of Public Health, Expanded Edition*. Baltimore, MD: Johns Hopkins University Press.

Rothman, David J. 1991. *Strangers by the Bedside: A History of How Law and Bioethics Transformed Medical Decision Making*. New York: Basic Books.

Rothman, David J. 1992. "Rationing Life." *New York Review of Books* 39 (5) (March 5): 32–37. http://www.nybooks.com/articles/archives/1992/mar/05/rationing-life (accessed January 10, 2011).

Russell, Betrand. 1977. *Education and the Social Order*. London: Unwin Paperbacks.

Russert, Britt. 2009. "'A Study in Nature': The Tuskegee Experiments and the New South Plantation." *Journal of Medical Humanities* 30 (3): 155–171.

Ryan, Michael. 1836. *Manual of Medical Jurisprudence, Second Edition*. London: Sherwood, Gilbert, and Piper. http://www.archive.org/details/amanualmedical j00ryangoog (accessed January 18, 2012).

Sachs, Benjamin. 2010. "Lingering Problems of Currency and Scope in Daniel's Argument for a Society Obligation to Meet Health Needs." *Journal of Medicine and Philosophy* 35 (4): 402–414.

Sacks, Oliver. 1982. *Awakenings*. Revised edition. London: Picador.

Salholz, Eloise. 1990. "Blaming the Voters; Hapless Budgeteers Single Out 'Greedy Geezers.'" *Newsweek* 116 (18) (October 29): 36.

Sass, Edmund. 2005. "The History of Polio: A Hypertext Timeline." http://www.cloudnet.com/%7Eedrbsass/poliotimeline.htm (accessed January 19, 2012).

Savulescu, Julian. 2001. "Harm, Ethics Committees, and the Gene Therapy Death." *Journal of Medical Ethics* 27 (3): 148–150.

Savulescu, Julian, and Anders Sandberg. 2008. "Neuroenhancement of Love and Marriage: The Chemicals between Us." *Neuroethics* 1 (1): 31–44.

Savulescu, Julian, and M. Spriggs. 2002. "The Hexamethonium Asthma Study and the Death of a Normal Volunteer in Research." *Journal of Medical Ethics* 28 (1): 3–4.

Schiff, Nicholas D. 2003. "Hope for 'Comatose' Patients." *Cerebrum* 5 (4): 7–24.

Schmidt, Harald. 2007. "Whose Dignity? Resolving Ambiguities in the Scope of 'Human Dignity' in the Universal Declaration on Bioethics and Human Rights." *Journal of Medical Ethics* 33 (10): 578–584.

Schoenle, Paul W., and W. Witzke. 2004. "How Vegetative Is the Vegetative State? Preserved Semantic Processing in PVS Patients—Evidence from 400 Event-related Potentials." *Neuro Rehabilitation* 19 (3): 29–34.

Schrag, Zachary M. 2010. *Ethical Imperialism: Institutional Review Boards and the Social Sciences: 1965–2009*. Baltimore, MD: Johns Hopkins University Press.

Shapin, Steven. 1994. *A Social History of Truth: Civility and Science in Seventeenth-Century England*. Chicago: University of Chicago Press.

Shapin, Steven. 1996. *The Scientific Revolution*. Chicago: University of Chicago Press.

Shapin, Steven, and Simon Schaffer. 1985. *Leviathan and the Air Pump: Hobbes, Boyle, and the Experimental Life*. Princeton, NJ: Princeton University Press.

Shenk, David. 2010. *The Genius in All of Us: Why Everything You've Been Told about Genetics, Talent, and IQ Is Wrong*. New York: Random House.

Shenk, David. 2011. "Is There a Genius in All of Us?" *BBC News Magazine*, January 12. http://www.bbc.co.uk/news/magazine-12140064 (accessed June 26, 2011).

Shuchman, Miriam. 2005. *The Drug Trial: Dr. Nancy Olivieri and the Science Scandal That Rocked the Hospital for Sick Children*. Toronto: Random House Canada.

Singer, Peter. 1983. *Hegel: A Very Short Introduction*. New York: Oxford University Press.

Singer, Peter. 1986. All Animals are Equal. In *Applied Ethics*, ed. Peter Singer, 215–228. New York: Oxford University Press.

Singer, Peter. 1993. *Practical Ethics*. 2nd ed. New York: Cambridge University Press.

Singer, Peter. 1994. *Rethinking Life and Death: The Collapse of Our Traditional Ethics*. New York: St. Martin's Griffin.

Singer, Peter. 2005. "Ethics and Disability: A Response to Koch." *Journal of Disability Policy Studies* 16 (2): 130–133.

Singer, Peter. 2009. "Happy Nonetheless." *New York Times*, December 28, MM34. http://www.nytimes.com/2008/12/28/magazine/28mcbryde-t.html?_r=1&ref=magazine (accessed March 24, 2010).

Skloot, Rebecca. 2011. *The Immortal Life of Henrietta Lacks*. New York: Broadway Paperbacks.

Snell, N. J. 2001. "Death of a Healthy Research Subject after an Inhalation Study—Old Lessons to Be Re-learned." *International Journal of Pharmaceutical Medicine* 15 (4) (August): 157–168.

Somerville, Margaret. 2000. *The Ethical Canary: Science, Society and the Human Spirit*. New York: Viking.

Somerville, Margaret. 2006. *The Ethical Imagination: Journeys of the Human Spirit*. Toronto: Anansi Press.

Sox, Colin M., William O. Cooper, Thomas D. Koepsell, David L. Di Guiseppe, and Dimitri A. Christakis. 2003. "Provision of Pneumococcal Prophylaxis for Publicly Insured Children with Sickle Cell Disease." *Journal of the American Medical Association* 290 (8): 1057–1061.

Specter, Michael. 2010. "A Deadly Misdiagnosis." *New Yorker* (November 15): 48–53.

Spike, Jeffrey, and Jane Greenlaw. 1995 "Ethics Consultation: Persistent Brain Death and Religion: Must a Person Believe in Death to Die?" *Journal of Law, Medicine & Ethics* 23 (3): 20–23.

Steen, Grant R. 2011. "This Is Not News." *The Scientist* (letters) 25 (1): 12. http://classic.the-scientist.com/2011/1/1/12/1/ (accessed January 18, 2012).

Steger, Manfred B., and Ravi K. Roy. 2010. *Neoliberalism: A Very Short Introduction*. New York: Oxford University Press.

Sullivan, William M. 2000. "Medicine under Threat: Professionalism and Professional Identity." *Journal of the Canadian Medical Association* 162 (5): 673–675.

Swick, Herbert M. 2000. "Toward a Normative Definition of Medical Professionalism." *Academic Medicine* 75 (6): 612–616.

Taylor, Charles. 1979. *Hegel and Modern Society*. New York: Cambridge University Press.

Taylor, Jill B. 2006. *My Stroke of Insight: A Brain Scientist's Personal Journey*. New York: Viking.

Ter Meulen, Ruud, and Fabrice Jotterand. 2009. "Individual Responsibility and Solidarity in European Health Care." *Journal of Medicine and Philosophy* 33 (3): 191–197.

Thomasma, David C. 1990. Anencephalics as Organ Donors. In *Biomedical Ethics Reviews, 1989*, ed. James M. Humber and Robert F. Almeder, 25–56. Clifton, NJ: Humana Press.

Thomasma, David C. 1997. "The Asbury Draft Policy on Ethical Use of Resources." *Cambridge Quarterly of Healthcare Ethics* 8 (2): 249.

Thomasma, David C. 1997. "Bioethics and International Human Rights." *Journal of Law, Medicine & Ethics* 25: 295–306.

Thomasma, David C. 1998. "Stewardship of the Aged: Meeting the Ethical Challenge of Ageism." *Cambridge Quarterly of Healthcare Ethics* 8 (2): 148–149.

Thomasma, David C., and Eric H. Lowey. 1997. "A Dialogue on Species-specific Rights: Humans and Animals in Bioethics." *Cambridge Quarterly of Healthcare Ethics* 6 (4): 435–444.

Thomasma, David C, Tommi Kushner, and Steven Hellig. 1999. "From the Editors." *Cambridge Quarterly of Healthcare Ethics* 8 (3): 263–264.

Thomasma, David C., Kenneth C. Micetich, John Brems, and David Van Thiel. 1999. "The Ethics of Competition in Liver Transplantation." *Cambridge Quarterly of Healthcare Ethics* 8 (3): 321–330.

Tilburt, Jon. 2011. "Shared Decision Making, after MacIntyre." *Journal of Medicine and Philosophy* 36 (2): 148–169.

Titmuss, Richard M. 1982. *The Gift Relationship: From Human Blood to Social Policy*. New York: Vintage Books.

Tremain, Shelley. 2005. Foucault, Governmentality, and Critical Disability Theory. In *Foucault and the Government of Disability*, ed. S. Tremain, 1–26. Ann Arbor: University of Michigan Press.

Trevelyan, Barry, Mathew Smallman-Raynor, and Andrew D. Cliff. 2005. "The Spatial Dynamics of Poliomyelitis in the United States: From Epidemic Emergence to Vaccine-Induced Retreat, 1910–1971." *Annals of the Association of American Geographers* 95 (2): 269–293.

Truog, Robert D. 1997. "Is It Time to Abandon Brain Death?" *Hastings Center Report* 27 (1): 29–37.

Truog, Robert D., and Franklin G. Miller. 2008. "The Dead Donor Rule and Organ Transplantation." *The New England Journal of Medicine* 359 (7): 674–675. http://www.nejm.org/doi/full/10.1056/NEJMp0804474?query=TOC (accessed June 20, 2011).

Truog, Robert D., and W. M. Robinson. 2001. "Correspondence." *New England Journal of Medicine* 345 (8): 616–618. http://www.nejm.org/doi/full/10.1056/NEJM200108233450813 (accessed February 22, 2012).

UNESCO. 2005. Universal Declaration on Bioethics and Human Rights. http://unesdoc.unesco.org/images/0014/001461/146180e.pdf (accessed December 18, 2010).

U.S. Senate Special Committee on Aging. 1991. *Who Lives, Who Dies, Who Decides: The Ethics of Health Care Rationing*. Hearing before the Special Committee on Aging, 102nd Congress, 1st Session. Washington, DC: U.S. Government Printing Office.

Uttal, William R. 2001. *The New Phrenology*. Cambridge, MA: MIT Press.

Venter, Craig J. 2010. "We Have Learned Nothing from the Genome," *Der Spiegel* online (July 29). http://www.spiegel.de/international/world/0,1518,709174-2,00.html (accessed May 29, 2011).

Veatch, Robert. 1993. "From Forgoing Life Support to Aid-in-dying." *Hastings Center Report* 23 (6): S7–S8. http://www.questia.com/googleScholar.qst?docId=5002196576 (accessed June 20, 2011).

Verghese, Abraham. 2005. "The Calling." *New England Journal of Medicine* 352 (18): 1844–1847.

Vonderlehr, Raymond A. 1936. "Untreated Syphilis in the Male Negro: A Comparative Study of Treated and Untreated Cases." *Journal of the American Medical Association* 107 (11) (September 12): 856–860.

Vuorisalo, Timo, and Olli Arjamaa. 2010. "Gene-culture Coevolution and Human Diet." *American Scientist* 98 (2): 140–142. http://www.americanscientist.org/issues/page2/2010/2/gene-culture-coevolution-and-human-diet (accessed September 22, 2010).

Wackers, Ger L. 1994. *Constructivist Medicine*. Maastricht, NL: Universitare Pers Maastricht.

Wade, Nicholas. 1999. "Patient Dies during a Trial of Therapy Using Genes," *New York Times*, September 29. http://www.nytimes.com/1999/09/29/us/patient-dies-during-a-trial-of-therapy-using-genes.html (accessed June 21, 2011).

Wade, Nicholas. 2009. "Genes Show Limited Value in Predicting Diseases." *New York Times*, April 15, A1. http://www.nytimes.com/2009/04/16/health/research/16gene.html (accessed July 4, 2011).

Wade, Paul A., and Trevor K. Archer. 2006. "Epigenetics: Environmental Instructions for the Genome." *Environmental Health Perspectives* 114 (3) (March 2): A140–A141. http://www.ncbi.nlm.nih.gov/pmc/articles/PMC1392246 (accessed September 22, 2006).

Waldby, Catherine, and Robert Mitchell. 2006. *Tissue Economies: Blood, Organs and Cell Lines in Late Capitalism*. Durham, NC: Duke University Press.

Walker, Margaret U. 1993. "Keeping Moral Space Open." *Hastings Center Report* 23 (2): 33–40.

Walker, Rebecca L. 2009. "Respect for Rational Autonomy." *Kennedy Institute of Ethics Journal* 19 (4): 339–366.

Wallace, John R. 1965. "Sortal Predicates and Quantification." *Journal of Philosophy* 62 (1): 8–13.

Walzer, Michael. 1983. *Spheres of Justice: A Defence of Pluralism and Equality*. New York: Basic Books.

Warner, John H. 1985. "Review: James H. Cassedy, American Medicine and Statistical Thinking, 1800–1860." Medical History 29 (4): 449–451. http://www.ncbi.nlm.nih.gov/pmc/articles/PMC1139990/pdf/medhist00073-0115b.pdf (accessed June 17, 2011).

Watson, James D. 1980. *The Double Helix: A Personal Account of the Discovery of the Structure of DNA*, ed. Gunther Stent. New York: Norton.

White, Michael J., and John Griffin. 1992. *Stephen Hawking: A Life in Science*. New York: Penguin.

Wiggins, Osborne P., and Michael A. Schwartz. 2005. "Richard Zaner's Phenomenology of the Clinical Encounter." *Theoretical Medicine and Bioethics* 26 (1): 73–87.

Wijdicks, E. F. M. 2001. "Reply to Critics." *New England Journal of Medicine* 345 (8): 618–619.

Wildes, Kevin William. 1993. "Moral Authority, Moral Standing, and Moral Controversy." *Journal of Medicine and Philosophy* 18 (4): 347–350.

Williams, Bernard. 1978. Introduction. In *Isaiah Berlin, Concepts and Categories: Philosophical Essays*, ed. Henry Hardy, xiii–xx. New York: Viking.

Wilson, J. M. G., and G. Junger. 1968. *Principles and Practice of Screening for Disease*. Public Health Papers No. 34. Geneva, Switzerland: World Health Organization. http://whqlibdoc.who.int/php/WHO_PHP_34.pdf (accessed January 18, 2012).

Wise, Sarah. 2004. *The Italian Boy: A Tale of Murder and Body Snatching in 1830s London*. New York: Henry Holt and Co.

Witten, Mark. 2010. "Brainwashed: Rethinking Man's Genetic Makeup." *The Walrus* (November): 18–20.

Wittgenstein, Ludwig. 1922. *Tractatus Logico-Philosophicus*, trans. C. K. Ogden. London: Routledge & Kegan Paul Ltd. http://www.brainyquote.com/quotes/quotes/l/ludwigwitt147256.html (accessed November 23, 2009).

Wolbring, Gregor. 2001. Where Do We Draw the Line? Surviving Eugenics in a Technological World. In *Disability and the Life Course: Global Perspectives*, ed. Mark Priestly, 38–49. Cambridge, UK: Cambridge University Press.

Woo, Joseph S. 2002. "A Short History of Amniocentesis, Fetoscopy and Chorionic Villus Sampling," *A Short History of the Development of Ultrasound in Obstetrics and Gynecology*. http://www.ob-ultrasound.net/amniocentesis.html (accessed June 21, 2011).

Wood, James. 2010. "The Fun Stuff: My Life as Keith Moon." *New Yorker* (November 29): 57–63.

World Records Academy. 2010. "Most Expensive Medicine—World Record Set by Soliris." February 23. http://www.worldrecordsacademy.org/business/most_expensive_medicine_world_record_set_by_Soliris_101573.htm (accessed February 2, 2011).

Young, Jenny. 2004. "Choosing Self-termination in a Rehabilitation Setting following High Lesion Spinal Cord Injury." M.A. thesis, Medical College of Wisconsin Graduate School of Bioethics. Milwaukee.

Zellen, Doris T. 2000. "Gene Therapy in Crisis." *Trends in Genetics* 16 (6): 272–275.

Zaner, Richard. 2005. "A Work in Progress." *Theoretical Medicine and Bioethics* 26 (1): 89–104.

Legal Citations

Bouvia v. Superior Court, 179 Cal. App. 3d 1127, 1135-36, 225 Cal. Rptr. 297. (Ct. App. 1986), review denied (Cal. June 5, 1986).

Buck v. Bell (1927) 274 U.S. 200.

Cruzan v. Director, Missouri Department of Health (1990) 497 U.S. 261.

In re Conservatorship of Wanglie (1991) No. PX-91-283 (Minn. Dist. Ct. Hennepin Co., July).

In the Matter of Quinlan (1976) 70 N.J. 10, 355 A. 2d. 647.

Jacobson v. Commonwealth of Massachusetts 197 U.S. 11 (1905).

National Research Act 1974 (July 12) Pub. L. 93-348.

Patient Self-determination Act (1990). *Omnibus Reconciliation Act of 1990*, Pub L No. 101-508 (November 5, 1990), § 4206 and 4751.

Regina v. Latimer (2001) 1 S.C.R. 3, 2001 SCC 1, §40.

RICO, The Racketeer Influenced and Corrupt Organizations Act of 1970, 18 U.S.C.

Roe v. Wade (1973) 410 U.S. 113.

Salgo v. Leland Stanford Jr. University Board of Trustees (1957) Civ. No. 17045. First Dist. Div. One.

United States v. Holmes, 26 F. Cas. 360; (1842), 369 (C.C.E.D. Pa 22 April 1842).

William A. Hyman v. Jewish Chronic Disease Hospital (1965) 268 N.Y.S. 2nd 397.

Index

Basic Bioethics

Arthur Caplan, editor

Books Acquired under the Editorship of Glenn McGee and Arthur Caplan

Peter A. Ubel, *Pricing Life: Why It's Time for Health Care Rationing*

Mark G. Kuczewski and Ronald Polansky, eds., *Bioethics: Ancient Themes in Contemporary Issues*

Suzanne Holland, Karen Lebacqz, and Laurie Zoloth, eds., *The Human Embryonic Stem Cell Debate: Science, Ethics, and Public Policy*

Gita Sen, Asha George, and Piroska Östlin, eds., *Engendering International Health: The Challenge of Equity*

Carolyn McLeod, *Self-Trust and Reproductive Autonomy*

Lenny Moss, *What Genes Can't Do*

Jonathan D. Moreno, ed., *In the Wake of Terror: Medicine and Morality in a Time of Crisis*

Glenn McGee, ed., *Pragmatic Bioethics*, 2nd edition

Timothy F. Murphy, *Case Studies in Biomedical Research Ethics*

Mark A. Rothstein, ed., *Genetics and Life Insurance: Medical Underwriting and Social Policy*

Kenneth A. Richman, *Ethics and the Metaphysics of Medicine: Reflections on Health and Beneficence*

David Lazer, ed., *DNA and the Criminal Justice System: The Technology of Justice*

Harold W. Baillie and Timothy K. Casey, eds., *Is Human Nature Obsolete? Genetics, Bioengineering, and the Future of the Human Condition*

Robert H. Blank and Janna C. Merrick, eds., *End-of-Life Decision Making: A Cross-National Study*

Norman L. Cantor, *Making Medical Decisions for the Profoundly Mentally Disabled*

Margrit Shildrick and Roxanne Mykitiuk, eds., *Ethics of the Body: Post-Conventional Challenges*

Alfred I. Tauber, *Patient Autonomy and the Ethics of Responsibility*

David H. Brendel, *Healing Psychiatry: Bridging the Science/Humanism Divide*

Jonathan Baron, *Against Bioethics*

Michael L. Gross, *Bioethics and Armed Conflict: Moral Dilemmas of Medicine and War*

Karen F. Greif and Jon F. Merz, *Current Controversies in the Biological Sciences: Case Studies of Policy Challenges from New Technologies*

Deborah Blizzard, *Looking Within: A Sociocultural Examination of Fetoscopy*

Ronald Cole-Turner, ed., *Design and Destiny: Jewish and Christian Perspectives on Human Germline Modification*

Holly Fernandez Lynch, *Conflicts of Conscience in Health Care: An Institutional Compromise*

Mark A. Bedau and Emily C. Parke, eds., *The Ethics of Protocells: Moral and Social Implications of Creating Life in the Laboratory*

Jonathan D. Moreno and Sam Berger, eds., *Progress in Bioethics: Science, Policy, and Politics*

Eric Racine, *Pragmatic Neuroethics: Improving Understanding and Treatment of the Mind–Brain*

Martha J. Farah, ed., *Neuroethics: An Introduction with Readings*

Books Acquired under the Editorship of Arthur Caplan

Sheila Jasanoff, ed., *Reframing Rights: Bioconstitutionalism in the Genetic Age*

Christine Overall, *Why Have Children? The Ethical Debate*

Yechiel Michael Barilan, *Human Dignity, Human Rights, and Responsibility: The New Language of Global Bioethics and Bio-Law*

Tom Koch, *Thieves of Virtue: When Bioethics Stole Medicine*